T0383795

Health Disparities, Disasters, and Crises

Health Disparities, Disasters, and Crises: Approaches for a Culture of Preparedness presents a roadmap to help guide the actions needed to address health disparities introduced as part of the pre-planning, planning, and mitigation phases of natural and technological disasters.

With contributions from 30 scholars in disaster management in public health, this text explores how the intersectionality of health disparities of different socioeconomic and racial/ethnic groups and how social determinants help shape exposure, and vulnerability to pandemic disasters and crises. Supported by examples from across the world, chapters are supplemented with case studies of best practices, graphs, and tables. Each of the seven parts address different topics, including how disasters affect the poor, medically underserved, and racial/ethnic groups, the impact of health disparities, and the growing link between global health, disaster planning/mitigation, and global security.

Written for the benefit of undergraduate and graduate students, working professionals, and academics in the US and abroad, *Health Disparities, Disasters, and Crises: Approaches for a Culture of Preparedness* provides the best overall understanding of professional disaster management and safety for all citizens. It is also an ideal text for graduate and undergraduate courses in public health, public policy, medicine and nursing, healthcare administration, emergency management, emergency preparedness, homeland security, epidemiology, sociology, and medical sociology.

Roland J. Thorpe Jr. holds joint appointments in medicine and neurology at the Johns Hopkins University School of Medicine. He is an Associate Professor of Health, Behavior and Society at the Johns Hopkins Bloomberg School of Public Health. He serves as the Director of the Program for Research on Men's Health at the Hopkins Center for Health Disparities Solutions. Dr. Thorpe's research focuses on racial and socioeconomic health disparities, particularly among US men.

DeMond S. Miller is a Professor of Sociology, Professor of Disaster Science and Emergency Management, and coordinates the Program in Healthcare Management and Administration. He serves as the Program Director in Disaster Science and Emergency Management. Dr. Miller's primary areas of research specialization are environmental sociology (disaster studies), sustainable disaster recovery, disaster equity studies, emergency services and response, community development, community-based research, technological disasters, international irregular migration, and acts of terror as disasters.

Health Disparities, Disasters, and Crises

Approaches for a Culture of Preparedness

Edited by
Roland J. Thorpe Jr.
DeMond S. Miller

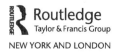

NEW YORK AND LONDON

Cover image: Getty Images

First published 2024
by Routledge
605 Third Avenue, New York, NY 10158

and by Routledge
4 Park Square, Milton Park, Abingdon, Oxon OX14 4RN

Routledge is an imprint of the Taylor & Francis Group, an informa business

ISBN: 978-0-367-67731-2 (hbk)
ISBN: 978-1-003-14024-5 (ebk)

DOI: 10.4324/9781003140245

Typeset in Times New Roman
by codeMantra

Roland J. Thorpe, Jr.
This book is dedicated to Dorothy Thorpe, Lucille Thorpe, Nora Buckner, and Roland J. Thorpe, Sr.

DeMond S. Miller
To those who continue to inspire me through their life lessons and examples….
John Wesley Craft, Sr. and Myrtis Ruth Bell Craft

Contents

Figures

Tables

Contributors

Muhammad Abid, MBBS, MCPS (Pakistan), DTCD (Austria), FFPHM (UK), is a consultant in public health, global health, infectious disease epidemiology, emergency preparedness, disaster management, vaccine-preventable diseases, disease surveillance, and health systems. He was trained in public health in the UK and then worked as a consultant in Public Health England in Oxford for many years. He is working as a Professor at the Institute of Public Health, College of Medicine and Health Sciences, United Arab Emirates University (UAEU), UAE for the last six years. Professor Abid is a Fellow of the Faculty of Public Health, UK and acts as an International Continuous Professional Development Advisor. His main areas of research interest include infectious diseases, immunization, blood-borne diseases such as viral hepatitis, HIV/AIDS, tuberculosis, and antimicrobial resistance. Over the years, he has been an author of many scientific publications in peer-reviewed journals.

Fikri Abu-Zidan, MD, PhD, is an international expert in Statistics, Research Methodology, Acute Care Surgery, Disaster Medicine, and Point-of-Care Ultrasound. He graduated (MD) from Aleppo University (Syria) in 1981; gained the FRCS, Glasgow, Scotland in 1987; earned his PhD in Trauma and Disaster Medicine from Linkoping University (Sweden) in 1995; and obtained his Postgraduate Diploma of Applied Statistics from Massey University (New Zealand) in 1999. He is currently serving as a Statistics and Research Methodology Consultant for the Research Office at the College of Medicine and Health Sciences at United Arab Emirates University. He has made major contributions to trauma management, education, and research in Kuwait, Sweden, New Zealand, Australia, and United Arab Emirates. He has more than 460 publications in books and refereed international journals. He presented more than 700 invited lectures and scientific abstracts and received more than 40 national and international awards for clinical research and educational activities.

DeBorah Ahmed, MA, is the Executive Director of the Better Family Life Cultural, Educational, and Business Center. This organization helps to unite families and empower communities in the Metropolitan St. Louis area. She is an award-winning Black History Visionary with outstanding achievements in public service, uplifting the urban St. Louis community, and her contributions in the area of social justice.

Faris El Akbani, BA, a Media Planner at Publicis Media, has contributed to growing research on community structure theory. Currently pursuing a career in advertising, El Akbani is interested in society's impact on media during this digital age. Additionally, he is fascinated by how both digital and traditional media continue to motivate social, economic, and political changes in the world's increasingly media-saturated society.

Samar Mohammed Alhaj, MD is a Junior Medical Doctor from the Ahfad University for Women, Khartoum, Sudan. She is a Researcher at Global Health Focus (GHF). Her research interests cut across Global and Public Health, specifically women's health related issues, food security, and tobacco harm reduction. Samar is a recent Knowledge-Action-Change Scholar.

Adaobi Anakwe, PhD, MPH, is an Assistant Professor in the Drexel School of Public Health. Her research focuses on social determinants and life course perspectives on women, men, and family health including structural, cultural, and environmental factors affecting health. She is also interested in community-focused engagement that contextualizes and examines disparities in health outcomes among US minority populations and developing economies in the US and sub-Saharan Africa.

Hillary Kay Ang, MD, completed her Doctor of Medicine and her Bachelor of Science in Physical Therapy degrees from the University of Santo Tomas (Philippines). Her research interests include allied health science, preventive medicine, and physical rehabilitation.

Paul Archibald, DrPH, LCSW-C (MD), LCSW (NY), MAC, is an Associate Professor and Master of Social Work Program Director in the Social Work Department at the College of Staten Island, City University of New York. Dr. Archibald is a public health social worker with over 20 years of clinical practice and training focused on the prevention and treatment of behavioral and physical health outcomes among persons exposed to chronic trauma and stressors. He utilizes an intersectional approach to survey the role of stress and trauma in the contribution of trauma-and-stress-related health disparities. His research is buttressed by the social model of disability, which holds that people experience disability due to societal barriers that expose them to inequities and a poor sense of belonging. He is a firm believer in the Ubuntu principle of health focused on the premise that "it takes a whole community to make a community whole!"

Ouma Atieno Sarah, MD, is a Junior Medical Doctor and a feted early career researcher with a particular focus in Psychiatry, Mental Health Policy & Advocacy, and Global Health. Besides clinical work, Dr. Ouma is currently working on using Human Centered Design to deliver community mental health services, research, and mental health policy and advocacy. She is a radical feminist who believes in the centering of African womxn's and minority groups' rights for the achievement of equity and equality.

Rhonda BeLue, PhD, CQM/OE, is a Professor of Public Health at the University of Texas, San Antonio and Associate Dean for Community Engagement and Partnerships. Her work focuses on improving healthcare access and promoting healthy behaviors in families and organizations in Black/BIPoC communities in the US and the global south. She has dedicated her career to the elimination of health inequities and advocating for social justice. She takes a holistic approach to advocating for social justice, including community-based participatory research approaches to addressing health disparities and participating in and supporting Black, indigenous , and diverse cultural arts activities, and serving local organizations that serve African American and BIPoC communities. She has also worked as a local public health practitioner in Nashville, TN. She holds a Master of Statistics and a PhD in Health Policy Analysis & Management from Cornell University and Graduate Certificates in Organizational Leadership and Development from St. Louis University.

Omar Bird, PhD is the new Director/Coordinator for the new Office of Health Equity in the Department of Health for the state of Hawaii. As a critical public social scientist, Omar has worked on projects that support Hawaii residents by working on state policy to expand long-term care services and support systems for the elderly, increasing awareness and expanding food options for Hawaii's keiki during the pandemic, and organizing local academics and policymakers to advance equitable local policy via the scholar strategies network. Throughout the pandemic, Omar has developed a COVID-19 mutual aid network for graduate students and often provides free public talks with members of the community.

Marino A. Bruce, PhD, MSRC, MDiv, is a sociologist and population health scientist who examines the full range of factors, including faith, religion, and spirituality, that influence cognitive and physical functioning among Black males over the life course and across generations. He is an Associate Dean for Research and a Clinical Professor at the University of Houston Tilman J. Fertitta Family College of Medicine. He also serves as the Founding Director of UHPH Collaboratories – synergistic interdisciplinary research and training units within UH Population Health, a university-wide initiative at the University of Houston driving improvements in quality of life. Dr. Bruce is co-editor of two books, *Men's Health Equity* and *Racism: Science and Tools for the Public Health Professional*, and co-author of more than 110 peer-reviewed articles and book chapters. His work has been featured on numerous global media outlets, including *USA Today*, The Today Show, US News and World Report, and *Time Magazine*.

Avantika D. Butani, MPH, BA, is a healthcare professional at Atlantic Health System and co-authored *Reduction of Infant Mortality through Neonatal Nursing Education* in 2021. A SMART Recovery Facilitator and Peer Health Educator, Butani advocates and investigates best policy reform methods for health education promotion within corporate environments.

Len E. Clark, DPA CEM, is a career emergency manager. He served at the local, county, state, and federal levels of government and in healthcare. Dr. Clark has helped to develop and launch both the emergency management undergraduate and graduate programs at Rowan University. Dr. Clark earned a Doctorate in Public Administration from the University of Baltimore. His dissertation was the first statewide evaluation of the Implementation of the National Incident Management System in New Jersey, and he contributed to DHS/FEMA's textbook on the topic. Dr. Clark's professional career spans over 30 years and includes the management of over 24 federally declared disasters and multiple large-scale emergencies requiring multi-agency cooperation throughout the US. Dr. Clark is a veteran of the US Coast Guard Reserve and deployed twice for Operation Guarding Liberty (NYC on 9/11) and Operation Enduring Freedom.

Alyssa Coleman, MPH, is a PhD candidate in the Department of Health Management and Policy at St. Louis University. She is interested in program evaluation and health equity.

Derron G. Cooney is a Research Assistant at Rowan University with scholarly interests in Sociology, Disaster Science, and Emergency Management. He is a resident of Gloucester City, NJ. In addition, Derron is a first responder for the North Wildwood Police Department.

Miranda Crowley, MPA, BA, was a Communication Studies major with a Women, Gender, and Sexuality Studies minor at The College of New Jersey. She was a panelist at the 2018 New Jersey Communication Association Conference, presenting on the socio-political consequences of news convergence. Crowley has also co-authored several community structure theory studies on both US multi-city and cross-national levels, some published, others accepted at academic conferences, including the biannual Kentucky and DC conferences on health communication and the annual conference of the International Communication Association.

Nicola Davis Bivens, EdD, is a Professor of Criminology at Johnson C. Smith University, where she also serves as the Program Coordinator and is the 2023 recipient of the school's Par-Excellence Teaching Award, 2022 Sit Lux Faculty Award, and 2012 CATO Par-Excellence Teaching

Award. She is also a Researcher at the HBCU Criminal Justice Research Hub at Texas Southern University. In 2018, she received the York County (South Carolina) Office of Emergency Management Service Award for her work during Hurricane Florence. For 30 years, Dr. Davis Bivens has studied, worked, or taught in the field of public safety and emergency management. Her scholarship has appeared in the *Studia z Polityki Publicznej* [*Public Policy Studies Journal*], *Journal of Education and Social Policy, Journal of Applied Security Research, Journal of Justice Studies, Paradigm Shift: An Interdisciplinary Journal on the African American Experience, Field Educator*, and the *Journal of Criminal Justice and Law Review*.

Fredrick Echols, MD, is the Founder and Chief Executive Officer, of Population Health and Social Justice Consulting, LLC. (PHSJC) and was previously the health commissioner and acting health director for the city of St. Louis. Before his positions in the city of St. Louis, Dr. Echols was the Director of Communicable Disease, Emergency Preparedness, Vector & Veterinary Programs for St. Louis County and before that he served as the Chief of Communicable Diseases for the Illinois Department of Public Health.

Anthony T. Estreet, PhD, MBA, LCSW-C, LCADC, is the National Association of Social Workers (NASW) CEO and a highly esteemed social work leader. Dr. Estreet, who has more than two decades of experience in the social work profession, has made significant contributions to the field through his academic and professional endeavors. He has published extensively in peer-reviewed journals, is a prolific national conference presenter and keynote speaker, and has co-edited a groundbreaking book on African-centered clinical interventions in social work mental health practice. In addition to his academic work, he has held several leadership positions within the social work profession, such as clinical director, treatment facility chief executive officer, and senior executive consultant. Dr. Estreet's dedication, extensive knowledge, and expertise continue to be invaluable in advancing the profession and improving the lives of those who rely on social workers for advocacy and support.

Dabney P. Evans, PhD, MPH, is an Associate Professor of Global Health at the Emory Rollins School of Public Health. She is a mixed-methods researcher focused on the health and human rights of women and girls. Dr. Evans received her MPH degree in 1998 from Emory University and her doctoral degree in Law from the University of Aberdeen (UK) in 2011. She is the Director of the Center for Humanitarian Emergencies in the Rollins School of Public Health and the Emory University Institute of Human Rights. As one of the first faculty to include health and human rights in the public health curriculum, Dr. Evans is an established teacher and trainer. Her teaching and training activities have touched over 19,000 learners from 171 countries. She is an editor of the text, *Rights-Based Approaches to Health*, has published over 40 book chapters, scholarly articles and commissioned works; she has made over 200 peer-reviewed and invited presentations.

Leslie Green, PhD, MS, BS, is an Assistant Professor of Consumer Affairs in the School of Family and Consumer Sciences at Texas State University. She received her PhD in Housing and Consumer Economics at the University of Georgia. Dr. Green also holds an MS degree in Consumer Sciences and a BS degree in Family and Consumer Sciences with an emphasis in Family Finance from Utah State University. She is an Accredited Financial Counselor® through the Association for Financial Counseling and Planning Education. She has served on the board of directors for both the Association for Financial Counseling and Planning Education and the Housing Education and Research Association. Dr. Green teaches Introduction to Research Methods for Family and Consumer Sciences and Personal and Family Financial Counseling. Her research interests involve the economic well-being of families and individuals.

Saria Hassan, MD, MPH, is an Assistant Professor at the Emory School of Medicine and Rollins School of Public Health. She is a physician and an implementation scientist with an interest in reducing the inequitable effects of climate change on the health of populations locally and globally. Her work utilizes implementation and systems science approaches to address the needs of people living with chronic non-communicable diseases (NCDs) in the setting of climate-induced disasters. Dr. Hassan has an NIH/NHLBI-funded career development grant working with Federally Qualified Health Centers in Puerto Rico and the US Virgin Islands. She has previously worked with the Pan American Health Organization to address disaster preparedness for NCDs in the Caribbean. Dr. Hassan received her MD from Harvard Medical School and completed her Medicine and Pediatrics training at the Yale School of Medicine. She received her MPH from the London School of Tropical Medicine and Hygiene.

Hui Liew, PhD, is an Associate Professor at the University of Nebraska at Kearney, Kearney, Nebraska, US. She obtained her master's and doctorate degrees in predictive analytics and sociology from Northwestern University and Mississippi State University. The focus of her research is on aging, medical sociology/demography, substance abuse, health inequality, and quantitative methodology.

Kemba Noel-London, PhD, MAT, is a social epidemiologist and athletic trainer who puts an emphasis on evidence-based care and exploring the intersection of sports medicine and public health. She is also an experienced Head Athletic Trainer with a demonstrated history of working in the health, wellness, and fitness industry. She serves as a member of several athletic training and diversity-related organizational boards.

Don Eliseo Lucero-Prisno III, MD, PhD, is a global health scientist whose works focus on health equity. He is also known for his global work in advancing science and research, particularly in the developing world, and in addressing global research inequity. His scientific work is hinged on creating evidence to influence global health policy and practice, improve the health of populations and achieve global health equity. Don is the Editor-in-Chief of Public Health Challenges (Wiley) and is the Deputy Editor-in-Chief of BMC Global Health Research and Policy. He teaches with the London School of Hygiene and Tropical Medicine and the University of the Philippines Open University. He finished his PhD at Cardiff University, MPH at the Royal Tropical Institute in Amsterdam, MSc in Health Economics Policy and Law in Global Health at Erasmus University in Rotterdam, The Netherlands, and his BSc in Psychology (cum laude), and Doctor of Medicine from the University of the Philippines.

Wilson Majee, PhD, MPH, is an Associate Professor with the Departments of Health Science and Public Health at the University of Missouri, Columbia. His overarching research goal is to explore, identify, and implement place-based approaches to health and well-being for those living in resource-limited communities. The history of community health efforts in impoverished and rural areas has largely been a tale of short-term, top-down, funded projects that disappear when grant funding ends, leaving communities jaded and underserved. Wilson works to create sustainable, real-world community health initiatives that live on after grants end because they are derived from and driven by the community members themselves. His work closes knowledge and practice gaps using a socioecological approach to multi-level individual-, family- and place-based factors affecting health and well-being. The interdisciplinary nexus of community leadership development, community engagement, and health promotion is the center of his work.

Keith C. Norris, MD, PhD, is an internationally recognized clinician-scientist and health policy leader who has been instrumental in shaping clinical practice guidelines for chronic kidney disease, developing policy initiatives to address health disparities, and increasing diversity in the biomedical sciences. He is a Professor and Executive Vice Chair for Equity, Diversity, and Inclusion for the UCLA Department of Medicine and Co-Director of the UCLA Clinical and Translational Science Institute Community Engagement Research Program. For 30 years, he has worked to promote community-partnered research. At present, he serves as PI or Multi-PI for 6 NIH research and training grants. As an elected member to the National Academy of Medicine, he has co-authored over 470 articles in peer-reviewed journals and over 30 book chapters.

Joseph Christian Obnial, MD, is currently an Associate Editor for Public Health Challenges by Wiley. He earned his Doctor of Medicine and his Bachelor of Science in Physical Therapy, cum laude, from the University of Santo Tomas (Philippines). He is a member of the Royal Society of Tropical Medicine and Hygiene and the Philippine Physical Therapy Association. His current fields of interest include global health, health policy, and health systems in low- and middle-income countries.

Goodness Ogeyi Odey is a Nigerian public health practitioner and researcher who strongly believes every young person and marginalized group deserves access to the correct information and services to make informed decisions, prevent unplanned futures, and maximize their potential. Goodness is the Regional Lead of Women in Global Health Leadership at Global Health Focus, Africa, where she mentors young women in the African network to actively participate in evidence-based research toward health systems strengthening and sustainable development in African communities. In 2022, Goodness received the prestigious Princess Diana Award for her excellent work advancing health equity in Africa through research, advocacy, and health intervention. She is also an International Conference on Family Planning (ICFP2022) Trailblazer Awardee for her commitment and essential leadership in promoting Sexual Reproductive Health and Rights, especially for young people in Nigeria. She is currently pursuing an MSc in Health Policy, Planning and Financing at the London School of Hygiene and Tropical Medicine (LSHTM) and London School of Economics and Political Science (LSE).

John C. Pollock, PhD, MPA, BA, is a Professor in the Departments of Communication Studies and Public Health, The College of New Jersey. Authored or edited books include *Tilted Mirrors: Media Alignment with Political and Social Change – A Community Structure Approach* (2007); *Media and Social Inequality: Innovations in Community Structure Research* (2013); *Journalism and Human Rights: How Demographics Drive Media Coverage* (2015); (with Mort Winston) *Making Human Rights News: Balancing Participation and Professionalism* (2017); (with Douglas Vakoch) *COVID-19 in International Media: Global Pandemic Responses* (2021); and (with Douglas Vakoch and Amanda Caleb) *COVID Communication: Exploring Pandemic Discourse* (2023). Grant recipient from the Social Science Research Council, the National Cancer Institute, and the United Nations Foundation, as well as a Senior Fulbright Scholar (Argentina, 2010), Pollock has spent over two decades advancing community structure theory, exploring the impact of society on media, examining health communication, and human rights issues.

Monica Ponder, PhD, is an Assistant Professor of Health Communication & Culture in the Department of Communication, Culture and Media Studies within the Cathy Hughes School of Communications at Howard University. Dr. Ponder's research interests examine organization-level approaches to public health and crisis communication practice, particularly those centering a radical Black feminist lens. She is the creator of The Henrietta Hypothesis, an interdisciplinary model for public health crisis communication. This scholarship offers crisis communication recommendations for public health and healthcare organizations seeking to understand, reach, and engage historically marginalized and racialized groups during public health emergencies. She is also the Co-Principal Investigator of Project REFOCUS (Racial Ethnic Framing of Community-Informed and Unifying Surveillance) developed to monitor and address how stigma and racism affect COVID disparities with the goal of creating a more effective response to COVID-19 and other public health crises in a community.

Len Price, Jr., LCSW-C, LCADC, is a PhD candidate in the School of Social Work at Morgan State University. He has over 15 years of experience working in the field of behavioral health, with over five years of clinical experience practicing as a Licensed Clinical Social Worker and as Licensed Clinical Alcohol and Drug Counselor. He has worked with special populations in the areas of addiction, treatment foster care, crisis intervention services, direct patient care within hospital settings and within the criminal justice system. Moreover, Mr. Price has certifications, clinical practice skills, and specialized training that focuses on the prevention and treatment of behavioral health issues such as trauma, grief and loss counseling, gambling disorders, mobile crisis prevention and intervention services, and domestic/intimate partner violence.

Robert Robinson, MPH, BA, currently pursues education in the field of nursing, specifically emergency medicine and critical care. Robinson previously worked with the city of Passaic, New Jersey, public health department. Subsequently, during and after the trauma of COVID-19, he has worked in the emergency room at Clara Maass Hospital, Belleville, New Jersey, from January 2022 to the present (June 2023). That assignment has given Robinson hands-on experience with varieties of physicians and nurses and with all aspects of patient care, increasing his comprehension of patient needs in a public health setting.

Sawsan Salah, MPH, is a PhD candidate in Biobehavioral Health at Penn State University. She is interested in maternal-child health disparities.

Clare V. Schuchardt, MPH, RN, is currently a PhD candidate in Nursing Innovation at Arizona State University. She is interested in children's health and provider mental health.

Mohamud Sheek-Hussein, DrPH, MD, MPH, DTM&H, FFPH (UK), is a consultant of international public health, infectious disease epidemiology, tropical medicine, vaccine-preventable diseases, health disparities, and health equity; currently, he is a Professor of Global Public Health and Infectious Diseases at the Institute of Public Health, College of Medicine and Health Sciences, UAE University-Al Ain, UAE. He holds a Doctor of Public Health from the School of Public Health, University of Texas, Houston-USA (2004); an MD from the University of Parma, Italy (1984); an MPH from Columbia University, New York-USA (1987); and a DTM&H from the Liverpool School of Tropical Medicine (UK). His main areas of research interest include infectious diseases, immunization, mother and child health, and blood-borne diseases, such as viral hepatitis, HIV/AIDS, liver cancer, tuberculosis, and malaria. During the past 40 years, he gained teaching and clinical expertise in health care systems, public health services, infectious disease surveillance, and emergency preparedness. He has published more than 40 papers in peer-reviewed journals.

Kelly D. Taylor, PhD, MPH, is a behavioral scientist with a background in community psychology, epidemiology, and evaluation methodology. She completed her postdoctoral fellowship in AIDS prevention at the University of California, San Francisco, Center for AIDS Prevention Studies. Her primary research interests are in research capacity building in low resource settings, health disparities, and psychosocial determinants of health in developing countries, particularly the role of health-seeking behavior among key populations at risk for HIV. She is also interested in the treatment of HIV and other chronic diseases such as hypertension and diabetes. Dr. Taylor's emphasis is in sub-Saharan Africa, and she has worked professionally in Ghana, Kenya, Mozambique, Nigeria, Senegal, and South Africa.

Jacqueline Veronica Velasco, MD, obtained her Doctor of Medicine, cum laude, from the University of Santo Tomas (Philippines) and a Bachelor of Science in Health Sciences from Ateneo De Manila University (Philippines). Her research interests include health policy, virology, and global health.

Paulene Miriel Viacrusis, BSc, is currently completing her Doctor of Medicine degree from the University of Santo Tomas (Philippines) and acquired her Bachelor of Science in Basic Human Studies, magna cum laude, from the same university. She has an interest in health technology and public health research.

1 Health, Inequalities, and Building a Culture of Preparedness

Roland J. Thorpe, Jr. and DeMond S. Miller

Disasters can spawn new or exacerbate root causes that produce disparities in health and health care. The genesis of *Health Disparities in an Age of Disasters and Crises: Responding with a Culture of Preparedness* predates the COVID-19 pandemic. Prior to this global disaster, calls for creating a culture of preparedness began just before the turn of the century and were more codified into legislation and laws with President George W. Bush's Homeland Security Presidential Directive-8 that asserted a bold vision that would

> …help ensure the preparedness of the Nation to prevent, respond to, and recover from threatened and actual domestic terrorist attacks, major disasters, and other emergencies, the Secretary, in coordination with the heads of other appropriate Federal departments and agencies and in consultation with State and local governments, shall develop a national domestic all-hazards preparedness goal.
>
> (HSPD-8, 2005, § 1)

However, the "natural disaster" Hurricane Katrina was not so natural after all. Root causes of social disparities in health before the hurricane were linked to poverty, poor housing, lack of access to health care, and discrimination. At the intersection of emergency management, public health, and the emergence of a culture of preparedness is the critical role that preparation for disasters plays in guarding against furthering social disparities in health as communities recover. Several hearings and investigations concluded that a re-emphasis on the role of preparedness was needed. Finally, the extensive report, *The Federal Response to Hurricane Katrina: Lessons Learned–Chapter Six: Transforming National Preparedness*, asserts the primary recommendation of developing a culture of preparedness. The culture of preparedness remains a strategic priority linked to national security as the underpinning of a National Preparedness System with a shared vision for preparedness as directed by the Homeland Security Presidential Directive 8 (HSPD-8, 2005). In the directive and further amplified by The Federal Response to Hurricane Katrina Report, the President called for the creation of a comprehensive National Preparedness System, starting with a "national domestic all-hazards preparedness goal" (HSPD-8, 2005, § 1) to incorporate the private sector, non-governmental organizations, faith-based groups, and communities, including individual citizens. The desired end-state of our National Preparedness System must be to achieve and sustain risk-based target levels of capability to prevent, protect against, respond to, and recover from major events to minimize the impact on lives, property, and the economy (United States, 2006, pp. 66–67) from an all-hazards perspective.

The COVID-19 pandemic has heightened our awareness to the number of different inequities that permeate society. Moving from notion to implementation of achieving health equity and social justice globally is paramount. Natural disasters, such as the current global pandemic, provides a

DOI: 10.4324/9781003140245-1

unique opportunity for scientific contributions to consider approaches that can benefit all in the darkest of circumstances. More specifically, gaining a better understanding of efforts at all levels while focusing on long-term recovery, resource allocation, and collaboration across a variety of sectors in society are critical for a preparedness for future disasters.

While addressing the social determinants of health has been a popular approach to reducing or eliminating the stark disparities in health and healthcare, this approach is further complicated when occurring simultaneously and in the aftermath of disasters such as COVID-19 (Wang & Tang, 2020). Our history of mitigating the effects of disasters has involved operating and requiring much from nimble infrastructures that did or were not able to communicate across sectors. Hence, we found ourselves trying to combat a disaster with less-than-ideal tools or a workforce that was not fully prepared or cognizant of the root causes of the challenges presented. Scholars, public health officials, and emergency managers must be able to clearly understand and situate health-related disasters as part of a more extensive system that recognizes root causes with implications for mitigation via a culture of preparedness.

As social disasters, civil unrest, interlocking risks, and dangers in the global community serve to propel unaddressed root causes (Chapman *et al.*, 2021; Miller, 2021), this volume highlights the ongoing challenges that lie at the root of health disparities and their impacts.

To understand inequalities during the COVID-19 pandemic, we must understand how risks and differential exposure to infection, differential susceptibility, and differential consequences of COVID-19 impact groups in society (Burström & Tao, 2020) and highlight the reality of the pre-existing social vulnerability. Authors herein note that no single dimension of vulnerability fueled the social catastrophe of global infection rates based on the interaction of multiple dimensions—race/ethnicity, income, social isolation, family structure, housing—that ultimately created the differential outcomes. For example, in the United States, the negative impacts of the COVID-19 pandemic were in large part borne by the African American community, the poor, renters, the unemployed, and the undereducated and, likewise, the literature on the long-term efforts to enhance resilience so that the social burdens of the impacts of future disasters are mitigated. An uneven distribution of vulnerabilities can impose different stresses across populations and lead to overall underinvestment in prevention and preparedness—thus, a lack of preparedness.

Health Disparities in an Age of Disasters and Crises: Responding with a Culture of Preparedness presents chapters that address how the intersection of emergency preparedness, emergency response, and health inequalities can lead to an integrated response. The chapters provide key insights into the interconnectedness of public health and emergency management and response systems.

As we move beyond socially constructed divides that place emphasis on variations in legal, cultural, and organizational contexts that exist from nation to nation, we will always have differences in health care systems, traditions, and official standards that govern practices. However, in the 21st century, we have a unique opportunity to rebuild public health systems that respond to the crises of our times. In essence, Quinn S.C. (2006, 204) notes, "[i]f we do not use this moment to address the underlying vulnerabilities of poor and minority communities, we will only perpetuate the social determinants that manifest themselves in health disparities and human suffering".

References

Burström, B., & Tao, W. (2020). "Social Determinants of Health and Inequalities in COVID-19." *European Journal of Public Health*, 30(4), 617–618. https://doi.org/10.1093/eurpub/ckaa095.

Chapman, C., Miller, D. S., & Salley, G. (2021). "Social Disruption of the Tourism and Hospitality Industries: Implications for post-COVID-19 Pandemic Recovery." *Worldwide Hospitality and Tourism Themes*, 13(3), 312–323. https://doi.org/10.1108/WHATT-02-2021-0038.

Miller, D. S. (2021). "Abrupt New Realities Amid the Disaster Landscape as One Crisis Gives Way to Crises." *Worldwide Hospitality and Tourism Themes*, *13*(3), 304–311. https://doi.org/10.1108/WHATT-02-2021-0037.

Quinn, S. C. (2006). Hurricane Katrina: A Social and Public Health Disaster." *American Journal of Public Health*, *96*(2), 204. https://doi.org/10.2105/AJPH.2005.080119.

The White House, Homeland Security Presidential Directive-8: National Preparedness ["HSPD-8"] (Washington, DC, December 17, 2003). Presidential Policy Directive / PPD-8: National Preparedness.

United States, Executive Office of the President, & United States, Assistant to the President for Homeland Security and Counterterrorism. (2006). *The Federal Response to Hurricane Katrina: Lessons Learned*. Washington, DC: White House.

Wang, Z., & Tang, K. (2020). "Combating COVID-19: Health Equity Matters." *Nature Medicine*, *26*, 458.

2 Inclusive Preparedness and Emergency Response for Disasters Yet to Come

Derron G. Cooney and DeMond S. Miller

Introduction

The failure to ensure the health and inclusive preparedness for those most vulnerable to disasters remains a significant issue during and after a disaster. It is essential to examine the past occurrences and the deficiencies in public health during disasters with a focus on disasters looming in the near future with a fundamental objective of preserving human lives. Accessible health care during a crisis can often be overlooked, even in areas with a greater population of vulnerable citizens and communities with a large population of individuals with functional needs. For example, functional need(s) individuals "are more likely to be adversely affected in emergencies, planning, and implementation of mitigation strategies and should incorporate these segments of the population to reduce the public health impact of emergencies" (Schroeder & Bouldin, 2019). It is estimated that in the United States, half of the population is believed to have an access issue or functional need concern (Schroeder & Bouldin, 2019). Many other demographics are disproportionately affected by not having access to health care services and basic needs to survive a disaster. Unfortunately, many of the groups who struggle at this time of disaster are individuals who are aging, low-income minorities, and single parents. One recent research study concluded that in November 2021,

> ...the Centers for Disease Control reported 1.9 times higher mortality rate for the Black population and 2.1 times higher mortality rate for the Latino population compared to the White population. Between 2019 and 2020, life expectancy dropped three years for the Latino population, 2.9 years for the Black population, and 1.2 years for the White population
>
> (Chandran & Schulman, 2022)

These numbers increase when presented with many different kinds of disasters. Moving forward with a focus on mitigation is critical. Proper measures are needed to meet the challenges posed by disasters. As such, the focus shifts to mitigation strategies that offer increased levels of protection and are effectively employed to afford inclusion from the onset and during the planning process. More disasters are bound to happen throughout the United States. What can be done to give adequate health care and resources to these groups most alienated by these impacts? Even following recent disasters, the need for health care accessibility and availability has not increased anywhere near enough to include the demographics most in need. Future disasters will continue to expose these problems if the necessary solutions are not presented and implemented. This chapter contains recommendations to enhance practices for proper and fair inclusion of groups for future disasters. Incorporating more voices in the disaster planning and mitigation processes is important, not only in the United States but worldwide. Now, more than ever, an inclusive approach to disaster

DOI: 10.4324/9781003140245-2

preparedness is vital to the long-term sustainability of resilience. It often occurs when basic human needs for survival are not met in a time of catastrophe and chaos and when support from public health is needed the most.

The Need for More Voices

In the emerging world of disasters and crises, it is essential to have a robust health system that is integrated with the emergency preparedness system. FEMA (n.d.) finds that while many community organizations focus on meeting the diverse needs of people with disabilities, other groups work on reducing disaster risk; however these issues are not always integrated. Many efforts to support the disaster-related needs of people with disabilities focus on preparedness and response, not long-term risk reduction. Bringing these issues together and focusing on risk reduction promotes community resilience. Clearly, while special needs populations can be expected to consume more resources in the event of a major regional disaster, there are no shortcuts to effective community disaster planning. When local health resources are rendered scarce or dysfunctional after a disaster, chronic conditions become acute, especially among racially and ethnically diverse segments of the most vulnerable groups of victims—children, elders, the infirm, and the impoverished (Andrulis et al., 2007; Institute of Medicine, 2010, p. 135; Mokdad et al., 2005). Unfortunately, efforts to enhance health system surge capacity increasingly proceed side by side with efforts to curtail health care expenses, making community-wide planning processes that invoke infrequently used social capital increasingly crucial (Felland et al., 2008; Institute of Medicine, 2010, p. 135; Koh & Cadigan, 2007). The effects of such a mismatch between health needs and resources after a major disaster can be truly devastating, as shown by the well-chronicled events that followed in the wake of Hurricane Katrina (Berggren & Curiel, 2006; Institute of Medicine, 2010, p. 135; Johnston & Redlener, 2006). The current COVID-19 pandemic and disasters that have already occurred, including Hurricane Katrina, offer insight into the complex intersections of multiple vulnerabilities and how they are intertwined. Without risk reduction measures taken to "prevent, protect against, quickly respond to, and recover from health emergencies, particularly those whose scale, timing, or unpredictability threatens to overwhelm routine capabilities" (Nelson et al., 2007), to save lives that may be lost and enhance health care outcomes following an event. Health preparedness is essential to the older population, with higher mortality and morbidity rates for elderly individuals. Older adults living alone are considered a higher at-risk group even before a disaster; the risk exponentially increases during and succeeding the event. There have been billions of dollars used toward programs and projects to attempt to improve this facet of the preparedness world, but they have been unsuccessful. This has been a controversial topic whether the United States has the health preparedness needed for current and future disasters. "Income and race on insurance coverage was devastating as low-income minorities with bad health had 68% less odds of being insured instead of uninsured or insured for part of the year than high-income Whites with good health" (Lee et al., 2021). Hurricane Katrina and COVID-19 illustrate the systemic lack of preparedness in the United States. COVID-19 clearly illustrates multiple failures to prepare and respond correctly to this pandemic disaster.

While it is difficult to prepare for such a disaster on a global scale, the negative impacts of this event were exasperated by citizens not having simple health resources. The focus on other issues in the United States had overshadowed the possibility of a pandemic and health preparedness. For example,

in the past two decades, the United States alone has spent countless billions on homeland security and counterterrorism to defend against human enemies, losing sight of the demonstrably far greater threat posed by microbial enemies; terrorists don't have the capacity to bring Americans' way of life to a screeching halt, something Covid-19 accomplished handily in a matter of weeks

(Osterholm & Olshaker, 2020)

Many leaders in the health industry had been forewarned of a major pandemic that would be occurring soon; sadly, they were correct, and many have suffered as a result of this inadequate preparation. These demographics are known to struggle the most without adequate health care and resources. The response during COVID-19 was unacceptable; many vulnerable older adults were at risk, and one Texas Lieutenant Governor suggested rationing their health care and sacrificing for the U.S. economy (Maxfield & Pituch, 2021). This is just one example of many instances in which politicians did not respect how at-risk older individuals are during these disasters. However, even when there was an emphasis on physical health and resources, the citizens forgot about the negative mental effects that isolation can create for people. Many research projects argue that "the psychological stress of the pandemic was highlighted in a nationwide survey conducted March 25 to 30, 2020, which revealed that approximately 45% of Americans report that COVID-19 worry or stress has had a negative impact on mental health" (Panchal et al., 2020 via. Maxfield & Pituch, 2021). The impacts on the people affected by a disaster are sometimes more mental problems that occur during, and often following, a disaster. Nurses and other medical personnel reported the failure to prepare for this pandemic; the health care industry has always been focused on profit rather than the health of the U.S. citizens (Svetvilas, 2020). Underprivileged groups often suffer the consequences of the healthcare system focusing on profit instead of inclusion.

COVID-19 has especially affected minority populations, with the Black population accounting for nearly 33% of hospitalized cases and Latinos for 23% so far. Native Americans have also been hard hit. The data has been a wakeup call in the industry.

(Castellucci, 2020)

The proper strategies and resources are not being provided to these communities in preparation for other infections or diseases. Before COVID-19, the Navajo Nation had many people who did not have sufficiently healthy living conditions: many had no running water or electricity. In addition, many in the community have pre-existing conditions or other illnesses that increased their vulnerability without access to the proper facilities needed to treat this minority population. Well before COVID-19, African- Americans have historically disproportionate higher rates of chronic diseases such as asthma, hypertension and diabetes—underlying conditions that exacerbated the mortality rate for this group during the height of the COVID-19 pandemic.

Health disparities among African Americans arise from an interplay of racial, social, and gender disparities in which the main social determinants of health are racism, poverty, educational level, environmental and living conditions (e.g., housing and exposures within the environment), access to healthy foods, violence, and inequities in criminal justice

(Noonan et al., 2016 via. Webber-Ritchey & Lane-Cordova, 2021)

As a result, many of these majority-black cities were being thumped by this pandemic with many areas having higher infection and death rates. Many in these areas already have pre-existing conditions, such as diabetes and/or hypertension, that increase the possibility of contracting the disease and impacting the recovery chances. "Lower income households further exacerbated under COVID when racial/ethnic minorities and low-income individuals are more likely to be susceptible to infection and mortality and less likely to get timely treatment and vaccination" (Lee et al., 2021). According to the numbers that were presented in bigger cities like Milwaukee, St. Louis,

Chicago, and New York City, which is home to a large African-American population, have had soaring infection rates (Millett et al., 2020; Webber-Ritchey & Lane-Cordova, 2021). Hurricane Katrina illustrated how the lack of health preparedness can impact groups of people for decades to come. Many citizens, structures, and businesses have still not recovered from this disaster and remain displaced. The government distrust during and after Hurricane Katrina regarding the well-being of lower-income individuals and the minority population is still prevalent. It is well-known that Louisiana is a very vulnerable state where there is constant flooding and repeated natural disasters. In addition, "Louisiana is among the states with the highest rates of chronic health conditions such as asthma, cardiovascular disease, diabetes, obesity, and cancer," and New Orleans led the country pre-Katrina in childhood asthma (Lichtveld et al., 2020). Many of these health issues arise from either not having enough money for health care, not having plans sufficient enough for their family, and/or not having the health resources provided in their low-income communities. Low-income individuals, single parents, and the aging population once again struggle in these disasters; this is a trend throughout time that has been recognized, but needs to be something we prepare for in the future.

> Tragically, the federal government's health policy response failed to rise to the level of need in the Gulf Coast region. Although the Bush administration had approved a temporary Medicaid expansion after the 9/11 attacks to ensure that low-income survivors were covered, it rejected a similar approach after Katrina and maintained restrictive eligibility rules. As a result, thousands of uninsured evacuees who attempted to sign up for coverage were turned away in their moments of greatest need.
>
> (Huelskoetter, 2015)

Even years before Hurricane Katrina devastated Louisiana and Mississippi, these states were already falling behind in the public health preparedness field from government acts like this one.

The health disparity and health inclusiveness margin continued to widen compared with other states in the United States. While Katrina made landfall, both states currently had the highest "uninsured rates" in the nation while also, "an annual public health survey ranked Mississippi and Louisiana the nation's two least healthy states in 2004" (Huelskoetter, 2015). If these citizens do not have health insurance and the proper health needs before disaster strikes, it can dramatically hinder their chances of responding to and recovering from such an event.

> When Katrina struck, about 22 percent of Louisiana residents and 23 percent of New Orleans residents were living in poverty ($16,090 for a family of three). Over 900,000 people or 21 percent of all residents in Louisiana, had no health insurance. Tied to these poverty and uninsurance rates, Louisiana also had some of the poorest health statistics in the country with high rates of infant mortality, chronic diseases such as heart disease and diabetes, and AIDS cases, and lower than average childhood immunization rates.
>
> (Kaiser, 2006, p. 1)

For example, after Medicaid[1] expansion following the terror attacks of 9/11, health care remained a challenge for many people. The reforms set boundaries on the ability to receive Medicaid, leaving many without the ability to properly treat illnesses. Only 19% of Louisiana pre-Katrina was covered in the Medicaid program even though the consensus in the country determined that they were one of the poorest states and the unhealthiest (Kaiser, 2006). How can citizens build healthy resilient communities to recover from assaults of natural disasters without proper assistance?

Building Resilient Healthcare Infrastructure

Clearly, the long-term goal is for every community to have specific plans for its vulnerable and functional needs populations as part of a comprehensive disaster plan for community crisis and disaster management via a concerted effort of public and private entities concerned with the health and well-being of the community as a whole. Looking back on COVID-19 pandemic and Hurricane Katrina, there should have been many changes in healthcare institutional preparedness following the lessons learned following the hurricane to enhance resilience for future disasters.

Disasters oftentimes serve to unveil the weaknesses of critical infrastructure, in this chapter's example, healthcare infrastructure preparedness, at a time when policymakers tend to prioritize evacuation, many were not committed to elevating the status or improving the issue. The United States needs to enhance access and availability of health resources to vulnerable populations, low-income individuals, and single parents. As noted throughout the chapter, the need to give these groups proper resources is essential in preparation for a disaster and recovery. As part of a well-designed response plan, recovery planning, in addition to the maintenance of life, is a critical aspect of building resilient communities that can be taken before a disaster occurs. The widespread media coverage following Hurricane Katrina clearly illustrated how the United States' disaster response was sorely lacking in its capabilities to care for its younger, older, functional needs citizens, dispossessed, food insecure, and carless (transportation insecure) groups. In essence, if a community's members are not able to "bounce back," such communities will find sustained recovery and long-term resilience-building challenging as they enter the recovery stage of disaster management. In such cases, the impacts of future disaster shocks will be far more devastating. Many years later, some of Hurricane Katrina's hardest-hit areas continue to live with complicated recovery issues exposing them to future hazards.

For the citizens who reside in the vulnerable states near the Gulf of Mexico, disasters frequently wreak havoc. Furthermore, these states struggle with healthcare access in urban and rural areas. Even the people in New Orleans still have problems getting adequate healthcare over a decade later. "Respondents who are worried that 'health care services might not be available if they need them' has dropped from 85 percent in 2006, it remains extremely high at 54 percent today," and there are still many who "report skipping medical care or prescribed drugs due to costs, especially among the uninsured" (Huelskoetter, 2015). Since Hurricane Katrina, improvements have continued; however, gaps in the healthcare infrastructure persist as evidenced by the response to COVID-19. Once again, a major disaster befell the region and that region, like many other regions, struggled to meet the needs of the most vulnerable. Many health preparedness plans were not established thus,

> [i]ntersecting with baseline vulnerability, a lack of resources to prevent and limit disease spread, including PPE, physical distancing, handwashing, testing, and access to effective and affordable vaccines, is amplifying the burden of addressing the immediate social determinants of COVID-19 in LMICs
>
> (Ho & Dascalu, 2021; McMahon et al., 2020)

Preparing for disasters can be done through many different practices. When considering public health preparedness, one of the best-regarded practices is the "Project Public Health Ready." This program is "a criteria-based public health preparedness program that assesses local health department capability and capacity to prepare for, respond to, and recover from public health emergencies" (Summers & Ferraro, 2017). Examining how capable an area is regarding its public health resources and the citizens' vulnerability helps identify a plethora of possible obstacles a region faces during a disaster. The Project Public Health Ready's main goals include local health departments' engagement in planning processes that develop "*a written all-hazards plan, a workforce development and training plan, and documentation of exercises or real-event responses*" (Summers & Ferraro, 2017). PPHR offers insights into health issues that many local health departments often overlook when creating preparedness plans. Finding out how many citizens have functional needs or health access could be consequential to the number of fatalities and injuries responding to or recovering from a disaster. The recovery aspect of a disaster is often one of the more overlooked parts of emergency management plans. Another reason the PPHR is considered one of the best is its ability to work with local, state, and federal governments to achieve their goals; this is often considered one of the most challenging parts of creating sound public health preparedness plans.

> PPHR is a tool and a framework that local health departments use to enhance preparedness capacity and capability rather than a prescriptive set of standards that must be met singularly. National reviewers undergo a training and assessment process before scoring applications to help ensure consistency across and among review teams
>
> (Summers & Ferraro, 2017)

When the PPHR can have this consistency throughout the country, it maximizes possible resources for each disaster or crisis that can strike vulnerable areas and citizens. As with any public health program, it can be challenging to reach other local and state jurisdictions; in response, the National Association of County and City Health Officials has developed alternative cohort models in conjunction with the CDC to allow the PPHR cost to be Public Health Emergency Preparedness reimbursable; it is currently using PPHR criteria to address healthcare infrastructure preparedness and response (Summers & Ferraro, 2017). "Since 2004, more than 500 LHDs have been recognized as meeting all the PPHR requirements individually or working collaboratively as a region" (PPHR, 2022, Par. 2).

Conclusion

As disasters continue, they serve as opportunities to address past issues as a way to save lives. An inclusive approach to emergency preparedness must include multiple stakeholder groups of a community in all aspects of emergency management, with members of the community engaged, to the extent possible, in every aspect of the preparedness, mitigation, response, short-term recovery, and long-term recovery processes. In fact, input from people with different functional needs and health needs can enhance policies, responses, and recovery processes. Much of the focus on health and inclusive preparedness often disregards the many resources different demographics require to respond sufficiently and recover. Unfortunately, the financial side of emergency response overshadows the actual physical needs in times of disaster.

Measures to address challenges to a robust and inclusive disaster preparedness system are underway. With building a resilient healthcare system in vulnerable communities based on lessons learned and best practices following Hurricane Katrina and COVID-19, Project Public Health Ready offers an indispensable model for cooperation among local and regional health departments. More work must be done in implementing inclusive preparedness to address the gaps in services, accessibility, and affordability of efforts to build resilient healthcare infrastructures and communities. Disasters will continue to occur. An inclusive process of planning and ensuring an inclusive response execution will bring us a step closer toward a more inclusive and responsive society focused on recovery.

Note

1   To obtain entry into the Medicaid program the person applying had to go through a long documentation process proving they could meet the strict boundaries, which include people considered low-income along with, "certain people with disabilities, children, the elderly, pregnant women, or very-low-income parents" (Huelskoetter, 2015). Furthermore, other low-income individuals who were not disabled and did not have children were denied this service (Huelskoetter, 2015). The long process deterred many from applying for healthcare assistance in one of the most vulnerable states in the country.

References

Andrulis, D. P., Siddiqui, N. J., & Gantner, J. L. (2007). Preparing Racially and Ethnically Diverse Communities for Public Health Emergencies. *Health Affairs, 26*, 1269–1279.

Berggren, R. E., & Curiel, T. J. (2006). After the Storm—Health Care Infrastructure in Post-Katrina New Orleans. *The New England Journal of Medicine, 354*, 1549–1552.

Castellucci, M. (2020). What We've Learned: Even the Brightest and Most-prepared Hospital CEOs Couldn't Have Been Ready for the Initial Wave of COVID-19, but Now They've Learned a Few Things. *Modern Healthcare, 50*(36), 14.

Chandran, M., & Schulman, K. A. (2022). Racial Disparities in Healthcare and Health. *Health Services Research, 57*(2), 218–222.

Felland, L. E., Katz, A., Liebhaber, A., & Cohen, G. R. (2008). Developing Health System Surge Capacity: Community Efforts in Jeopardy. Research Brief No. 5. Center for Studying Health System Change: 2008. [accessed March 9, 2010].

FEMA. (n.d.). Guide to Expanding Mitigation Making the Connection to People with Disabilities. https://www.fema.gov/sites/default/files/documents/fema_r2-making-connection-people-disabilities.pdf.

Ho, A., & Dascalu, I. (2021). Relational Solidarity and COVID-19: An Ethical Approach to Disrupt the Global Health Disparity Pathway. *Global Bioethics, 32*(1), 34–50.

Huelskoetter, T. (2015, August 20). *Hurricane Katrina's Health Care Legacy.* Center for American Progress. Retrieved May 25, 2022, from https://www.americanprogress.org/article/hurricane-katrinas-health-care-legacy/

Institute of Medicine (US) Forum on Medical and Public Health Preparedness for Catastrophic Events. Medical Surge Capacity: Workshop Summary. Washington (DC): National Academies Press (US) (2010). G, Vulnerable Populations in Disasters: Health Effects and Needs. Retrieved from: https://www.ncbi.nlm.nih.gov/books/NBK32854/

Johnston, C. & Redlener, I. (Eds.) (2006). Hurricane Katrina, Children, and Pediatric Heroes: Hands-on Stories by and of Our Colleagues Helping Families during the Most Costly Natural Disaster in US History. American Academy of Pediatrics. Itasca, IL: Elk Grove Village.

Kaiser Commission on Medicaid and the Uninsured: Key Facts. (2006). Kaiser Family Foundation's Washington, DC. Retrieved from https://www.kff.org/wp-content/uploads/2013/01/7442.pdf

Koh, H. K., & Cadigan, R. O. (2007). Disaster Preparedness and Social Capital. In: Kawachi, I., Subramanian, S. V., & Kim, D., editors. *Social Capital and Health.* New York: Springer New York, pp. 273–285.

Lee, D.-C., Liang, H., & Shi, L. (2021). The Convergence of Racial and Income Disparities in Health Insurance Coverage in the United States. *International Journal for Equity in Health, 20*(1), 1–8.

Lichtveld, M., Covert, H., El-Dahr, J., Grimsley, L. F., Cohn, R., Watson, C. H., Thornton, E., & Kennedy, S. (2020). A Community-Based Participatory Research Approach to Hurricane Katrina: When Disasters, Environmental Health Threats, and Disparities Collide. *American Journal of Public Health, 110*(10), 1485–1489.

Maxfield, M., & Pituch, K. A. (2021). COVID-19 Worry, Mental Health Indicators, and Preparedness for Future Care Needs across the Adult Lifespan. *Aging & Mental Health, 25*(7), 1273–1280.

McMahon, D. E., Peters, G. A., Ivers, L. C., & Freeman, E. E. (2020, July 1). Global resource shortages during COVID-19: Bad news for low-income countries. *PLoS Neglected Tropical Diseases, 14*(7), 1–3. https://doi.org/10.1371/journal.pntd.0008412

Millett, G. A., Jones, A. T., Benkeser, D., Baral, S., Mercer, L., Beyrer, C., Honermann, B., Lankiewicz, E., Mena, L., Crowley, J. S., Sherwood, J., Sullivan, P. S. (2020 Jul). Assessing differential impacts of COVID-19 on black communities. *Annals of Epidemiology*, *47*, 37–44. doi: 10.1016/j.annepidem.2020.05.003. Epub 2020 May 14. PMID: 32419766; PMCID: PMC7224670.

Mokdad, A. H., Mensah, G. A., Posner, S. F., Reed, E., Simoes, E. J., & Engelau, M. M. (2005 Nov). When Chronic Conditions Become Acute: Prevention and Control of Chronic Diseases and Adverse Health Outcomes During National Disasters. *Preventing Chronic Disease.* Spec No: A04. Epub 2005 Nov 1.

Nelson, C., Lurie, N., Wasserman, J., & Zakowski, S. (2007). Conceptualizing and Defining Public Health Emergency Preparedness. *American journal of public health*, *97*(Suppl 1), S9–S11. https://doi.org/10.2105/AJPH.2007.114496

Osterholm, M. T., & Olshaker, M. (2020). Chronicle of a Pandemic Foretold. *Foreign Affairs*, *99*(4), 9–24.

PPHR. (n.d.). *Project Public Health Ready (PPHR)*. NACCHO. Retrieved July 27, 2022, from https://www.naccho.org/programs/public-health-preparedness/pphr

Schroeder, J., & Bouldin, E. D. (2019). Inclusive Public Health Preparedness Program to Promote Resilience in Rural Appalachia (2016–2018). *American Journal of Public Health*, *109*, S283–S285.

Summers, S. K., & Ferraro, M. J. (2017). Project Public Health Ready: History and Evolution of a Best Practice for Public Health Preparedness Planning. *American Journal of Public Health*, *107*, S138–S141.

Svetvilas, C. (2020). National Nurse Survey Exposes Hospitals' Knowing Failure to Prepare for a Covid-19 Surge. *National Nurse*, *116*(4), 6–7.

Webber-Ritchey, K. J., & Lane-Cordova, A. D. (2021). Health Disparities and COVID-19 Pandemic: Increasing Clinical Research Participation among African Americans. *Journal of Health Disparities Research & Practice*, *14*(2), 53–63.

3 Racialized Healthcare Inequities as Determinant of COVID-19 Disaster Risks and Outcomes

Moving Toward COVID-19 Disaster Recovery

Paul Archibald, Marino A. Bruce, Keith C. Norris, and Roland J. Thorpe, Jr.

Introduction

On March 13, 2020, the coronavirus disease 2019 (COVID-19) pandemic was declared a disaster for all states, tribes, territories, and the District of Columbia by former President Trump (The White House, 2020). This decision was supported by Section 501 (b) of the Robert T. Stafford Disaster Relief and Emergency Assistance Act, 42 U.S.C. 5121–5207 (the "Stafford Act"), which was enacted in 1988 to provide systematic structure to state and local governments' federal natural disaster assistance to their citizens (United States Department of Homeland Security, 2021). As state and local governments are scrambling to assist their communities during this disaster, the COVID-19 pandemic as a disaster risk to populations has a social dimension that must be understand in order to reduce risk and increase resilience (Seddighi, 2020). For instance, it has been shown that there is not an equal distribution of COVID-19 risk. COVID-19 risks tend to be higher in zip codes with lower socioeconomic status (SES) and increased populations of Blacks compared with zip codes with higher SES and decreased populations of Blacks (Akanbi, Rivera, Akanbi, & Shoyinka, 2021; Chen & Krieger, 2021; Palacio & Tamariz, 2021; Whittle & Diaz-Artiles, 2020).

In addition, this reality of the COVID-19 pandemic among the U.S. population unearthed the deep-rooted and unsurprising inequities in the U.S. health care system. The inequities are caused by pervasive policies and practices that promote an unequal distribution of economics, education, resources, and ultimately power and resources among communities based on race, place, gender, socioeconomic status, and other factors. This chapter will describe how these racialized inequities inherent in the U.S. health care system has influenced the COVID-19 disaster risk, and outcomes and are not solely a political or social issue but also a public health issue. We use Bonilla Silva's (1997) framework of racialized systems to provide some explanation for the disproportionate impact of COVID-19 on the Black community. We use the National Disaster Recovery Framework (NDRF) and the National Response Framework (NRF) to guide our discussion on the COVID-19 disaster recovery process for the Black population. We provoke a call to service for public health professionals to develop a social justice and health equity approach to public health. This public health social justice approach views everyone as valuable with equal rights and opportunities, including the right to optimal health. Then, and only then, we will be able to promote successful COVID-19 pandemic disaster recovery.

Disaster Recovery, COVID-19 Disaster Risk, and Public Health

The NDRF and the NRF are frameworks used to identify disaster response actions (United States Department of Homeland Security, 2011). The NRF framework are the short-term recovery activities that address the life-saving/sustaining measures intended to neutralize the immediate

DOI: 10.4324/9781003140245-3

life-threatening events. The NDRF then provides the long-term tools to promote the early integration of recovery methods into the early response phase extending to post-disaster recovery. Hence, both the NDRF and the NRF are helpful tools used to guide our discussion on the COVID-19 disaster recovery process. However, to be able to fully examine the scope of COVID-19 disaster recovery process, we must discuss the COVID-19 disaster risk and its relationship to public health. The COVID-19 disaster risk can be best explained using the formula, risk = disaster × vulnerability × exposure (Seddighi, 2020). The relationship among COVID-19 (as the disaster), vulnerability, and exposure in the Black community can be best understood using public health social justice lens. For instance, the promotion of health care is the foundation of social justice for public health. In this view, everyone deserves an opportunity to achieve and maintain good health. Public health is grounded in principles of prevention and early intervention as approaches to the establishment and maintenance of health and wellbeing. The World Health Organization (WHO) (1948) defined health as "the state of complete physical, mental and social wellbeing and not merely an absence of disease or infirmity." This conceptualization of health seemed to suggest that other dimensions of health co-exist with the presence of disease and infirmity. The measurement of health using this paradigm later served as the catalyst for the development of what is known today as the social determinants of health (SDoH). SDoH are the "structural determinants and conditions and circumstances in which people are born, grow up, live, work and age…" (WHO, 2019). SDoH has been gaining increased attention in public health as they have been found to be associated with the causes of differential health outcomes among Black people (Noonan, Velasco-Mondragon, & Wagner, 2016). Some major SDoH include racism, poverty, education, housing, zip code, neighborhood conditions, access to healthy foods, health care access, environmental exposures, community violence, and criminal justice.

WHO (1986) protest that everyone should have access to a wholesome-healthy life. However, this has not been realized for Black people due to the lack of health equity and illuminated during this COVID-19 pandemic (Chen et al., 2020; Krieger, Waterman, & Chen, 2020; Wolf et al., 2020; Woolhandler & Himmelstein, 2020). The Healthy People 2020 defines health equity as the "attainment of the highest level of health for all people" (US Department of Health and Human Services, 2010). Being able to achieve health equity requires that everyone's life is valued equally with an emphasis on comprehensively addressing historical and current injustices, health and health care disparities, and all structural inequalities. This would mean that a successful COVID-19 pandemic disaster recovery process for the Black population would promote practices that enhance their health equity which would minimize their risk to the hazards of the pandemic (United States Department of Homeland Security, 2011). Promoting health equity among the Black population would also strengthen their ability to withstand and recover from the COVID-19 pandemic, building on their resiliency.

Racism as a Factor in the COVID-19 Disaster Recovery Process

A successful COVID-19 pandemic disaster recovery process includes an assessment of the risks that serve as recovery challenges to the Black population, such as exposure to racism. There are numerous conceptualizations of racism in the public health literature. However, race is not rooted in biology, but it is a sociopolitical, economic, and cultural construct that has developed through time and context (Barrett & Roediger, 2012). In Ta-Nehisi Coates' book, *Between the World and Me*, he writes in the form of a letter from a father to a son, and coined the phrase "race is the child of racism, not the father" (p. 7). In this context, if race is the child and not the father, then race was birthed from racism. In developing a biopsychosocial model of racism, Clark and colleagues (1999) identified that these conceptualizations could be catalogued into two categories: attitudinal or behavioral. Attitudinal racism refers to attitudes and beliefs that are held about a group of people while behavioral racism is the action taken to block a group of people from equal access to resources. All of these are based on the phenotypic characteristics or ethnic affiliation of the targeted group. Echoing the premise of that conceptualization, racism is also understood through Ostrom's (1969) adapted socio-psychological ABC model. The ABC model of racism proposes three components that are manifested by the racist perpetrator on the targeted group based on their ethnic affiliation or phenotypic characteristics. The *A* represents the *affective* component, which are prejudicial feelings toward a group of people. The *B* is the *behavioral* component, representing the discriminatory acts toward a group of people. The *C* encompasses the *cognitive* component, incorporating the stereotypes or beliefs about a group of people. Stereotypes (cognition) rationalize prejudice (beliefs), leading to discrimination (behavior) (Dovidio & Gaertner, 1996).

Bonilla-Silva (1997) argued that racism should be viewed beyond an ideology and more in terms of racialized social systems that are hierarchically structured and based on racial categories that are socially constructed to benefit one group over another. This racialization framework takes into consideration the initial or historical social formation and intent of the racial categories that informs the contemporary racial hierarchical structure. Racial phenomena, such as stereotypes, prejudices, and discrimination, then become crystalized over the course of social systems' existence producing racial inequities—that ultimately affect health outcomes. Several theoretical frameworks and studies have been developed to explain the effects of racialized systems on health among Black adults. Gabbidon and Peterson (2006) coined the *living while Black* phenomenon, which posits that the social cost of being Black in the United States influences health status. Geronimus, Hicken, Keene, and Bound (2006) theorized the *weathering hypothesis* that states that Black adults' exposure to socioeconomic and sociodemographic inequalities and racism subjects them to higher allostatic load—defined as the accumulated physiological burden of adaptation to chronic stress (McEwen, 2000).

Most recently, the field of public health has also recognized racism as a racialized social system. Dr. Camara Phyllis Jones, past president of the American Public Health Association from 2015 to 2016, launched a National Campaign Against Racism and identified racism as a social system stating:

> Racism is a system of structuring opportunity and assigning value based on the social interpretation of how one looks (which is what we call "race"), that unfairly disadvantages some individuals and communities, unfairly advantages other individuals and communities, and saps the strength of the whole society through the waste of human resources.

(p. 231)

This is important as Paradies and colleagues (2015) evaluated data from 293 studies published between 1983 and 2013 and found an extensive association of self-reported racism with poor health behaviors and negative physical health outcomes.

Racialized System of Health

The use of socially identified race to stratify people in America impacted all facets of life, including health. Racialized health systems were developed from the social relations and practices based on racial distinctions prevalent across the health care systems (Bonilla-Silva, 1997). The United States' Black population's racialized health began with the *middle passage*, the human trafficking transport from Africa to the New World, and continued through the *seasoning process*, named by the White plantation owners as the initiation into New World slavery (Buxton, 1840). It has been estimated that approximately 12.5% of slaves died in the middle passage, 4.5% died on the shore while waiting to be sold, and one-third died during the seasoning process while attempting to adjust to the New World. This accounted for an average mortality rate of 50% (Klein, Engerman, Haines, & Shlomowitz, 2001). Slavery in the United States officially lasted from 1619 to 1865, nearly 250 years, and with it, a system of oppression, marginalization, suffering, and low life expectancy. That history continues to underline the current health disparities and mortality rates of the Black population. This has been proven in several studies showing that the real contributing causes of mortality rates among Black persons were the racialized social systems in the United States. Woolf, Johnson, Fryer, Rust, and Satcher (2008) revealed that 880,000 deaths per year would be avoided if the United States had a smaller income gap similar to other Western European nations. Hemenway (2010) found that if social policies in the United States, during the periods of 1991 to 2000, were in place to equalize the mortality rates of Blacks and Whites, 686,202 deaths would have been averted; only 176,633 deaths were prevented due to the medical innovations during that period. Galea, Tracy, Hoggatt, Dimaggio and Karpati (2011) found that 245,000 deaths in the United States could be traced back to low education; 162,000 were attributable to racial segregation; 133,000 were caused by poverty at the individual level; and 119,000 might be attributed to inequality in income.

These findings are not novel as it has been noted as early as the 1850s when Dr. James McCune Smith argued to the medical profession that one's health was not primarily a consequence of innate constitution, but a reflection of their intrinsic membership in groups created by the social relations of the society (Krieger, 1987; Link, 1967; Smith, 1859). This argument was scientifically reinforced in 1899 when W.E.B DuBois conducted the first sociological study of Blacks in America. Results from this work demonstrated that racial differences in mortality could be explained by social contextual factors impacting Black life in Philadelphia during the late 19th century (DuBois, 1899). This comprehensive study used multiple methods, including participant observation, survey data collection, and secondary data analysis, to document how discrimination, oppression, and White supremacy contributed to the elevated levels of despair, disease, and death in Philadelphia's Seventh Ward. Brown and Fee (2003) describe how W.E.B. Dubois further clarified this position at the Eleventh Atlanta University Conference stating:

> We might continue this argument almost indefinitely going to one conclusion, that the Negro death rate and sickness are largely matters of condition and not due to racial traits and tendencies…With the improved sanitary condition, improved education and better economic opportunities, the mortality of the race may and probably will steadily decrease until it becomes normal.
> (p. 273)

The groundbreaking work of DuBois was largely ignored by the social and health scientists for the better part of a century as the scientific community focused on establishing biological explanations for racial differences in outcomes (Zuberi, 2001). The salience of Black health emerged nonetheless as DuBois published an edited volume in 1906, *The Health and Physique of the Negro American*, that documented racial health disparities in the United States. A key finding from this work was that 45% of the mortality among the Black population was preventable. These findings fueled the effort for health advocacy and social justice as Booker T. Washington launched a national campaign to improve the health of Black Americans (Patterson, 1939). It initially started as a movement called *Health Improvement Week*, but evolved into a massive 35-year national campaign called *National Negro Health Week (NNHW)* (Quinn & Thomas, 2001). It was observed from Sunday to Sunday during the first week of April, to commemorate Booker T. Washington's birthday on April 5. Brown (1937) reported that the main objective of NNHW's public health community mobilization effort was to "stimulate the people as a whole to cooperative endeavor in clean-up, educational, and specific hygienic and clinical services for general sanitary improvement of the community and for health betterment of the individual, family, and home" (p. 555).

These efforts coupled with social movements to establish Blacks as full citizens of the United States pushed notions of Black biological, intellectual, and moral inferiority from the mainstream to the margins throughout the 20th century. The report of the 1985 Secretary of the U.S. Department of Health and Human Services (US DHHS) Task Force on Black and Minority Health, known as the Heckler Report, was the first government-sanctioned assessment of racial health disparities (Heckler, 1985). Findings from the task force were similar to DuBois' as they indicated that Black persons had not benefited equitably from the advanced scientific knowledge of the health systems. This mortality inequity was linked to six leading causes of preventable *excess deaths* for the Black population (42% excess death compared with the White population): cancer, cardiovascular disease, diabetes, infant mortality, chemical dependency, and homicide/unintentional injury. Results from this report led to the creation of the Office of Minority Health in the U.S. Department of Health and Human Service with the mission to improve the health of racial and ethnic minority population. Health disparities and minority health were recognized as important focus areas at the federal level and some states established April as minority health month for health promotion and disease prevention among their underserved populations. Momentum for national recognition of April as Minority Health Month was accelerated by the Health People 2010 initiative in 2001 and received the support of the U.S. Congress in 2002 (Harris, 2018).

1918 Influenza Pandemic Parallels the COVID-19 Pandemic

Public health advocacy for the Black population in early–20th century America was more than a scientific enterprise. It was essential for survival for this population during the influenza pandemic of 1918. This infectious disease pandemic exposed an estimated 2% to 5% of the human population that accounted for 675,000 in the United States. At the onset of the influenza epidemic, despite efforts by Black public health activists such as W.E.B DuBois and Booker T. Washington, Black communities continued to be riddled with racist policies that advanced their poor health status (DuBois, 1906; Gamble, 2010; Patterson, 1939). According to Gamble (2010), it was a common thought that the Black population had a lower incidence of influenza exposure. However, inaccurate data collection from the Black population due to poor access to medical care may have added to the underreporting of cases. Nonetheless, the Black population had a greater rate of mortality despite a reported lower incidence and morbidity rate (Økland & Mamelund, 2019). The disproportionate exposure to influenza was determined to be caused by several factors that were prevalent in the Black population: higher risk for pulmonary disease, malnutrition, social and economic disparities, racial residential segregation, burden of urban density (e.g., unsanitary living environments), and poor access to health care (Gamble, 2010).

The COVID-19 pandemic has re-awakened the public health community to the same racialized systems that were unmasked during the 1918 influenza pandemic. This is illustrated daily by the COVID Racial Data Tracker, which is a collaboration between the COVID Tracking Project and the Boston University Center for Antiracist Research gathering comprehensive COVID-19 data relative to race and ethnicity in the United States (COVID Tracking Project, 2021). The COVID Racial Data Tracker reports data on COVID-19 racial disparities and showed that as of March 7, 2021, COVID-19 had killed approximately 73,462 Black people in the United States. The COVID Racial Tracker also found that Black people accounted for 15% of the COVID-19 deaths, although they constitute only 13% of the U.S. population. Additionally, Black people were dying at a rate of 178 per 100,000 people compared with White people who were dying at a rate of 124 per 100,000.

This data demonstrated that Black people's COVID-19 mortality rate was 1.4 higher than that of their White peers.

This dismal picture of the plight of the Black population during this pandemic has been shown in several studies, highlighting the role of racialized systems in the United States (Chen et al., 2020; Krieger et al., 2020; Shierholz, 2020; Wolf et al., 2020; Woolhandler & Himmelstein, 2020). During the early stages of the first wave of the COVID-19 pandemic, a study found that 89% of patients hospitalized for COVID-19 had an underlying chronic medical condition, such as hypertension (49.7%), obesity (48.3%), chronic lung disease (mainly asthma) (34.6%), diabetes (28.3%), and cardiovascular disease (CVD) (27.8%) (Garg et al., 2020), all chronic conditions due to which Black adults are currently disproportionately affected, excluding CVD (CDC, 2019). Another study conducted by Krieger and colleagues (2020) stratified zip code social conditions to examine the mortality surge of COVID-19 exposure during the early stages of the pandemic (first two weeks of April). They revealed the association of inequities caused by racialized systems and COVID-19 mortality rate. COVID-19 mortality was 1.1 higher in poorer zip codes than other zip codes, 1.7 higher for zip codes with household crowding; 3.1 higher in zip codes with racialized economic segregation; and 1.8 higher in zip codes with people of color. This raises the question: what are the social, structural, and clinical drivers of racial inequities in COVID-19 morbidity and mortality that produces differential exposure, transmission, and susceptibility among the Black population?

Racial Vulnerabilities in the COVID-19 Pandemic Disaster

The vulnerabilities of a population must also be taken into consideration when examining the COVID-19 pandemic disaster recovery process to also include an assessment of the risks and vulnerabilities that serve as recovery challenges to the Black population, such as exposure to racism. Vulnerability in this context refers to the historical and contemporary, cultural, social, environmental, political, and economic variables that influence the conditions of a group of people. The level of vulnerability increases the risk of exposure to COVID-19 as a result of marginalization, oppression, and lack of access to resources (Bankoff, 2004; Schiele, 2007).

Differential Susceptibility

The pandemic has led to increased unemployment, which has heightened food insecurity, and reduced access to care, both of which may increase COVID-19 susceptibility (National Conference of State Legislatures, 2020). Food insecurity could potentially lead to micronutrient deficiency and lower the baseline level of immune function, leading to increased susceptibility to COVID-19 infection and a worse clinical course, while reduced access to care could delay diagnosis and treatment, further increasing susceptibility to poor COVID-19-related health outcomes (Pereira & Oliveira, 2020). Food insecurity has increased during the pandemic due to an increase in acute and chronic under- or unemployment (Shierholz, 2020), leaving many households incapable of securing basic food and supplies, following the massive rush to hoard and stockpile groceries and other necessities. In addition, school closures have left many children from low-income families incapable of accessing free school meals, a major source of mitigating food insecurity. These pandemic-related ramifications have led to as much as a 2–3-fold increase in food-insecure households with children. Food insecurity can lead to micronutrient deficiency. The one micronutrient that most closely regulated the immune system and could be linked to COVID-19 susceptibility is deficiency of vitamin D, which is also more common in African Americans. Patients with low vitamin D levels were noted to be more than 1.7 times more likely to test positive for COVID-19 than persons with normal vitamin D levels (Meltzer et al., 2020). Several studies have reported higher-level care for COVID-19 patients was reduced with the administration of vitamin D (Castillo et al., 2020; Meltzer et al., 2020), but the unequivocal evidence for the role of vitamin D in COVID-19 prevention or treatment remains undetermined. Vitamin D has several immune-regulatory functions, including macrophage activation via toll receptors and modulation of inflammatory mediators via its influence on oxidative stress pathways and nuclear factor-erythroid-2-related factor 2 (Nrf2) (Mohan & Gupta, 2018; Norris et al., 2018). Thus, vitamin D plays an important role in immune regulation, inflammation, cellular immunity, and oxidative stress responses (Berridge, 2015; Jones, 2006; Mohan & Gupta, 2018), reinforcing its important role as a key mediator of immune function, especially in the setting of increased stress. Vitamin D deficiency may exacerbate the vicious cycle of increasing oxidative stress, leading to increased inflammation, and vice versa (Mohan & Gupta, 2018), thereby leading to differential susceptibility to COVID-19 in groups at risk for vitamin D deficiency, such as African Americans. It is important to note the risk of vitamin D deficiency during the pandemic is further amplified by the requirement to shelter at home and the wearing of face masks, both reducing exposure to sunlight and the conversion of pre-vitamin D to Vitamin D. In the absence of vitamin D supplementation, the risk for vitamin D deficiency is increased and vitamin D supplementation should be recommended during the pandemic at doses of 1,000–4,000 IU per day (Ames, Grant, & Willett, 2021).

The structural inequities that have been amplified by the pandemic have disproportionately levied job loss, transportation disadvantage, health insurance loss, and even access to telemedicine among people and communities of color further exacerbating disparities in health care and amplifying the differential susceptibility to COVID-19 infections and associated adverse outcomes (Johnson & Goodnough, 2020; Kim et al., 2020; J.-H. Kim et al., 2020). Despite some public health insurance programs extending access to their plans during the pandemic (Gangopadhyaya & Garrett, 2020), it is estimated that in addition to the nearly 30 million Americans being uninsured before the pandemic (Tolbert, Orgera, Singer, & Damico, 2019), over 7 million recently unemployed workers have now become newly uninsured (Woolhandler & Himmelstein, 2020). Further, the COVID-19 pandemic has introduced broad transportation system challenges from reduced public transit service to lessened ability to rely on others for fear of contracting the virus. This has led to many people of color who were already more likely to struggle with transportation prior to the pandemic even more likely to find themselves at a disadvantage of susceptibility to and delayed care for COVID-19 infections (Chen et al., 2020). Indeed, transportation barriers have been associated with higher odds of a positive COVID-19 test with up to 40% of U.S. adults reporting delays in medical care at varying times during the pandemic (Chen et al., 2020). Finally, the COVID-19 pandemic's toll on the labor market and transportation has reshaped how and where people access health care, with a disproportionate impact on communities of color (Chen et al., 2020).

John Henryism

The COVID-19 pandemic has had a substantive adverse impact on the Black community, leading to an acute superimposed set of psychosocial stresses on top of the chronic stresses that the community suffers from, in a race-based, casteist society. One form of an adaptive behavioral response is active coping in response to excessive psychosocial and/or environmental stressors. This has been well characterized in the African American community and has been termed John Henryism. This form of active adaptive coping was named after John Henry, an African American folk hero whose prowess as a steel-driver was highlighted in a race he won against a steam powered rock drilling machine, only to die in victory with hammer in hand as his heart gave out from stress. In clinical terms, John Henryism is defined as prolonged, high-effort coping in response to difficult psychosocial environmental stressors and reflects how such active coping (especially by Black men) in a racial, casteist society interacts with low socioeconomic status to adversely influence the health of African Americans (James, 1994). A more contemporary social theory interpretation of John Henryism would be the adverse health impact of the additional effort and coping required by a Black man striving to compete in an unequal society. The baseline high level of daily energy required to manage the psychological stress generated by these highly intertwined psychosocial stressors (e.g., chronic financial strain, job insecurity, racial or social discrimination) and the associated stress superimposed when coupled with high-effort coping can lead to significantly increased sympathetic nervous system activation contributing to elevated blood pressure and other "stress-related" health problems.

The COVID-19 pandemic is a stark example of an intense and difficult psychosocial environment that disproportionately affects African Americans and has thus created for many an acute state superimposed on a chronic state of John Henryism. This has been characterized as too many Black Americans are "trying to make a way out of no way—the Black American story" and this pervasive state for Black Americans (yet hidden from the view of much of America) is now visibly highlighted through the COVID-19 pandemic (Johnson & Martin, 2020). Thus, John Henryism represents an adaptive response to excess stressors that leads to an early expression and/or exacerbation of many disease states. However, the impact of the societal stresses on Black Americans can be manifest in other ways beyond John Henryism.

Weathering

The increased focus on COVID-19-related racial and ethnic disparities along with a parallel increase in a national movement toward racial and social justice has prompted the medical community to re-evaluate how it defines and operationalizes race. The clearer recognition of race as a social construct being a risk factor for racism (Jones, 2002), and racism being linked to biology may have implications for COVID-19 disparities. The biology of racism is often wrongly conflated with the biology of race.

Broadly, the biologic impact of the multitude of excess stressors that society has levied upon Black Americans through the many dimensions of historic and contemporary racism has been termed weathering (Geronimus et al., 2006). Weathering is a term used to describe the health disadvantage from a cumulative lifetime exposure to adverse socioeconomic conditions (e.g. food insecurity, living in substandard housing, inadequate access to health care) as well as discrimination and institutionalized racism (Geronimus et al., 2006). These stressors on oppressed groups are expressed as biologic differences in allostatic load (physiologic consequences of chronic exposure to stress), inflammatory, neuroendocrine, immune, and other markers across racial groups (Geronimus, 1992; Geronimus et al., 2006; McEwen, 1998; Thames, Irwin, Breen, and Cole, 2019). Weathering is often detected clinically by an increase in allostatic load, typically measured through parameters, such as the level of blood pressure, HbA1C, and C-reactive protein, lipids, and, when available, measures of the hypothalamic–pituitary axis (Duru, Harawa, Kermah, & Norris, 2012; Seeman, Singer, Rowe, Horwitz, and McEwen, 1997). An increase in allostatic load is strongly associated with premature mortality risk (Duru et al., 2012; Seeman et al., 1997).

Many authorities have considered race-based health outcomes to be a proxy for socioeconomic status (SES) with a common White supremacy narrative that many racial and ethnic minority groups have worse health outcomes because of lower SES and they have low SES because they are inherently inferior. While there are strong associations between self-reported race and SES in a discriminatory race-stratified society, the association of race and health is linked to so much more than SES: it is not race per se, but the historic and contemporary race-based inequities in the structures and systems in our society that lead to group-level differences in SES. The heightening of many socioeconomic and discriminatory adversities during the COVID-19 pandemic has led to a disproportionate increase in stress and likely accelerated weathering for many living in communities of color.

Racial Exposure in COVID-19 Pandemic Disaster

During the early stages of a COVID-19 public health assessment, exposure pathways are evaluated (Mizukoshi, Nakama, Okumura, and Azuma, 2021; Seddighi, 2020). During this process, location-specific situations are identified using the following questions: (1) who at a given location is exposed to COVID-19; and (2) what are the conditions necessary for the exposure to occur? This helps to identify points of exposure and the populations that are potentially more at risk of exposure. To add to this, Frohlic and Potvin (1999) present arguments demonstrating the social constructionist view of exposure based on lifestyle choices affected by the available opportunities and resources that are defined by SDoH. Therefore, a careful examination of exposure in the Black population is necessary for our understanding of the COVID-19 pandemic disaster recovery process.

Differential Exposure

Since March 2020, much of the United States has enacted "Safer at Home" orders and closure or restrictions of non-essential services in response to the COVID-19 pandemic. Alongside health care workers, many low-income and previously marginalized residents instantly became "essential" to the fabric of America—a status they have rarely experienced since its founding. In early reports about the COVID-19 outbreak, Black Americans were less likely to believe they would get sick from the virus and were less concerned or prepared for the pandemic compared with their Whites peers (Wolf et al., 2020). In sharp contrast to these beliefs, subsequent reports described widespread racial and ethnic disparities in COVID-19 deaths, heavily weighted toward Black, Hispanic, and Indigenous persons (Health, 2020; Staff, 2020). The disparities that COVID-19 has exposed are not new health disparities, but they are more stark, pervasive, and are not subsiding. Now, nearly a year later, the racial and ethnic disparities in COVID-19 hospitalizations and deaths persist with Black, Hispanic, and Native American communities suffering from COVID-19 infection, hospitalizations, and death rates nearly 2–3 times higher than those of their White peers (CDC, 2020a, 2020b). Unfortunately, the initial US$2 trillion 'stimulus' bill from the U.S. government offered no health insurance subsidies or coverage for the many Americans who are no longer working, nor did it provide support for the many essential workers who are disproportionately people of color (Woolhandler & Himmelstein, 2020).

The inequities in the differential exposure to COVID-19 infections and subsequent morbidity and mortality are grounded in the maldistribution of resources that influence viral exposure and transmission as well as overall health and access to health care. The many structures and systems that directly and indirectly influence health comprise the SDoH, and include education, employment, transportation, criminal and environmental justice, food security, income, health insurance, access to health care, and more. This is critical as it is estimated that as much as 50–80% of health tracks back to SDoH and where people live (Hood, Gennuso, Swain, and Catlin, 2016). The inequitable distribution of the SDoH through racialized laws, policies, and practices represents a highly complex reinforcing and interactive network and is termed structural racism. Structural racism helps to maintain the unequal distribution of resources and reinforce discriminatory beliefs and stereotypes perpetuating racial and ethnic health disparities. Importantly, structural racism persists in governmental and institutional policies even when many individuals are not explicitly racially prejudiced (Williams, Lawrence, & Davis, 2019) This means without active approaches to dismantle structural racism, it continues unabated.

Managing prevention and care for patients and families with complex health issues (e.g., chronic disease, mental health issues, substance abuse, and now COVID-19) has become increasingly complicated. While each community has a unique mix of greater and fewer SDoH, including health care systems, the highly limited resources in most racial and ethnic minority communities make the need to connect patients to life-sustaining resources beyond the clinical walls of a health-setting critical to treating many minority patients with complex health problems. While challenging to do, if effective, such strategies can lead to improved health outcomes (Institute for Clinical Systems Improvement, 2014).

As a primarily airborne infectious disease, the transmission of COVID-19 is highly influenced by key exposure risks, such as occupation, transportation, and housing density. Being an employee in jobs with high-density, close exposure to many people and often poor circulation, such as a sanitation worker, front-line retail worker, or factory worker, increases exposure to and likelihood of contracting the COVID-19 infection. While adherence to wearing a mask, washing your hands, and watching your distance is recommended, watching one's distance can be challenging when structural factors, such as type of employment, high-density working conditions with poor circulation, public transportation service, and high-density housing settings all conspire to increase the risk of exposure and transmission (Wong & Li, 2020).

Short- and Long-Term COVID-19 Pandemic Disaster Recovery Solutions

Several short-term COVID-19 pandemic disaster recovery solutions have been initiated. To allow health plans to reduce or eliminate cost-sharing for COVID-19 testing and treatment, Federal Notice 2020-15 (High Deductible Health Plans and Expenses Related to COVID-19) was activated on March 11, 2020. This policy includes high deductible health plans, which, prior to this policy, were prohibited from covering such services until after enrollees met their health plan deductibility needs (Fendrick & Shrosbree, 2020). Another short-term COVID-19 pandemic disaster recovery solution was the Coronavirus Aid, Relief, and Economic Security Act on March 27, 2020 that extended coverage to any COVID-19 testing or screening in-person visit (Fendrick & Shrosbree, 2020). In addition, the Families First Coronavirus Response Act (March 18, 2020) that enabled private insurance plans to provide first-dollar coverage of telehealth services for COVID-19 care also required all plans to cover future COVID-19 vaccines without cost-sharing (Fendrick & Shrosbree, 2020).

While these are important steps, these acts operate through health care insurance plans leaving the most vulnerable and many low-income working families without health insurance whose members are mostly persons of color, still exposed to the health and health care cost ravages of COVID-19.

To help close that gap, several policies have been introduced that could also be important long-term COVID-19 pandemic disaster recovery solutions, but unfortunately, they have not been enacted including: (1) the Worker Health Coverage Protection Act that would allow some unemployed workers to maintain their previous employer-sponsored health coverage, (2) the Health Care Emergency Guarantee Act (2020) to achieve universal coverage without cost-sharing and fully protecting Americans from financial costs of medical care, (3) the Medicare Crisis Program (2020) to ensure health coverage for unemployed workers and their families through Medicare, and expand coverage to other low-income individuals through Medicaid; eliminate medical costs for COVID-19-related care, and (4) Medicare for All Act (2019) designed to eliminate cost concerns and financial liability for patients with COVID-19 and all other conditions through universal first-dollar coverage (Gaffney, Himmelstein, & Woolhandler, 2020). Additional long-term COVID-19 pandemic disaster recovery solutions should examine reinvesting in public health infrastructure (Gaffney et al., 2020), expansion of employer diversity, and equity and inclusion initiatives to include employee and family health and wellbeing as a central outcome (Sherman, Kelly, & Payne-Foster, 2020).

More Ready Access to Racial and Ethnic Demographic Data on COVID-19 Infection and Mortality

An immediate need is transparent and facile access to racial and ethnic demographic data on COVID-19 infection, hospitalizations, and mortality as well as COVID-19 vaccination. One source of such data at the national level is the Kaiser Family Foundation (https://www.kff.org/coronavirus-covid-19/issue-brief/latest-data-covid-19-vaccinations-cases-deaths-race-ethnicity/) that collects and analyzes data on COVID-19 infection, hospitalizations, and mortality ND vaccinations by race/ethnicity. This is critical for monitoring and hopefully preventing racial disparities related to COVID-19 and, especially, COVID-19 vaccines, given the disproportionate impact of the pandemic on minoritized communities. It is important to have all states participate and all reporting use the same metrics to not mislead the public and eliminate disinformation campaigns. As of February 1, 2021, less than half of the states have reported vaccination by race or ethnicity, limiting the ability to ascertain disparities and make corrective action when needed. Table 3.1 provides an illustration of a COVID-19 Disparities Index and dashboard that could be created to help target public health messaging and allocation of community-level COVID-19 prevention and treatment resources (Maul & Joshi, 2021).

Expanding Access to Health Care Nationwide

The COVID-19 pandemic has revealed critical gaps in the U.S. health care system, including, but not limited to, major inequities in access to and quality of care and shortages of primary care providers (Geyman, 2021). Short-term solutions include expanding the workforce by strategies, such as increasing the scope of advance nurses' practice (Feyereisen & Puro, 2020) to changes in health care policies (Gaffney et al., 2020; Geyman, 2021).

With over 30 million Americans uninsured and over 40 million more underinsured pre-COVID-19 and with those figures now about 50% higher due to the impact of the pandemic on the economy, a safety net is insufficient and a major reform is needed (Gaffney et al., 2020; Geyman, 2021).

Table 3.1 Sample COVID-19 Disparities Index Dashboard

Risk Group (e.g., Race/Ethnicity)	*% COVID-19 Infections by Subgroup (e.g., >65 years)*	*% Population by Subgroup (e.g., >65 years)*	*COVID-19 Disparities Index*
White	A	B	A/B
Black or African American	C	D	C/D
Hispanic or Latinx	E	F	E/F

Sample COVID-19 Disparities Index can be used to monitor COVID-19 infections, hospitalizations, and/or deaths by different risk groups at different population levels, such as county, state, national, or other.

Three potential reform alternatives include: (1) to enhance and expand upon on the 2010 Affordable Care Act; (2) to implement the public option; and (3) to revisit the single-payer option with some form of a National Health Insurance (Gaffney et al., 2020; Geyman, 2021; McMorrow, 2021). Thus, we face a new normal in U.S. health care accompanied by increasing support to prioritize public interest through some form of a single-payer system to achieve affordable, accessible, and comprehensive health care for all Americans. It has also become clear that only such an egalitarian approach can overcome the deeply embedded structural racism that perpetuates inequities in the SDoH as well as the existing system of health care. Over a decade ago, Victor Fuchs predicted that following a major event such as war, a depression, or large-scale civil unrest, a change in the political climate would usher in a form of National Health Insurance (Fuchs, 2010). We are in the midst of both a pandemic and major civil unrest so now is the time to push for the needed political will to enact such a change (Woolhandler & Himmelstein, 2020).

Reducing Administrative Barriers to Accessing Key Social Services (e.g., Supplemental Nutrition Assistance Program [SNAP] and Temporary Assistance for Needy Families [TANF])

An estimated 40 million U.S. residents lost their jobs in the first two months of the coronavirus disease 2019 (COVID-19) pandemic and of those who lost their jobs, 31% reported food insecurity and 33% reported eating less due to financial constraints (Raifman, Bor, & Venkataramani, 2021). In response, the Federal Government expanded unemployment insurance benefits in both size (US$600/week supplement) and access to SNAP and TANF programs (Raifman et al., 2021; Saloner, Gollust, Planalp, & Blewett, 2020). The degree of food insecurity has varied during the pandemic based on the receipt of unemployment insurance and access to safety net programs. Since the pandemic, unemployment insurance enrollment increased from 9.2% to 17.1%, SNAP from 20.1% to 24.3%, and TANF from 1.7% to 2.6% (Raifman et al., 2021; Saloner et al., 2020). As the final wave of the survey ahead of the federal supplement to unemployment insurance was ending, food insecurity and eating less during the pandemic were more common among non-White persons, lower-income households, younger persons, and sexual or gender minorities. Overall, the receipt of unemployment insurance, as well as SNAP and/or TANF can lead to significant reductions in food insecurity (Raifman et al., 2021; Saloner et al., 2020).

Invest in Culturally Responsive Community Care

In times of crisis, creating new or engaging existing partnerships with community are critical to enhance health surveillance, response, and recovery as well as social resilience, and adaptive capacity, which ultimately are required to overcome the crisis at hand and to strengthen health system responses to further outbreaks (Wells et al., 2013). Indeed, efforts to address the multiple impacts the pandemic will have on society should include community-informed decision-making to strengthen evaluation approaches and tie evidence to policymaking (Zhu, Grande, Jones, & Tipirneni, 2020). Strategies for culturally responsive community care during COVID-19 may require several steps but should include a high level of engagement and partnership between communities and governmental/academic/industry entities. An adaptation of seven community-engaged steps suggested by Carson and colleagues to consider during COVID-19 include: (1) ensuring community engagement in emerging COVID-19 protocols and priorities; (2) focus engagement on disproportionately affected communities for early identification and response to disparities; (3) practice honesty, humility, and humanism, especially in newly partnered activities that are occurring remotely; (4) support and create opportunities for bi-directional knowledge exchange; (5) maintain commitment to a community-partnered health, research, and policy workforce; (6) ensure accessibility in engagement; and (7) include funding for community participation in emerging COVID-19 health, research, and policy activities (Carson et al., 2020).

Social Justice and Health Equity Model

Justice and equity require an assessment of needs to understand the resources needed to help those with the least. Policies grounded in equality and not equity, superimposed on a race-based, caste-based society ensures the perpetuation of group-level disparities. Indeed, a recent analysis of relief funding by county found that Black communities disproportionately received the same level of relief funding as other counties despite having greater health care and financial needs (Kakani, Chandra, Mullainathan, & Obermeyer, 2020). These findings highlight how structural racism persists and maintains inequities despite anti-discrimination laws having led to many post-civil rights policies, yet have a "disparate impact" on Black populations, even if the policies do not explicitly use information based on race (Kakani et al., 2020). To achieve public health social justice, it will be critical to provide more transparent and facile access to racial and ethnic demographic data on COVID-19 vaccination.

A more immediate and specific approach to moving toward equity and providing COVID-19 pandemic disaster recovery methods is the use of a COVID-19 vaccine equity index (VEI) through a dashboard of high-risk subgroups (Maul & Joshi, 2021). For example, to hold individual counties accountable for vaccination equity, a state could use the sample VEI, as illustrated in Table 3.2, to determine the quantity and location of future weekly first-time vaccine allocation decisions. VEI thresholds could be developed to activate immediate conversations between local and state officials to modify strategies to improve vaccination rates of specific groups. Providing VEI transparently to the public could improve trust and better engage local stakeholders. Data integrity and quality are critical to such approaches. Many states and health systems have such data, and census-level data for VEI can be used when individual-level data are not adequate for use in a social vulnerability/inequity index (captures community-level SDoH, such as education, income, housing density, employment, criminal justice). And even if individual-level data are available, the social vulnerability/inequity index can be used as a group-level adjustment to capture community-level socioeconomic inequities. Other risk group dashboards might include migrant worker status, gender identity, sex, incarceration, and more (Maul & Joshi, 2021).

In summary, the COVID-19 pandemic disaster has highlighted the plight of racism and its impact on racial and ethnic minority communities in the United States, leading many to attempt to make positive changes with a vision of one day eliminating America's enduring unspoken caste system (Bonilla-Silva, 2006). At a macro level, the WHO has outlined three major principles of action to address the unequal distribution of the SDoH, the systemic injustices that underlie health

Table 3.2 Sample Vaccine Equity Index (VEI)

Risk Group (e.g., Race/Ethnicity)	% Vaccinated by Subgroup (e.g., >65 years)	% Population by Subgroup (e.g., >65 years)*	VEI
White	A	B	A/B
Black or African American	C	D	C/D
Hispanic or Latinx	E	F	E/F

Sample VEI can be adapted as a dashboard for monitoring different risk groups and for different population levels (e.g., county, state, or national).

* Census track social vulnerability/inequity index can be used when individual-level data is not adequate and/or as an adjustment to capture community-level socioeconomic inequities.

disparities, and aid in a successful COVID-19 pandemic disaster recovery for the Black commu-nity (Organization, 2008). These include: (1) reorganizing the structure of society to enhance each individual's living and working conditions to allow them to achieve their full health potential; (2) re-aligning the distribution of power, resources, and money in a more fair and equitable manner; and (3) educating not only health care workers but the broader society on how inequities in the distribution of the SDoH drive the disparities we consistently state we want to eliminate. Then and only then can we realize a successful COVID-19 pandemic disaster recovery by: (1) overcoming the physical and emotional impact of the COVID-19 pandemic; (2) establishing an economic base that instills confidence in individual and community viability; and (3) integrating the knowledge of all community members on the racialized health care inequities that is driving the consequences of the COVID-19 pandemic (United States Department of Homeland Security, 2011). A successful COVID-19 pandemic disaster recovery is more than returning the Black community to pre-disaster circumstances. Ultimately, only through the elimination of structural racism and the associated inequities in the distribution of the SDoH can the vision of true health equity lead to minimiza-tion of risk of the COVID-19 pandemic exposure for the Black population. If accomplished, the Black community will be strengthened and able to withstand and recover from future pandemic-disasters—demonstrated by their post-disaster conditions.

Acknowledgments

This work was supported by grants from the National Heart, Lung, and Blood Institute (1R25HL126145, 1K01H88735, HHSN268201800012I), National Institute for Diabetes and Digestive and Kidney Diseases (1P30DK092950), National Institute of Aging (K02AG059140, P30AG021684, P30AG059298), National Institute on Minority Health and Health Disparities (U54MD000214), and the National Center for Advancing Translational Sciences (UL1TR001881).

References

Akanbi, M. O., Rivera, A. S., Akanbi, F. O., & Shoyinka, A. (2021). An ecologic study of disparities in COVID-19 incidence and case fatality in Oakland County, MI, USA, during a state-mandated shutdown. *J Racial Ethn Health Disparities, 8*(6), 1467–1474. https://doi.org/10.1007/s40615-020-00909-1

Ames, B. N., Grant, W. B., & Willett, W. C. (2021). Does the high prevalence of vitamin D deficiency in African Americans contribute to health disparities? *Nutrients, 13*(2). https://doi.org/10.3390/nu13020499

Bankoff, G. (2004). *The historical geography of disaster: 'Vulnerability' and 'local knowledge' in western discourse*. Earthscan.

Barrett, J. E., & Roediger, D. (2012). How white people became white. In P. S. Rothenberg (Ed.) *White privi-lege: Essential readings on the other side of racism* (pp. 39–44). New York, NY: Worth Publishers.

Berridge, M. J. (2015). Vitamin D: A custodian of cell signalling stability in health and disease. *Biochem Soc Trans, 43*(3), 349–358. https://doi.org/10.1042/bst20140279

Bonilla-Silva, E. (2006). *Racism without racists: Color-blind racism and the persistence of racial inequality in the United States*. Rowman & Littlefield Publishers.

Bonilla-Silva, Eduardo. (1997). Rethinking racism: Toward a structural interpretation. *Am Soc Rev, 62*(3), 465–480.

Brown, R. (1937). The national Negro health week movement. *Negro Educ, 6*, 553–564.

Brown, T. M., & Fee, E. (2003). Voices from the past: The health and physique. *Am J Public Health, 93*(2), 272–276.

Buxton, T. F. (1840). *The African slave trade and its remedy*. S.W. Benedict.

Carson, S. L., Gonzalez, C., Lopez, S., Morris, D., Mtume, N., Lucas-Wright, A., … Brown, A. F. (2020). Reflections on the importance of community-partnered research strategies for health equity in the era of COVID-19. *J Health Care Poor Underserved, 31*(4), 1515–1519. https://doi.org/10.1353/hpu.2020.0112

Centers for Disease Control and Prevention (CDC). (02/10/2020a). Cases of Coronavirus Disease (COVID-19) in the U.S. Retrieved from https://www.cdc.gov/coronavirus/2019-ncov/cases-updates/cases-in-us.html

Centers for Disease Control and Prevention (CDC). (02/10/2020b). Provisional Death Counts for Coronavirus Disease (COVID-19): Data Updates by Select Demographic and Geographic Characteristics. Retrieved from https://www.cdc.gov/nchs/nvss/vsrr/covid_weekly/

Centers for Disease Control and Prevention (CDC). (2019). Health, United States, 2018: Data Finder. Retrieved from https://www.cdc.gov/nchs/hus/contents2018.htm?search=,Black_or_African_American

Chen, K. L., Brozen, M., Rollman, J. E., Ward, T., Norris, K., Gregory, K. D., & Zimmerman, F. J. (2020). Transportation Access to Health Care during the COVID-19 Pandemic: Trends and Implications for Significant Patient Populations and Health Care Needs. University of California Institute of Transportation Studies. Report No.: UC-ITS-2021-11 | DOI: 10.17610/T6RK5N https://escholarship.org/uc/item/22b3b1rc

Chen, J. T., & Krieger, N. (2021). Revealing the unequal burden of COVID-19 by income, race/ethnicity, and household crowding: US county versus zip code analyses. *J Public Health Manag Pract*, S43–S56. https://doi.org/10.1097/PHH.0000000000001263

Clark, R., Anderson, N.B., Clark, V. R., & Williams, D.R. (1999). Racism as a stressor for African Americans: A biopsychosocial model. *Am Psych, 54*(10), 805-816.

COVID Tracking Project (2021). The COVID racial data tracker: COVID-19 is affecting Black, indigenous, Latinx, and other people of color the most. Retrieved from https://covidtracking.com/race

Dovidio, J. F., & Gaertner, S. L. (1996). Affirmative action, unintentional racial biases, and intergroup relations. *J Soc Issues, 52*(4), 51–75. https://doi.org/10.1111/j.1540-4560.1996.tb01848.x

Du Bois, W. E. B. (1906). *The health and physique of the Negro American*. The Atlanta University Press.

Du Bois, W. E. B. (1899). *The Philadelphia Negro: A social study*. University of Pennsylvania.

Duru, O. K., Harawa, N. T., Kermah, D., & Norris, K. C. (2012). Allostatic load burden and racial disparities in mortality. *J Natl Med Assoc, 104*(1–2), 89–95. Retrieved from http://www.ncbi.nlm.nih.gov/pubmed/22708252, http://www.ncbi.nlm.nih.gov/pmc/articles/PMC3417124/pdf/nihms-394840.pdf

Entrenas Castillo, M., Entrenas Costa, L. M., Vaquero Barrios, J. M., Alcalá Díaz, J. F., López Miranda, J., Bouillon, R., & Quesada Gomez, J. M. (2020). Effect of calcifediol treatment and best available therapy versus best available therapy on intensive care unit admission and mortality among patients hospitalized for COVID-19: A pilot randomized clinical study. *J Steroid Biochem Mol Biol, 203*, 105751. https://doi.org/10.1016/j.jsbmb.2020.105751

Fendrick, A. M., & Shrosbree, B. (2020). Expanding coverage for essential care during COVID-19. *Am J Manag Care, 26*(5), 195–196. https://doi.org/10.37765/ajmc.2020.42920

Feyereisen, S., & Puro, N. (2020). Seventeen states enacted executive orders expanding advanced practice nurses' scopes of practice during the first 21 days of the COVID-19 pandemic. *Rural Remote Health, 20*(4), 6068. https://doi.org/10.22605/rrh6068

Frohlich, K. L., & Potvin, L. (1999). Collective lifestyles as the target for health promotion. *Can J Public Health, 90* (Suppl 1), S11–S14. https://doi.org/10.1007/BF03403571

Fuchs, V. R. (2010). Government payment for health care–causes and consequences. *N Engl J Med, 363*(23), 2181–2183. https://doi.org/10.1056/NEJMp1011362

Gabbidon, S.L., Peterson, S.A. (2006). Living while Black: A state-level analysis of the influence of select social stressors on the quality of life among Black Americans. *Journal of Black Studies, 37*(1), 83–102.

Gaffney, A., Himmelstein, D. U., & Woolhandler, S. (2020). COVID-19 and US health financing: Perils and possibilities. *Int J Health Serv, 50*(4), 396–407. https://doi.org/10.1177/0020731420931431

Galea, S., Tracy, M., Hoggatt, K. J., Dimaggio, C., & Karpati, A. (2011). Estimated deaths attributable to social factors in the United States. *Am J Public Health, 101*(8), 1456–1465.

Gamble, V. N. (2010). "There wasn't a lot of comforts in those days": African Americans, public health, and the 1918 influenza epidemic. *Public Health Reports, 125*(Suppl 3), 113–122.

Gangopadhyaya, A. and Garrett, A.B. (2020) Unemployment, Health Insurance, and the COVID-19 Recession. Urban Institute. https://doi.org/10.2139/ssrn.3568489

Garg, S., Kim, L., Whitaker, M., O'Halloran, A., Cummings, C., Holstein, R., … Fry, A. (2020). Hospitalization rates and characteristics of patients hospitalized with laboratory-confirmed coronavirus disease 2019—COVID NET, 14 States, March 1–30, 2020. *Morbidity and Mortality Weekly Report (MMWR)*. https://doi.org/10.15585/mmwr.mm6915e3, https://www.cdc.gov/mmwr/volumes/69/wr/mm6915e3.htm?s_cid=mm6915e3_w

Geronimus, A. T. (1992). The weathering hypothesis and the health of African-American women and infants: Evidence and speculations. *Ethn Dis, 2*(3), 207–221.

Geronimus, A. T., Hicken, M., Keene, D., & Bound, J. (2006). "Weathering" and age patterns of allostatic load scores among blacks and whites in the United States. *Am J Public Health, 96*(5), 826–833. https://doi.org/10.2105/ajph.2004.060749

Geyman, J. P. (2021). Beyond the COVID-19 pandemic: The urgent need to expand primary care and family medicine. *Fam Med, 53*(1), 48–53. https://doi.org/10.22454/FamMed.2021.709555

Harris, M. C. (2018). April Is National Minority Health Month. Retrieved from https://axesspointe.org/april-is-national-minority-health-month

Health. (2020). Health NYC: Age-adjusted rate of fatal lab confirmed COVID-19 cases per 100,000 people by race/ethnicity group as of April 6, 2020. Retrieved from https://www1.nyc.gov/assets/doh/downloads/pdf/imm/covid-19-deaths-race-ethnicity-04082020-1.pdf

Heckler, M. M. (1985). U.S. department of health and human services. Report of the secretary's task force report on black and minority health Volume I: Washington, DC: Executive summary. U.S. Government Printing Office. Retrieved from http://www.minorityhealth.hhs.gov/assets/pdf/checked/1/ANDERSON.pdf

Hemenway, D. (2010). Why we don't spend enough on public health. *N Engl J Med, 362*(18), 1657–1658.

Hood, C. M., Gennuso, K. P., Swain, G. R., Catlin, B. B. (2016). County health rankings: Relationships between determinant factors and health outcomes. *Am J Prev Med, 50*(2), 129–135. https://doi.org/10.1016/j.amepre.2015.08.024

Institute for Clinical Systems Improvement. (2014). Going beyond clinical walls: Solving complex problems. Retrieved from https://www.nrhi.org/uploads/going-beyond-clinical-walls-solving-complex-problems.pdf

James, S. A. (1994). John Henryism and the health of African-Americans. *Cult Med Psychiatry, 18*(2), 163–182. https://doi.org/10.1007/bf01379448

Johnson, A., & Martin, N. (2020). How COVID-19 hollowed out a generation of young black men. *ProPublica.* December 22, 2020.

Jones, C. P. (2002). Confronting institutionalized racism. *Phylon (1960–), 50*(1/2), 7–22. https://doi.org/10.2307/4149999

Jones, D. P. (2006). Redefining oxidative stress. *Antioxid Redox Signal, 8*(9–10), 1865–1879. https://doi.org/10.1089/ars.2006.8.1865

Kakani, P., Chandra, A., Mullainathan, S., & Obermeyer, Z. (2020). Allocation of COVID-19 relief funding to disproportionately black counties. *Jama, 324*(10), 1000–1003. https://doi.org/10.1001/jama.2020.14978

Kim, J, & Kwan, MP. (2020). The impact of the COVID-19 pandemic on people's mobility: A longitudinal study of the U.S. from March to September of 2020. *J Transp Geog, 93*(103039). https://doi.org/10.1016/j.jtrangeo.2021.103039

Klein, H. S., Engerman, S. L., Haines, R., & Shlomowitz, R. (2001). Transoceanic mortality: The slave trade in comparative perspective. *William Mary Q, 58*(1), 93–117.

Krieger, N. (1987). Shades of difference: Theoretical underpinnings of the medical controversy on black/white differences in the United States, 1830–1870. *Int J Health Serv, 17*(2), 259–278. https://doi.org/10.2190/dby6-vdq8-hme8-me3r

Krieger, N., Waterman, P. D., Chen, J. T. (2020). COVID-19 and overall mortality inequities in the surge in death rates by zip code characteristics: Massachusetts, January 1 to May 19, 2020. *Am J Public Health, 110*, 1850–1852. https://doi.org/10.2105/AJPH.2020.305913

Link, E. P. (1967). The civil rights activities of three great negro physicians (1840–1940). *J Negro Hist, 52*(3), 169–184.

Maul, A., & Joshi, M. (2021). The vaccine equity index — A tool to reduce racial disparities in COVID-19 vaccinations. *MedPage Today.* February 8, 202. Retrieved from https://www.medpagetoday.com/infectiousdisease/covid19/91104?xid=nl_secondopinion_2021-02-09&eun=g1096824d0r

McEwen, B. S. (1998). Protective and damaging effects of stress mediators. *N Engl J Med, 338*(3), 171–179. https://doi.org/10.1056/nejm199801153380307

McEwen B. S. (2000). Allostasis and allostatic load: implications for neuropsychopharmacology. *Neuropsychopharmacology, 22*(2), 108–124. https://doi.org/10.1016/S0893-133X(99)00129-3

McMorrow, S. (2021). Stabilizing and strengthening the affordable care act: Opportunities for a new administration. *J Health Polit Policy Law.* https://doi.org/10.1215/03616878-8970753

Meltzer, D. O., Best, T. J., Zhang, H., Vokes, T., Arora, V., & Solway, J. (2020). Association of vitamin D status and other clinical characteristics with COVID-19 test results. *JAMA Netw Open, 3*(9), e2019722. https://doi.org/10.1001/jamanetworkopen.2020.19722

Mizukoshi, A., Nakama, C., Okumura, J., & Azuma, K. (2021). Assessing the risk of COVID-19 from multiple pathways of exposure to SARS-CoV-2: Modeling in health-care settings and effectiveness of nonpharmaceutical interventions. *Environ Int, 147*, 106338. https://doi.org/10.1016/j.envint.2020.106338

Mohan, S., & Gupta, D. (2018). Crosstalk of toll-like receptors signaling and Nrf2 pathway for regulation of inflammation. *Biomed Pharmacother, 108*, 1866–1878. https://doi.org/10.1016/j.biopha.2018.10.019

National Conference of State Legislature. (2020). National Employment Monthly Update. Accessed February 4, 2021. Retrieved from https://www.ncsl.org/research/labor-and-employment/national-employment-monthly-update.aspx

Noonan, A. S., Velasco-Mondragon, H. E., & Wagner, F. A. (2016). Improving the health of African Americans in the USA: An overdue opportunity for social justice. *Public Health Rev, 37*, 12. https://doi.org/10.1186/s40985-016-0025-4

Norris, K. C., Olabisi, O., Barnett, M. E., Meng, Y. X., Martins, D., Obialo, C., … Nicholas, S. B. (2018). The role of vitamin D and oxidative stress in chronic kidney disease. *Int J Environ Res Public Health, 15*(12). https://doi.org/10.3390/ijerph15122701

Økland, H., & Mamelund, S. E. (2019). Race and 1918 Influenza Pandemic in the United States: A review of the Literature. *Int J Environ Res Public Health, 16*(14), 2487. https://doi.org/10.3390/ijerph16142487

Ostrom, T. M. (1969). The relationship between the affective, behavioral, and cognitive components of attitude. *Journal of Experimental Social Psychology, 5*(1), 12–30.

Palacio, A., & Tamariz, L. (2021). Social determinants of health mediate COVID-19 disparities in South Florida. *J Gen Int Med, 36*(2), 472–477. https://doi.org/10.1007/s11606-020-06341-9

Paradies, Y., Ben, J., Denson, N., Elias, A., Priest, N., Pieterse, A., Gupta, A., Kelaher, M., & Gee, G. (2015). Racism as a determinant of health: A systematic review and meta-analysis. *PloS One, 10*(9), e0138511. https://doi.org/10.1371/journal.pone.0138511

Patterson, F. (April–June, 1939). Statement concerning national Negro health week. *National Negro Health News, 7*, 13.

Pereira, M., & Oliveira, A. M. (2020). Poverty and food insecurity may increase as the threat of COVID-19 spreads. *Public Health Nutrition, 23*(17), 3236–3240.

Quinn, S. C., & Thomas, S. B. (2001). The national Negro health week, 195–1951: A descriptive account. *Minority Health Today, 2*(3), 44–49.

Raifman, J., Bor, J., & Venkataramani, A. (2021). Association between receipt of unemployment insurance and food insecurity among people who lost employment during the COVID-19 pandemic in the United States. *JAMA Network Open, 4*(1), e2035884–e2035884. https://doi.org/10.1001/jamanetworkopen.2020.35884

Saloner, B., Gollust, S. E., Planalp, C., & Blewett, L. A. (2020). Access and enrollment in safety net programs in the wake of COVID-19: A national cross-sectional survey. *PLoS One, 15*(10), e0240080. https://doi.org/10.1371/journal.pone.0240080

Schiele, J. H. (2007). Implications of the equality- of- oppressions paradigm for curriculum content on people of color. *J Social Work Education, 43*, 83–100. https://doi.org/10.5175/jswe.2007.200400478

Seddighi, H. (2020). COVID-19 as a natural disaster: Focusing on exposure and vulnerability for response. *Disaster Medicine Public Health Preparedness, 14*(4), e42–e43. https://doi.org/10.1017/dmp.2020.279

Seeman, T. E., Singer, B. H., Rowe, J. W., Horwitz, R. I., & McEwen, B. S. (1997). Price of adaptation–allostatic load and its health consequences: MacArthur studies of successful aging. *Arch Intern Med, 157*(19), 2259–2268. Retrieved from http://archinte.jamanetwork.com/data/Journals/INTEMED/17572/archinte_157_19_013.pdf

Sherman, B. W., Kelly, R. K., & Payne-Foster, P. (2020). Integrating workforce health into employer diversity, equity and inclusion efforts. *Am J Health Promot*, 890117120983288. https://doi.org/10.1177/0890117120983288

Smith, J. M. (1859). On the fourteenth query of Thomas Jefferson's notes on Virginia. *Anglo-African Magazine, 1*(8), 225–238.

Staff, A. (2020). The color of coronavirus: COVID-19 deaths by race and ethnicity in the U.S. Retrived from https://www.apmresearchlab.org/covid/deaths-by-race

Thames, A. D., Irwin, M. R., Breen, E. C., & Cole, S. W. (2019). Experienced discrimination and racial differences in leukocyte gene expression. *Psychoneuroendocrinol, 106*, 277–283. https://doi.org/10.1016/j.psyneuen.2019.04.016

The White House. (March 13, 2020). Letter from president Donald J. Trump on emergency determination under the Stafford act [Letter]. Retrieved from https://trumpwhitehouse.archives.gov/wp-content/uploads/2020/03/LetterFromThePresident.pdf

Tolbert, J., Orgera, K., Singer, N., Damico, A. (13 December 2019). Key facts about the uninsured population. *Kaiser Family Foundation.* Retrieved from https://www.kff.org/uninsured/issue-brief/key-facts-about-the-uninsuredpopulation/

United States Department of Homeland Security. (2021). Robert T. Stafford disaster relief and emergency assistance act, P.L. 93–288 as amended. United States Code, Title 42. The Public Health and Welfare, Chapter 68. Disaster Relief [42 U.S.C. 5121 et seq]. Washington, DC: Federal Emergency Management Agency. Retrieved from https://www.fema.gov/sites/default/files/documents/fema_stafford_act_2021_vol1.pdf

United States Department of Homeland Security. (2011). National disaster recovery framework: Strengthening disaster recovery for the nation. Washington, DC: FEMA. Retrieved from https://www.fema.gov/pdf/recoveryframework/ndrf.pdf

US Department of Health and Human Services, Office of Minority Health. (2010). National partnership for action to end health disparities. The national plan for action draft as of February 17, 2010. Retrieved from http://www.healthypeople.gov/2020/about/foundation-health-measures/Disparities#5

Wells, K. B., Tang, J., Lizaola, E., Jones, F., Brown, A., Stayton, A., … Plough, A. (2013). Applying community engagement to disaster planning: Developing the vision and design for the Los Angeles County community disaster resilience initiative. *Am J Public Health, 103*(7), 1172–1180. https://doi.org/10.2105/ajph.2013.301407

Whittle, R. S., & Diaz-Artiles, A. (2020). An ecological study of socioeconomic predictors in detection of COVID-19 cases across neighborhoods in New York City. *BMC Med, 18*(1), 271. https://doi.org/10.1186/s12916-020-01731-6

Williams, D. R., Lawrence, J. A., & Davis, B. A. (2019). Racism and health: Evidence and needed research. *Annu Rev Public Health, 40*, 105–125. https://doi.org/10.1146/annurev-publhealth-040218-043750

Wolf, M. S., Serper, M., Opsasnick, L., O'Conor, R. M., Curtis, L. M., Benavente, J. Y., … Bailey, S. C. (2020). Awareness, attitudes, and actions related to COVID-19 among adults with chronic conditions at the onset of the U.S. outbreak: A cross-sectional survey. *Ann Intern Med.* https://doi.org/10.7326/M20–1239

Wong, D. W. S., & Li, Y. (2020). Spreading of COVID-19: Density matters. *PLoS One, 15*(12), e0242398. https://doi.org/10.1371/journal.pone.0242398

Woolf, S. H., Johnson, R. E., Fryer, G. E. Jr, Rust, G., Satcher, D. (2008). The health impact of resolving racial disparities: An analysis of US mortality data. *Am J Public Health, 98*(9 suppl 1), S26–S28.

Woolhandler, S., & Himmelstein, D. U. (2020). Intersecting U.S. epidemics: COVID-19 and lack of health insurance. *Ann Intern Med.* https://doi.org/10.7326/M20-1491

World Health Organization (1948). Preamble to the Constitution of the World Health Organization as adopted by the International Health Conference. World Health Organization.

World Health Organization (1986). Ottawa charter for Health Promotion. Retrieved from https://www.who.int/teams/health-promotion/enhanced-wellbeing/first-global-conference

World Health Organization. (2019). Social determinants of health: Key concepts. Retrieved from http://www.who.int/social_determinants/thecommission/finalreport/key_concepts/en/index.html

World Health Organization (2008). *Closing the gap in a generation: Health equity through action on the social determinants of health.* World Health Organization.

Zhu, J. M., Grande, D., Jones, D. K., & Tipirneni, R. (2020). Health policy perspective: Medicaid and state politics beyond COVID. *J Gen Intern Med, 35*(10), 3040–3042. https://doi.org/10.1007/s11606-020-06117-1

Zuberi, T. (2001). *Thicker than blood: How racial statistics lie.* University of Minnesota Press.

4 Partnering with Black Organizations to Deliver Vaccine Education in Black Communities

*Rhonda BeLue, Sawsan Salah, Clare V. Schuchardt,
Kelly D. Taylor, Alyssa Coleman, Adaobi Anakwe,
Kemba Noel-London, DeBorah Ahmed, and Fredrick Echols*

Introduction

Disparities in vaccine coverage and uptake, particularly for minority populations, is a challenge that can threaten pandemic recovery. Per the Centers for Disease Control and Prevention (CDC), vaccine equity, which supports distribution and administration of vaccines to populations and communities most in need, considering their vulnerability to COVID-19, is an important goal (Hughes et al., 2021). Even though vaccine equity is an identified priority, efforts to achieve this goal have been slow and, in some regions, lacking. Across the United States, recent statistics show stark differences in who will receive the COVID-19 vaccine, with those at highest risk of morbidity and mortality from the virus at highest risk for poor vaccine coverage (Hughes et al., 2021; Ndugga et al., 2022). Specifically, counties with majority Black populations report lower coverage rates compared with counties with a larger White population (Ndugga et al., 2021; Recht & Weber, 2021).

The St. Louis (STL) region is historically racially divided by county as well as neighborhood boundaries. St. Louis County is predominantly non-Hispanic White (66.2%), with Black/African Americans comprising only 25.1% of the population, largely clustered in Northern neighborhoods with fewer resources. St. Louis City (STL city) holds a more even distribution of Black and White people (44.6% and 46.9% respectively), with Black people living in more impoverished and poorly resourced communities (Think Health St. Louis, 2021a). STL city's demographic distribution demonstrates the effect of historic segregationist policies that led to systemic disenfranchisement of its Black population, which continues to shape both the socioeconomic and health landscapes of its residents. Of particular importance is the famed "Delmar Divide." Areas located north of this major boulevard (hereafter referred to as North City) are not only predominantly Black, but disproportionately bear a greater burden of social and economic disadvantage in the region (including poverty, lower educational attainment, homelessness, and high unemployment rates) (Think Health STL, 2021b). People living in North City bear a greater burden of poor health outcomes from heart disease, cancer, lower/upper respiratory diseases, and unintentional injuries (CHNA, 2017). A closer look at this region in the context of the pandemic showed that North City was disproportionately impacted by higher COVID-19 case and death rates than other areas of the city (St. Louis, 2021).

A Social Need Vaccine Dissemination Approach Is Needed

The CDC social vulnerability index (SVI), defined as the "social and structural factors associated with adverse health outcomes" (Barry et al., 2021), was used to prioritize vaccine allocation and distribution in some areas of the United States. This approach was used to ensure equitable distribution of vaccines to those at highest risk of contracting or dying from the disease. Low-income

DOI: 10.4324/9781003140245-4

Black populations are more likely to work in low-income frontline jobs, which increases their risk of contracting the virus. This, coupled with less access to health care and high prevalence of comorbidities, increases their chances of experiencing complications of the COVID-19 virus if contracted (CDC, 2020).

STL city has a high vulnerability with an 0.78 SVI compared with St. Louis County with a 0.26 SVI, indicating significantly lower vulnerability (Office of the Assistant Secretary for Planning and Evaluation [ASPE], 2021). Similarly, the SocioNeeds Index® (SNI), which was created specifically for the St. Louis area (city and county), highlights the social vulnerability of specific locations within the greater metropolitan area and correlates with poor health outcomes observed in those places (Think Health STL, 2021b). Examination of the SNI (read on a scale from 1 to 100, with those closer to 100 at highest vulnerability) showed that in the city, there are five zip codes, all located in North City, with a high SNI (>90), indicating a high social vulnerability. Whereas, there was only one zip code in the county with a similar SNI. Furthermore, ten of the most vulnerable census tracts in the STL region are located in North City (Health Prism, 2021a; Think Health STL, 2021b). These data clearly demonstrate the need for equitable distribution of COVID-19 resources, given the highlighted social susceptibility and risk factors for poor outcomes in the communities that reside within these boundaries.

Despite these multilayered risk factors, vaccine coverage for STL city residents remains low overall, with vaccine coverage among the White population continuing to outpace that of Black population in the area. For instance, as of May 2021, although Black people accounted for 25% of COVID-19 cases and 12% of mortality, only 9% of Black residents were vaccinated compared with 18.3% of White residents (Ndugga et al., 2022). In addition, North City has a high concentration of vaccine deserts (Health Prism, 2021b). These vaccine coverage gaps and disparities underscore the need for an increased focus on identifying and addressing factors that hinder access to and uptake of the COVID-19 vaccine among Black residents in North City. It further necessitates an understanding of the (1) vaccine–allocation roll-out plan within the state; (2) public health infrastructure in place to disseminate vaccines; and (3) extent to which this planning structure may have negatively impacted vaccine dissemination, especially in North City.

Efforts to increase vaccine rollout and uptake are limited by several factors, including geographical location (lower vaccination rates in Southern and Western states than other regions), vaccine supply shortage, limited access to vaccination sites, complicated scheduling and appointment booking, and vaccine skepticism and hesitancy (https://www.nytimes.com/interactive/2020/us/covid-19-vaccine-doses.html). Further, equitable distribution of vaccines to the most vulnerable populations (especially in racial/ethnic minority and resource poor settings) remains slow. In Missouri, 63% of adults have received at least one shot of the COVID-19 vaccine, which lags far behind the national average of 74.7% (Mayo Clinic, 2022).

Vaccine rollout in Missouri was conducted in three phases: Phase 1 = long-term care facility staff, healthcare workers, and critical infrastructure workers; Phase 2 = vaccinate populations at increased risk of acquiring or transmitting COVID-19, and Phase 3 = vaccinate most vulnerable populations, including homeless and incarcerated populations (MODHSS, 2020). Vaccine coverage for racial and ethnic minorities was incorporated in Phase 2, which placed MO in the category of the 50% of states that explicitly included racial/ethnic minorities in their vaccine roll-out plan (Michaud et al., 2020). However, this did not necessarily mean that the state planned for equitable vaccine distribution, as coverage remains consistently lower in high-vulnerability counties than in low vulnerability counties (especially areas in North St. Louis City). Missouri lags far behind the national average in vaccine coverage (MODHSS, 2021). This can be attributed, in part, to a weak public health infrastructure, and to the continued disinvestment in public health.

The need for a thriving public health infrastructure became more evident during the pandemic. Missouri's public health infrastructure has been under-resourced for many years. In 2016, Missouri ranked second-to-last on public health funding, spending only US$5.90 per person compared with the national median of US$35.77 (Missouri Foundation for Health, 2021a) and continues to rank lower than most states post-2016. Further, the public health structure is fragmented, with 114 local public health authorities having different governance structures and receiving funding from multiple sources; resulting in an "under-funded, understaffed and poorly coordinated system" (Hughes, 2020). This further results in wide variations in the amount per person spending, and the quantity and quality of services delivered to local residents. This structure additionally hinders coordination between LPHAs and the broader health care system, a collaboration that became increasingly necessary during the pandemic. Additionally, for vaccine response efforts, the state bypassed its LPHAs to outsource this work to hospitals, consultants, and federal programs (Missouri Foundation for Health, 2021b). With the state's disinvestment in its public health sector, Missouri's most vulnerable populations will remain at highest risk of dying from the virus without needed vaccination.

Target Area

Our project focuses on the Promise Zone area in North City, St Louis, MO that is mostly Black (94.0%), and has had the highest COVID-19 rates and the lowest vaccine uptake rates in the city. Promise Zones are

> high poverty communities where the federal government partners with local leaders to increase economic activity, improve educational opportunities, leverage private investment, reduce violent crime, enhance public health and address other priorities identified by the community
> (https://www.hudexchange.info/programs/promise-zones/promise-zones-overview/)

As of the end of August 2021, Black residents of North Saint Louis were still disproportionately affected by COVID-19 infection, where 80% of new cases are among the African American community. North City has approximately 83,209 residents.

In this chapter, we present how

1 To build a sustainable community-based infrastructure to increase COVID-19 vaccine awareness, access, and knowledge in predominantly Black communities in St. Louis with the lowest vaccine rate.
2 To build a sustainable infrastructure to address ongoing health issues in the African American Community that pre-existed and has been exacerbated by COVID-19 (Figure 4.1).

The Partnership

To achieve the desired outcome of increasing COVID-19 vaccine knowledge and vaccine uptake, we used a multi-organization partnership model where (1) An academic institution, Saint Louis University (SLU), served as the coordinator of activities and creator/developer of culturally grounded vaccine education training/evaluation and corresponding materials (2) a local community-based organization, Better Family Life (BFL), that has historically served the Black population in our partnering community and has existing outreach programs that were repurposed for COVID-19 vaccine education outreach. For example, BFL conducts door-to-door and phone-banking outreach related

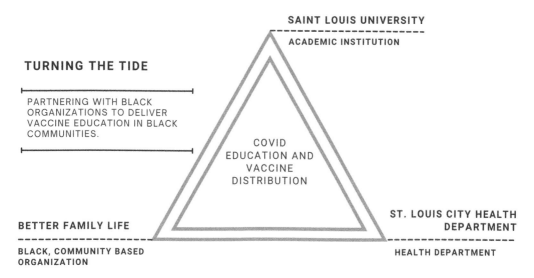

Figure 4.1 Organizational partnership chart

to food insecurity and violence de-escalation. Vaccine education was added to these initiatives. BFL also conducts 'Ground Zero' events in resource-limited neighborhoods where condoms and Narcan are distributed. Vaccine education was added to these events. Along with vaccine education, information on where and how to get vaccinated (including rides offered by BFL and SLU) were offered to increase vaccine uptake. Finally, out of general concern for the well-being of the community and the fact that individuals with comorbid conditions are more likely to have poor COVID-19-related outcomes, a general health assessment was included with all COVID-19 vaccine education information so that BFL could follow up with their clients regarding their overall health.

https://docs.google.com/forms/d/e/1FAIpQLSeoH-qLC9C-MSRKNe60SYAlme7OaVHG-joEmj8mDnq1s9SgfwQ/viewform

(3) The local city health department provided vaccinations at events hosted at BFL such as the annual Kwanzaa festival and the Black Business expo. Additional vaccine events were also held at local religious organizations and beauty and barbershops in our catchment area where the health department provided vaccinations and SLU and BFL staff provided COVID-19 vaccine education.

Working with a Local Black-Owned CBO to Conduct Vaccine Education

Local CBOs are essential for community-development and community engagement. Better Family Life, Incorporated (BFL) is a Black-founded and run not-for-profit, community-based organization that has served a predominantly Black community, which, for over 50 years, has been systematically and historically disenfranchised. BFL has over four decades of experience strengthening and promoting St. Louis families via holistic, resident-driven solutions focused on: (1) employment training and placement; (2) education; (3) housing and asset development; (4) community connection; and (5) youth, family, and clinical services rooted in cultural and racial awareness, pride, enlightenment, and integrity. BFL's centrally located facility sits in the heart of a community that has been 95% African American for the last 50 years, and is in the heart of the Promise Zone. One of BFL's goals, along with that of the Promise Zone initiative, is to reduce violent crime and increase economic opportunity in these communities. BFL provides direct social services to over 12,000 families per year, and indirect services (e.g., outreach activities, hosting community events, and information sessions) to an additional 10,000 per year.

The COVID-19 pandemic has heavily impacted the catchment area of BFL. The zip codes and residents in BFL's target service area have some of the highest case-rates of COVID-19 in the St. Louis region. This reflects the area's ongoing health disparities. This debilitating and deadly virus has had multiplicative deleterious health, social, and economic consequences. The economic sequelae of COVID-19 have included loss of productivity, loss of employment, disability, and mental health decline (Cutler & Summers, 2020).

BFL just completed a three-year pilot of de-escalation centers that swiftly and effectively disrupted cycles of violence in our focus communities. This project builds on the competencies and relationships yielded by this prior work, which was, at its core, focused on mediating symptoms of mental health crises that stem from racialized trauma, relentless toxic stress and complex barriers to social connection, and behavioral health services. They also bring to the table existing outreach events and community activities, such as the Kwanzaa Holiday Expo, that are well-attended and beloved by North City residents. COVID-19 vaccine education and access were incorporated into these existing activities during the partnership, and assisted in spreading the message about the COVID-19 vaccines in a trusted setting.

BFL holds a well-established trust and relationship with the Black community in North City, experience in education and outreach to the Promise Zone, and a local perspective on the project, as many of BFL's staff members live in North City as well as work there. Their partnership was critical in getting resources and information out to the Promise Zone communities.

Culturally Responsive Vaccine Education

The foundation of this course was a combination of two courses, Cultural Humility and Vaccine Communications. These courses were designed for the California contact tracing and case investigation workforce and were developed by the University of California, San Francisco and University of California, Los Angeles, with CBOs working with populations most impacted by COVID-19 (Brickley et al., 2021; Golston et al., 2021). The training was delivered via the Virtual Training Academy. Cultural Humility is a six-module course that has both asynchronous and live components with the following training topics: defining cultural humility; implicit bias, impacts, and response; effective communication; motivational interviewing; building collaborative relationships; and advocacy skills. Vaccine Communications includes vaccine basics; individual community barriers and enablers to vaccines; responding to frequently asked questions; health coaching for COVID-19 vaccination: tools to support decision-making and action.

While developing the California training workshops, it was clear that input from CBOs and their representatives were essential for an effective course. Using this model, we further refined and tailored the content based on feedback from the participants in the St. Louis course to reflect the local context of the pandemic. The training developed for the St. Louis community also included asynchronous learning delivered online and in-person didactic sessions that included the following learning approaches:

• Interactive lectures;
• Breakout groups with opportunities for role-play, skills building, and modeling activities.

Course participants were introduced to the core tenets of cultural humility and vaccine basics and how to apply them toward respectful and effective engagement. All sessions required learners to actively engage and practice skills in self-reflection, active listening, and providing asset-based recommendations.

Learning goals and objectives were presented at the outset of the course. The goals were tailored to reflect the needs of the local communities served and included:

• To confidently communicate about COVID-19 vaccines and vaccine efficacy
• To be knowledgeable about the vaccine, its effectiveness, and safety among local populations
• To translate knowledge regarding COVID-19 vaccines in plain language using common terms when engaging the local community
• To communicate with members of the community in a non-judgmental way about their vaccination status.

The first training occurred on September 15, 2021 and was hybrid (i.e., virtual and in-person). Thirteen members of the community attended the three-hour training including staff from BFL, members from Saint Louis University Training, and members from the St. Louis City Health Department. Prior to the training, attendees were required to complete a 4.5-hour, 4-module asynchronous training titled, *Making Contact: A training for COVID-19 contact tracers and case investigators* provided by the Association of State and Territorial Health Officials. This pre-work provided learners with foundations in (1) Public Health and COVID-19, (2) Case Investigation and Contact Tracing, (3) Conducting Effective Interviews, and (4) Monitoring and Support Services. Learners received a certificate of completion. The training consultant and a physician from the City Health Department led the training. Attendees held engaged discussions with training leaders to better understand aspects of the vaccine. Next, attendees worked in breakout groups to complete activities related to responding to frequently asked questions and using the health-coaching techniques.

Attendees answered an online pre- and post-training survey. The evaluation assessed attendees' knowledge of the following COVID-19 vaccine domains: basics, barriers to vaccination, techniques to remove barriers to vaccination, frequently asked questions about the vaccine, and action planning for vaccination. Additionally, the evaluation assessed training utility and recommendations for improvement.

COVID-19 vaccine knowledge was high at pre-training, ranging from 72% to 100% correct. In turn, just 25% of attendees reported a major improvement in their knowledge about COVID-19 vaccine at post-training. Approximately, 71% of attendees reported major improvements in knowing ways to talk to people about the COVID-19 vaccine and 71% strongly agreed that they learned something they will use in their work.

Attendees found the role-playing scenarios, health-coaching techniques, and session with a physician from the City Health Department as valuable parts of the training. Attendees found the required pre-training and limited time devoted to building trust and culturally specific language as the least valuable part of the training. Suggestions for improvement included increasing the amount of time spent in role-playing scenarios, removing the hybrid format, including information about failures related to vaccine misinformation and allocation, adding where people can get vaccinated locally, and including resources to help people get vaccinated such as transportation support.

Developing an African American Focused Education

Talking Points and Materials

The culturally responsive COVID-19 vaccine education highlighted the need for African American/Black community members. To develop Black–community focused education materials, the following activities were conducted.

Key Informant Interviews Were Conducted with BFL Community Outreach Staff

BFL staff generated a list of COVID-19 vaccine concerns expressed by BFL staff, clients, and other community members. The list covered everything from common misinformation and myths to culture-specific concerns stemming from a history of discrimination. These myths and questions were then taken and culturally acceptable answers were developed (Tables 4.1 and 4.2).

Research on African American/Black Scientists Involved in COVID-19 Vaccination Research

To address myths and issues related to mistrust, we highlighted the involvement of Black scientists and academics who had prominent roles in the development of the vaccines. We sourced videos from a culturally appropriate website (The Conversation/La Conversation) with videos discussing issues around the COVID-19 vaccine, tailored for the Black community and made by Black doctors, nurses, and other medical professionals. All of this information was linked to a project-specific website for all project participants, to browse according to their individual interests. It was also developed into culturally appropriate informational fliers.

Table 4.1 Common Myths and Questions

I heard that Black people died in the vaccine trials.
Black people weren't represented in the trials.
I don't want to be a lab rat.
The COVID vaccine can give you COVID.
Do the vaccines contain Microchips/nanobots?
I heard that getting the vaccine can make you shed (could refer to virus or to other components).
Is it safe for me to get the vaccine if I want to have a baby someday?
I don't want my DNA messed up.
There is sodium in the vaccine and I have high blood pressure.
I don't know what the ingredients are.
I am healthy so I don't need a vaccine.
They made the vaccine too fast and skipped FDA steps.
I already had COVID, so I'm immune. I don't need the vaccine.
We don't know if the vaccine works against the variants. It's not worth getting the vaccine.

Table 4.2 Focus Group Questions

How has COVID affected you? (Health, mental well-being, finances, can be on many dimensions)
If you feel comfortable sharing, have you had COVID or known anyone who has? What was that experience like?
What things do you do as far as COVID precautions?
What are your thoughts about the COVID vaccine?
Do you know people who have had the COVID vaccine?
If you have had the vaccine, why did you decide to get it?
If you have not been vaccinated, what information would you need to help you feel comfortable with being vaccinated?
How do you feel about other vaccinations?
What things do you want to know about the COVID vaccine? What are your questions?
What things do you do to stay healthy in general?
What are some health issues or concerns you had prior to the pandemic?

Focus Groups with Community Stakeholders

Focus groups consisted of nine African American individuals, mostly men who were mostly un-vaccinated for COVID-19. The participants were prompted into a discussion with a series of questions related to their experiences with COVID-19 pandemic, vaccinations, and related topics, their thoughts on the vaccine, and what information they would consider persuasive in making a decision whether to get vaccinated or not.

From the discussion, it was learned that the hesitation to get vaccinated stems from three main concerns: (1) the history of medical malpractice and racism toward Black people has led to decades of mistrust; (2) confusion regarding the mechanism by which the vaccine enters the body and what happens in the body afterward; (3) the overwhelming information from news and TV that does not always match up. During this session, when direct questions about the vaccine were asked, a healthcare professional was available to answer them openly.

Focus Group Follow-Up

Given what we learned from the focus groups, the educational materials, training, and infographics created were modified to better reflect specific community concerns. The infographics were modified to address major myths through charts and illustrations and included instructions on how to find a convenient vaccine location. The website URL was pasted on fliers, made into a QR code, and shared with community outreach workers for their reference.

https://covidvaccinesstl.wixsite.com/website

Overcoming Vaccine Hesitancy Narratives

Narrative and stories are powerful tools to relay health education messages, especially to resistant audiences. The Narrative Engagement Theory (Miller-Day & Hecht, 2013) that describes the qualities of culturally grounded and engaging stories needed to reach low awareness and/or resistant audiences was used as a basis for uncovering *Overcoming Vaccine Hesitancy* narratives among our partnering community. BFL identified several community members who went from being vaccine-hesitant to vaccinated. SLU staff interviewed identified community members to develop "overcoming vaccine hesitancy" stories to be used as education tools by project staff.

https://app.animaker.com/animo/UBaVjr5Y9UUOxjrr/
https://app.animaker.com/animo/MUjaVE9wyqESy3oc/

Tips and Best Practices

- Training is not one size fits all. It is vital to tailor educational materials to the audience. This requires understanding the local context and getting feedback from constituents.
- Include trusted members of the community to provide subject matter expertise.
- COVID-19 vaccination materials are most effective when culturally tailored to the partnering community. Tailored education materials should include information directly from community partners and clients.
- Include materials in many formats, but ensure that there is something for people to take with them and "digest" as it were, so that they can take the information and think about it to make an informed decision.

• Provide consistent and transparent coordination between all partners. While the focus of the project was to provide culturally grounded COVID-19 vaccine education, the culture of local government, CBO, and academic institutions differs and must be accounted for to maximize coordination and efficiency.

References

Barry, V., Dasgupta, S., Weller, D. L., Kriss, J. L., Cadwell, B. L., Rose, C.,... & Black, C. L. (2021). Patterns in COVID-19 vaccination coverage, by social vulnerability and urbanicity—United States, December 14, 2020–May 1, 2021. *Morbidity and Mortality Weekly Report, 70*(22), 818.

Brickley, D. B., Forster, M., Alonis, A., Antonyan, E., Chen, L., DiGiammarino, A., Dorian, A., Dunn, C., Gandelman, A., Grasso, M., Kiureghian, A., Maher, A. D., Malan, H., Mejia, P., Peare, A., Prelip, M., Shafir, S., White, K., Willard-Grace, R., & Reid, M. (2021). California's COVID-19 virtual training academy: Rapid scale-up of a statewide contact tracing and case investigation workforce training program. *Frontiers in Public Health, 9.* https://doi.org/10.3389/fpubh.2021.706697

Community, Work, and School. (2020, December 10). Centers for Disease Control and Prevention. Retrieved from https://www.cdc.gov/coronavirus/2019-ncov/community/health-equity/racial-ethnic-disparities/increased-risk-illness.html

COVID-19 Data. (2022, January 11). Stlouis-Mo.Gov. Retrieved from https://www.stlouis-mo.gov/covid-19/data/index.cfm

Cutler, D. M., & Summers, L. H. (2020). The COVID-19 pandemic and the $16 trillion virus. *JAMA, 324*(15), 1495. https://doi.org/10.1001/jama.2020.19759

Golston, O., Prelip, M., Brickley, D. B., Cass, A., Chen, L., Dorian, A., Gandelman, A., Keh, C., Maher, A., Myrick, R., Reid, M. J. A., White, K., Willard-Grace, R., & Shafir, S. (2021). Establishment and evaluation of a large contact-tracing and case investigation virtual training academy. *American Journal of Public Health, 111*(11), 1934–1938. https://doi.org/10.2105/ajph.2021.306468

HealthPrism™. (2021a, May 26). *State of Missouri covid-19 response St. Louis FQHC deep dive.* Retrieved January 15, 2022, from https://covidvaccine.mo.gov/equity/pdf/State%20of%20Missouri%20Health-Prism_STL%20FQHC_05262021_Final.pdf

HealthPrism™ - Missouri. (2021b, May 24). *State of Missouri COVID-19 response vaccine distribution analysis.* Retrieved January 15, 2022, from https://covidvaccine.mo.gov/equity/pdf/State%20of%20Missouri_HealthPrism_Vaccine%20Distribution%20Analysis_05242021_Final.pdf

Hughes, D. L, and Cindy, M. (2020). Financing The Infrastructure Of Accountable Communities For Health Is Key To Long-Term Sustainability. *Health Affairs* (Project Hope), *39*(4), 670–678. doi:10.1377/hlthaff.2019.01581

Hughes, M. M., Wang, A., Grossman, M. K., Pun, E., Whiteman, A., Deng, L.,,... & Toblin, R. L. (2021). County-level COVID-19 vaccination coverage and social vulnerability—United States, December 14, 2020–March 1, 2021. *Morbidity and Mortality Weekly Report, 70*(12), 431.

Making contact: A training for covid-19 contact tracers. (n.d.). ASTHO Learning. Retrieved January 15, 2022, from https://learn.astho.org/products/making-contact-a-training-for-covid-19-contact-tracers

Mayo Foundation for Medical Education and Research. (2022). *U.S. COVID-19 vaccine tracker: See your state's progress.* Mayo Clinic. Retrieved January 15, 2022, from https://www.mayoclinic.org/coronavirus-covid-19/vaccine-tracker/

Michaud, J., Kates, J., Dolan, R., & Tolbert, J. (2020, November 18). *States are getting ready to distribute COVID-19 vaccines: What do their plans tell us so far?* Retrieved January 15, 2022, from https://www.kff.org/coronavirus-covid-19/issue-brief/states-are-getting-ready-to-distribute-covid-19-vaccines-what-do-their-plans-tell-us-so-far/

Miller-Day, M., & Hecht, M. L. (2013). Narrative means to preventative ends: A narrative engagement framework for designing prevention interventions. *Health Communication, 28*(7), 657–670. https://doi.org/10.1080/10410236.2012.762861

Missouri Foundation for Health. (2020a, July 15). *Prioritizing public health infrastructure: Why improvement and innovation should be front and center*. Retrieved January 15, 2022, from https://mffh.org/news/prioritizing-public-health-infrastructure/

Missouri Foundation for Health. (2020b, July 21). *A Tale of Two Systems – the Shortchanging of Public Health*. Retrieved January 15, 2022, from https://mffh.org/news/a-tale-of-two-systems-the-shortchanging-of-public-health/

Ndugga, N. N., Hill, L. H., Artiga, S. A., & Haldar, S. H. (2022, January 12). *Latest data on COVID-19 vaccinations by race/ethnicity*. KFF. Retrieved from https://www.kff.org/coronavirus-covid-19/issue-brief/latest-data-on-covid-19-vaccinations-by-race-ethnicity/

Recht, H. R., & Weber, L. W. (2021, August 13). *Black Americans are getting vaccinated at lower rates than white Americans*. Kaiser Health News. Retrieved December 12, 2021, from https://khn.org/news/article/black-americans-are-getting-vaccinated-at-lower-rates-than-white-americans/

St. Louis County Public Health, City of St. Louis Department of Health, & St. Louis Partnership for a Healthy Community. (2017, December). *Community health status assessment*. Think Health STL.

Think Health St. Louis. (2021a, January 1). *Think health St. Louis:: Demographics :: County :: St. Louis*. Copyright (c) 2022 by Think Health St. Louis. Retrieved December 12, 2022, from https://www.thinkhealthstl.org/demographicdata

Think Health St. Louis. (2021b). *Think health St. Louis :: Indicators*. Copyright (c) 2022 by Think Health St. Louis. Retrieved from https://www.thinkhealthstl.org/index.php?module=indicators&controller=index&action=socioneeds

Vaccine hesitancy for COVID-19: State, county, and local estimates. (2021, June 16). ASPE. Retrieved from https://aspe.hhs.gov/reports/vaccine-hesitancy-covid-19-state-county-local-estimates

5 Toward Re-Enforcing Resilience in Crisis

African American Family Voices during the COVID-19 Pandemic

Adaobi Anakwe, Wilson Majee, Monica Ponder, and Rhonda BeLue

Introduction

The disproportionate burden of public health emergencies on minority populations, especially among African Americans (AAs) in the United States is not new. Historically, AAs have endured greater psychological distress, stress, and disruptions to social connections from public health emergencies such as natural disasters and pandemic events (Adepoju et al., 2021; Fothergill et al., 1999; Laditka et al., 2010; Lee et al., 2009). Yet, efforts toward ensuring that AAs receive more equitable, culturally aligned services during public health emergencies are not commendable. The AA family system exists in a fragile equilibrium, i.e., an adapted state necessary to thrive amid multilevel structures working to disrupt and systematically disadvantage this population. This inherently stressful state and the expectation to be resilient in the face of crises have been normalized in many AA families and communities (Anderson, 2019). Families play significant roles in ensuring the well-being of its members and function as a source of safety and support during crises (Jackson II et al., 2019).

The COVID-19 pandemic highlighted the effects of deeply rooted systemic racism and its far-reaching impact on AAs. Specifically, AAs bore a disproportionate burden of the effect of the pandemic, including higher mortality, morbidity, financial stress, and their cascading effects (Artiga, et al., 2020; Rossen, 2021). For AA families, this meant navigating a disproportionate burden of predisposing factors to, and negative consequences from, the disease that further threatened their fragile existence (Chaney, 2020; Davis et al., 2020). AA families experienced a disproportionate burden of the pandemics' direct effects (i.e., increased morbidity and mortality from the virus) (Rossen, 2021). They were also hard hit with indirect effects (i.e., financial hardship, poorer access to healthcare, inadequate food supply, and social isolation) (Fairlie et al., 2020; Lopez et al., 2020) and endured co-occurring crises due to racial tensions simultaneously occurring during the pandemic lockdown (Bright, 2020). These pandemic experiences and effects are discussed in detail later in the chapter. The pandemic highlighted the effects of the historical systemic disadvantage this population faces that necessitates an understanding of AA families as a pandemic response unit. This chapter focuses on creating a cultural understanding of how AA families navigate these emergencies. It also highlights how resources can be tailored to support post-pandemic recovery, foster resilience, and close the disparities gap using a family-strengths perspective.

The processes by which people receive and act on pandemic messages and how they experience the pandemic are culturally defined (Airhihenbuwa, 2020; Fothergill et al., 1999). Cultural codes, including respect for family heads, strong family and community affiliation and prioritization, and trust in information or knowledge provided by the community, shape how information is shared, received, and acted on (Nobles, 2007). By understanding the influences of family culture on pandemic experiences, interpretation, and action taking, the public health workforce can better target messaging and interventions in a culturally relevant manner that will foster resilience and spur action in preparation for future pandemics. Given the unique context of AA families during public

DOI: 10.4324/9781003140245-5

health emergencies, this chapter applies a culturally grounded lens to explicate how these families experienced the pandemic. We specifically discuss challenges they faced and how their sociocultural contexts influenced their experience of and response to the crisis. The chapter describes the process of risk resilience in AA households using the culturally defined PEN-3 framework.

The PEN-3 Conceptual Framework and Key Principles

The PEN-3 model is a cultural framework that is used to examine cultural meanings that are central to how people define their relationship with their social worlds. It has been applied in several contexts to frame people's health states and behaviors and it highlights the roles family systems play in influencing health behaviors (Airhihenbuwa et al., 2009; Iwelunmor et al., 2014) and in addressing chronic health conditions (e.g., HIV, cancer, hypertension, diabetes) and other behavioral health issues (Iwelunmor et al., 2014). The PEN-3 framework offers a strategy for organizing and synthesizing complex processes and relationships within cultural contexts to identify areas of strengths that should be promoted and challenges that can be addressed to create behavior change.

Cultural Identity (CI), Relationships and Expectations (RE), and Cultural Empowerment (CE) are the three interdependent domains that characterize the framework (Airhihenbuwa et al., 2009; Airhihenbuwa, 2007). The CI domain focuses on three areas – *person* (i.e., the individual that influences the health behavior most), *extended* (i.e., identifying kinship influences on health behaviors), and *neighborhood* (i.e., the role and context of community and values that shape health behaviors). The RE domain highlights three areas – *perceptions* (examining the beliefs and values of the people experiencing the condition), *enablers* (factors and/or resources that promote or hinder the behavior), and *nurturers* (the role of family and friends in making positive or negative changes). The CE domain that also consists of three areas – *positive* (examining the positive attributes of the culture that supports the behavior), *existential* (creates an understanding of the unique attributes of the culture), and *negative* (highlights aspects of the culture that contributes to poor behaviors).

We apply the framework to assess and create a cultural understanding on AA familial experiences of and responses to the COVID-19 pandemic. Using the framework also facilitates the identification of areas of focus to strengthen resilience and cultivate preparedness for future public health emergencies. First, we discuss the identity of the AA family and its cultural emergence. We then draw from a study we conducted with AA families to demonstrate how they experienced the pandemic within their cultural domain and highlight areas of emphasis for future pandemic planning.

A Cultural Understanding of the African American Family System (Cultural Identity)

According to Robert Hill, AA families are characterized by five unique strengths (1) strong achievement orientation; (2) strong work orientation; (3) strong kinship bonds; (4) adaptability of family roles; and (5) strong religious bonds (Hill, 1999). These strengths rest on the values of communalism and harmony, i.e., the belief that individual and collective identities and functioning occur within families and communities (Thomas, 2017). The emergence of these strengths can be traced to the historical origins of AA people, extended slavery, and the persistent will to thrive despite systemic disadvantage (Du Bois & Eaton, 1996; Littlejohn-Blake & Darling, 1993). AAs make meaning of their world through their freedom to navigate their environments, including neighborhood, schools, sporting events, and church. Through these media, AAs "develop individual and collective identity, give and receive advice, share group wisdom, celebrate victories and combat racism" (Davis et al., 2020).

The social positioning of Black people in the United States and the structural forces at work have shaped the cultural emergence of AA families and its functioning. AA family structure, which has emerged as predominantly single-female or grandparent-led, is entrenched in the long history of slavery and discriminatory practices (Littlejohn-Blake & Darling, 1993; Moras et al., 2018). Historically, AA females had a high labor-force participation, with inadequate employment opportunities for males, which narrowed the wage differential between males and females and increased the likelihood of marital instability (Moras et al., 2018; Ruggles, 1994). Government welfare programs, which favored single-mother-headed families, are thought to have inadvertently encouraged the break-up of AA families (Peterson, 2015). The incarceration crises further entrenched the culture of single parenting and perpetuates the absent father syndrome in these families. About one in four Black children have a parent who is incarcerated, and most are disproportionately male (Morsy & Rothstein, 2016). In other words, AA families (and their structures) emerged as a functional adaptation in response to adverse external conditions.

Despite this cultural emergence of the AA family system, and the persistent adverse conditions in which it continues to exist, parents within this system persevere in propagating teachings of strength, pride, self-confidence, spirituality, kinship, and resilience, especially in navigating multiple layers of systemic disadvantage. However, single-parent-female-headed AA households are more likely to endure financial instability and generational poverty making them more vulnerable to the adverse effects of public health emergencies (Laditka et al., 2010; Obinna, 2021).

Pandemic Experiences and Effects on the AA Family System

The pandemic posed a significant threat to the well-being of AA families because of financial insecurity, social disruption, caregiving burden, and confinement-related stress (Prime et al., 2020). Although previous research alluded to the centrality of family processes as a buffer against the risks posed by the pandemic, the literature examining these processes from a cultural perspective is emerging. By developing a cultural understanding on how the pandemic disrupted the fragile equilibrium of the AA family, we will not only mitigate risks associated with poor family well-being but utilize the strengths inherent in this family system to foster resilience through shared family beliefs.

Pandemic Direct Effects: Excess Mortality, Morbidity, and Its Consequences

Pandemic direct effects are defined here as the biomedical outcomes that were a consequence of contracting the virus such as morbidity or mortality. The AA population bore a disproportionate burden of the direct effects of the pandemic, including higher numbers of COVID-19 cases, deaths, and hospitalizations. For instance, in August 2020, Black individuals accounted for more cases and deaths relative to their share of the population, and Black people died at a rate that was two times higher than White people (Artiga et al., 2020). Beyond these immediate effects, studies have suggested that AA families will continue to bear a disproportionate burden of the long-term health consequences from contracting the disease (Andrasfay & Goldman, 2020). As noted by Lee and colleagues (Lee et al., 2009), familial experiences of death due to public health emergencies place the greatest psychological strain on AA families, and these families are less likely to show psychological resilience (Lee et al., 2009). AA men also had the highest mortality due to COVID-19 that further disrupted the economic stability of the home (Rushovich et al., 2021). In addition, AA women (who disproportionately play the role of primary caregivers) were burdened with providing care to family members who may suffer from long-term complications due to COVID-19 independent of their own health status (Crable, 2021; Obinna, 2021). This spill-over effect of the pandemics' direct effects creates significant challenges for families, particularly for women assuming both the responsibility of household head and primary caretaker. Although these disruptions to the AA family fabric are not new, their perpetuation continues to threaten their stability and resilience in a post-pandemic world (Crable, 2021).

Pandemic Indirect Effects: Socioeconomic Hardship and Loss of Access to Health-Promoting Resources

The indirect effects are used here to denote the secondary effects such as financial hardship, loss of social connection, and loss of access to health-promoting resources (healthcare, food) that AA families suffered because of the pandemic. Similar to the direct effects, AA families endured a disproportionate burden of financial hardships from the pandemic. AA families that are more likely than their White counterparts to work in low-wage and essential-duty jobs (homecare, warehouses, and other frontline service jobs), had higher exposures to the virus than White people (Centers for Disease Control and Prevention, 2020). Due to the instability inherent in these employment types, AAs also had a higher likelihood of pandemic-related job layoffs. In April 2020, 44% of at least one AA adult in a household reported losing their job compared with 38% of White adults (Ismail et al., 2021) worsening an already existing disparity in employment. Prior to the pandemic, AAs had a higher unemployment rate than White adults (31.8% vs 23.5%), and lower savings in their bank accounts (Farrell et al., 2020) compared with White households with a bank account. This lack of a financial buffer before the pandemic further placed AA households at risk for adverse effects from the pandemic, including homelessness, lack of food, lack of health access, and other direct effects (Centers for Disease Control and Prevention, 2020). When financial stresses occur, family functioning can be disrupted due to increased parental stress and hinder positive parenting practices that, in turn, can affect the parent–child and sibling relationship (Anderson, 2019; Prime et al., 2020). AA families that endured a greater burden of financial instability from the pandemic may become especially vulnerable to poorer functioning due to these stressors.

Because of school closures, AA parents had to take on additional roles of pseudo-teachers and instructors, to help their children with virtual learning. The structure of AA households (i.e., predominantly female-headed) suggests that these roles fell largely to single mothers and or grandmothers, further threatening the fragile equilibrium of the AA household.

Other Sociocultural Factors: Loss of Culturally Relevant Social Networks Affecting the Personal, Extended, and Neighborhood Domains

When families experience crises, the family system makes an effort to maintain its balance. Families often become flexible and adaptable to ensure that the well-being of household members is maintained (Sheridan et al., 2013). For AA families, this is typically achieved by leaning into the cultural strengths of the family system. Culturally, AA families congregate around food to grow cultural bonds that are historically nested in food as a means of emancipation (Du Bois & Eaton, 1996). However, due to the pandemic, families did not only have reduced access to food from store closures as a result of lockdown mandates, but they were unable to congregate around food (i.e., large family dinners), a significant part of AA family culture. Further, because religious gatherings were stopped, as a public health measure to slow the spread of the virus, AA families lost a key source of social support, i.e., the Black church. Typically, during crisis, AA families rely on their key support networks – family and church to tackle adversity (Chaney, 2020). However, with reduced access to these resources, AA families were once again tossed into the chaos of navigating the pandemic with minimal culturally relevant support systems.

Beyond these factors that compromised the AA family support system, these families endured additional crises during the pandemic lockdown. Racial tensions emanated from the killings of Black people through police violence (e.g., Breonna Taylor, George Floyd, Rayshard Brooks, Ahmaud Arbery, Makiyah Bryant) and a riot at the U.S. Capitol by right-wing White supremacists (Bright, 2020; Stelter, 2021). AA parents were doubly tasked with interpreting these predicaments for themselves and communicating to their children. Together, the crises strained the AA family system especially in managing the psycho-emotional consequences of deaths and powerlessness felt due to the inability to access the resources they needed to mitigate these effects, higher financial instability, job losses, homelessness, and a higher burden of childcare without the needed community support. In other words, AA families endured a greater overall burden of the pandemic due to their unique cultural niche as Black people living in a racially divided society.

Given these direct and indirect effects of COVID-19 on AAs, and to further interrogate the PEN-3 cultural framework, we use narratives from a pilot project that examined experiences of AA household heads during the COVID-19 pandemic. We hope to draw evidence-based insights on the unique challenges AA families faced, coping mechanisms used, and local solutions identified for cultivating resilience prior to, during, and after public health emergencies.

Case Study

The case study is based on a pilot qualitative research project that was conducted among 11 AA household heads in a small city in Midwestern United States. We provide findings from this research to support the narrative that pandemic experiences, especially in AA communities, are culturally defined. We further highlight the need to align pandemic preparedness efforts with cultural practices of the affected population.

Participants in this study identified as the household head and primary caregiver of a school-aged child (ages 5–17 years). Most participants were 46 years old or older (63.6%), female (either a mother or grandmother [81.2%]), single (i.e., never married, separated, divorced, or widowed [81.2%]), and 45% reported that they had experienced a reduction in their income due to the pandemic. Data for this project was collected through semi-structured interviews that consisted of nine questions that broadly examined AA families' awareness of COVID-19 and the strategies used to cope with the pandemic. Interviews were thematically analyzed following a data-immersion and familiarization process (Braun & Clarke, 2006). A detailed report on the methods used in this study and the demographic profile of participants are reported elsewhere (Anakwe et al., 2021).

Insights from African American Heads of Household

In line with the PEN-3 framework, we provide sample quotes categorized into the RE and CE domains of the PEN-3 model (Table 5.1). Consistent with previous literature, these domains were crossed in a 3×3 format to generate nine cells that identified positive and negative perceptions, positive and negative enablers, and positive and negative nurturers (Airhihenbuwa et al., 2014). While perceptions are important, we intentionally discuss findings with emphasis on the enablers and nurturers of pandemic experiences, and potential intervention points when planning for future public health emergencies. We focus on these two aspects to highlight areas with opportunities for targeted interventions.

Positive Versus Negative Enablers

The PEN-3 model, as applied to this chapter highlights the cultural role of AA families as an "intervention entry point" (Iwelunmor et al., 2014). Consistent with the literature on AA families' adaptive processes in the face of disruptions, these families rallied together to mitigate the disruptive effects of the pandemic (Walsh, 2015). Despite an overwhelming awareness to their susceptibility and vulnerability to the pandemic, AA family heads, leaned into cultural strengths such as spirituality and strong achievement orientation to cultivate resilience within their families, i.e., by believing that they will overcome any challenges the pandemic presented. However, these families experienced

Table 5.1 Sample Quotes Categorized into the RE and CE Domains of the PEN-3 Model

Domains	Positive	Existential	Negative
Perceptions	• COVID as a blessing *I think that's the blessing of it all is that I've been able to get to know myself and my son better than I have his whole life because I've always had to work nonstop through his life (033).*	• Whatever it takes attitude *I'm not letting anybody come over, and if they do come over I'm spraying it down, bleach water, and you gotta wash your hands all the way up to your elbows (032).*	• Inundating risk perceptions *I think about the fact that African Americans are being hit the hardest. I think about how to me it's concerning that we're hit the hardest as a people (037)* • Sudden and drastic changes *Everybody had to take either a week without pay or 10% salary cut for three months. (041)*
Enablers	• Access to resources *I have blood pressure medications and Walgreens was still available. So, we haven't really had any challenges (037) We have gotten telehealth. When I was sick, I was able to video with my primary care provider and get the script that I needed, get the order needed to get the COVID test, and I've done video psych sessions as well, so I've still been able to get what I needed through telehealth." (039). I always try to go out and keep buying a little bit at a time, a little here, a little there just keep up on our stock of food. (034)*	• Church/spirituality *Normally we're in church every Sunday and most of the week honestly for some reason or another, so that has been a lot of prayer on my end. That's the best coping I've found is counseling, meditation, praying (033). Well, like Sunday my church did something out of the box. Even though COVID's going on we, they had a caravan and it was like 20 people, you know, 20 cars and then when everybody got out of their car there was probably 30, 35 people, but they sat in my front lawn and sang praise and worship songs. My; my bishop, he prayed over us, they asked us how we were doing, they talked to my granddaughters, they talked to my grandson, they talked to me. (041)*	• Lack of food choices *So initially when everything was going on, you would go to the stores and there would be nothing, like all the bread would be gone, milk would be gone, you know. And with him (son), he's very specific in what he eats so that's been, that was kind of a challenge at the beginning.... his diet is extremely limited so that was really scary initially cause when I got to go I'd get there and there'd be things that he eats that would just be gone......And then when my hours got reduced at work before I was able to get put on unemployment, it, there were days that I wasn't, we had to stretch some things out like quite a bit just because Mommy wasn't gonna get paid until the next week so we had to just stretch what we had. (033)* • Diminished quality of healthcare *Well, I had a doctor's appointment by phone. I just checked in with him and I guess it's just on the honor system, cause they can't really, check your blood pressure or your sugar levels or your weight or anything like that so, I just kind of had a self-report to him, what I was noticing with my own health. (040)* • Lack of digital resources and access *I looked at the neighborhood I grew up in in St. Louis, it's 99% Black at the schools and the only other 1% is Hispanic. It's a 100% poverty rate and I'm looking at the school and be like who's learning at this school. They don't have computers, the families are poor, they don't have WiFi..., those families they don't, they're not learning anything right now. They're not connected online, ain't got no cell phone, no app. Now if they got a flip phone but they ain't got no smart phones, you know; if they got a smart phone, it's a neighborhood smart phone and they share it but now it's dangerous. (038)*

(Continued)

Table 5.1 (Continued)

Domains	Positive	Existential	Negative
		When I think about coping, I guess I'm just such at peace. I'm really at peace. I've been at peace with all of, through this whole time because I simply just keep myself in prayer. (034)	*My children are fighting more, not like they physically fight…. "Well, I'm watching this" (on the tablet). That's a fight every day. Like, I have to minimize the times that the kids use it. Then you don't want them to be on devices too long so I'm up to the point where taking them and hiding them up under my mattress. You got an eight-year old and you got a ten-year old and you have to work with them and then they fight amongst each other, then they fight with the 16-year old. They drive me insane. (032)*
Nurturers	• Parent–child crises communication *You don't want them to be scared, oh, I'm gonna die… you don't want them to be naïve either but then you don't want to scare them. I'm an adult and I'm scared. (032) I feel like we have the relationship with them (children) when we're having conversations around the dinner table and we're talking about those things that concern us and the things that we have to do different and acknowledging the sacrifices that we all have to make I think it, it makes it easier: (037)* • Bonding and understanding children *I think that we kind of need to push that reset button and kind of figure out what has value for us, what works for us, and as we see a lot of us we can work from home, so why don't we just make this the norm? (038).*	• Social interaction/ connection *It is hard to realize that, you want to be with family, to hang out. We're used to going to the movies or going out to dinner and those things are not happening. (037) Our belief in God. Our love for one another. Just trusting that this too shall pass. It's our situation today is not gonna be our future. We gonna get through this. That's what got us through day by day (041)*	• Lack of trust in information sources (word of mouth) *…all my information came from work and listening to the other nurses talk about it. (041)* • Pandemic unpreparedness *I think about how unprepared we were for it and I think we could have been better prepared if we had better things in place to implement when it finally did make it here, and that's neither here nor there now. Like the schools could have maybe started preparing in case we needed to shelter in place…. I think that (internet) should be a given during the school year, period, regardless of what's going on because we send these kids home with tablets or whatever; laptops, but if they can't get on the internet to access the things what good is having the tablet at home? (039)*

many negative enablers like diminished quality of healthcare, poorer food choice, and/or options and lack of digital access. These system-level challenges created additional hardship for these families.

Pandemic as a curse: Participants alluded to the pandemic as a curse in that it brought with it financial stress, tasked parents (who were already stressed) with homeschooling their children and obstructed social interaction and connection – a key element in AA family relational dynamics. The stress was, however, more pronounced in already income-vulnerable populations such as single-female-headed AA households. Participants in this study expressed that non-pharmaceutical intervention measures, put in place to curtail the spread of the pandemic, resulted in reduced household income. Household income reduction during unsettling times resulted in financial stress that made them feel exhausted, angry, and distracted. Additional demands from children for resources such as access to internet, which would otherwise have been provided in school settings, further exacerbated some of this stress.

Lack of access to resources: AA families disproportionately bore the impact of the indirect effects of the pandemic. Participants lacked adequate access to healthcare and food during the pandemic. Participants expressed frustration with virtual healthcare services and inability to schedule in-person hospital appointments for health conditions unrelated to COVID-19. While some families had their healthcare needs met through telehealth, others, whose healthcare needs required in-person visits such as for domestic accidents, routine management of multiple conditions, and children with behavioral health needs, felt that telehealth diminished the quality of healthcare they would have received otherwise.

Lack of food products in stores and limited financial resources due to pandemic-related job layoffs were important food insecurity factors discussed. Participants felt that the response time to ensure that they had adequate food amid the lockdown was low and this caused them to go hungry. Food choice also became an important factor in food access. Participants' experiences suggest that even though food may have been available, they lacked the variety that would support a healthy lifestyle or meet the nutritional needs for specific household members.

This lack of access to healthcare and food resources was further exacerbated by the digital divide – which refers to the growing gap in internet access between the underprivileged members of society, especially between the urban and rural poor and the urban and suburban wealthy populations who have access (van Dijk, 2006). Participants felt disempowered to meet the needs of their children because they (a) lacked access to the required technolo gy to support their children's education and engagement and (b) lacked the technology savviness to navigate these spaces safely (Anakwe et al., 2021). This lack of access to digital resources not only impacted engagement with children and social networks, but also stymied access to other essential resources such as healthcare and engaging in academic activities that shifted to online formats. For participants, these effects emphasized an overall lack of pandemic preparedness at the local, state, and national level, and were a reminder of the social consequences they endure due to systemic factors.

Positive Versus Negative Nurturers

Despite the negative enablers AA families encountered, cultural safety nets such as kitchen table discussions, emerged as useful tools to help families navigate conversations that emanated from experiencing the pandemic. Communication is a valuable part of family life and helps to assure its members' well-being (Prime et al., 2020). During crises, communication is key to help family members manage their fears and expectations and can also serve as a source of resilience. AA household heads used the dinner table as a place to share these values.

Culturally, kitchen table discussions serve not only as a point for strengthening family cohesion but also provide a space for household heads to share and preserve history (McCoy, 2011). Further, the pandemic enabled parents to bond with their children through focusing on shared values. Interconnected relationships between family members suggest that multiple-layered stressors experienced during the pandemic can impede the functioning of one member, which in turn can disrupt the functioning of the whole system (Masten & Obradovic, 2008; Prime et al., 2020). As such, intentional approaches toward active bonding between family members during crisis can also be a positive adaptation used to cultivate resilience. However, even though families keyed into their cultural strengths to weather the pandemic storm, Anderson (2019) cautions about the cons of constantly expecting AA families to lean inward to cultivate resilience. A constant expectation to remain resilient in the face of systemic barriers could unintentionally foster greater and more damaging vulnerabilities in the future, especially in a post-pandemic world (Anderson, 2019). Thus, there is a need to identify other resilience-building mechanisms that are cognizant of these inherent vulnerabilities and actively utilize equitable approaches to eliminate the systemic factors that create them.

Considerations for Improving Pandemic Preparedness and Cultivating Resilience for Future Public Health Emergencies

Familial experiences of the pandemic occurred on a complex continuum nuanced by the social situation of each family. For instance, while some families continued to have access to healthcare through telehealth, others either lacked access completely or felt that telehealth diminished their quality of care. Future preparedness efforts will require eliminating negative enablers and promoting the positive nurturers. Building resilience requires removal of negative enablers. Negative enablers both directly and indirectly limit access to social supports and services known to facilitate resilience (Anderson, 2018). Negative enablers can disrupt prosocial family processes that build resilience and buffer families against the stress brought on by the COVID-19 pandemic (Prime et al., 2020).

Addressing the Negative Enablers

Availability of food options as an indicator of food insecurity: The pandemic has highlighted that for vulnerable families, food choice should also be considered an important indicator of food security (Anakwe et al., 2022). Ability to purchase food online can increase access to a wider variety of foods and increase food choice. As consumers' preference shifts to purchasing food online, having digital access is central to addressing food insecurity (George & Toner, 2021). However, if the digital divide is not addressed in AA communities, it can become an additional determinant of health that will hinder resilience in future pandemics.

Telemedicine should be culturally aligned to AA family needs: As the rapid shift to telemedicine continues to be advocated for, our study suggests that this mode of healthcare delivery should not be one-size-fits-all (Anakwe et al., 2022). This model may not be suitable for specific populations with unique healthcare needs including those requiring in-person access for their health management and families with children with behavioral health needs. Chang et al. (2021) demonstrated that disparities in access to and utilization of telehealth services are dependent on the socioeconomic characteristics of the populations served. Particularly, racial and ethnic minority populations who are more likely to belong to high social vulnerability groups are less likely to have access to telehealth (Chang et al., 2021). Further, Chang and colleagues noted that providers serving this population were more likely to defer to telephone services (i.e., without video capturing options) to provide care, limiting the range of health services providers can offer. This telephone-only option, as suggested by our study participants, diminished their quality of care. Disparities in access can continue to impact the health of this population especially as reliance on telehealth becomes more common place. Our study calls to the U.S. government to aggressively invest in broadband internet services in resource-limited communities.

Harnessing the Positive Nurturers to Cultivate Resilience

Utilizing culturally trusted sources of information: Although how crisis information is received, shared, and acted on is culturally defined (Airhihenbuwa, 2020), typically a one-size-fits-all communication approach is used during public health emergencies. This approach tends to be inattentive to the sociocultural contexts and inherent vulnerabilities of minority populations. For AA families, pandemic messaging should utilize culturally trusted sources such as community-based organization, churches, and barbershops, to disseminate information. More efforts should be focused on ensuring that these community resources have the tools to receive, process, and disseminate accurate information to this population. Intentional partnerships developed between governments, schools, and community organizations can be a useful alliance during public health emergencies to assure community trust and engagement with preparedness efforts. One approach could be creating Black Leadership Advisory Boards created through local and state governments (Majee et al., 2022).

The kitchen table as an intervention point for AA families: Congregating around food at home is a cultural practice used to promote family cohesion, connection, and well-being. By promoting this culture, especially during public health emergencies, families can utilize cultural safety nets to cope with the changes and challenges crises bring. Household heads play important roles in ensuring this safe space for honest communication that may not only modulate reaction to crises but strengthen recovery and resilience (McCoy, 2011). However, their (household heads) own well-being should also be prioritized during these crises. As noted by Conger (2020), poor caregiver well-being, as experienced by many AA heads of households during the pandemic, may serve as a conduit for social disruptions to the family (Conger, 2020). More needs to be done to support parents, household heads, and/or primary caregivers as they serve as primary responders to their families during public health emergencies.

Creating a culture of preparedness: Unpreparedness on the part of institutions, state, and the nation created heightened perceptions of vulnerability. Given the social vulnerability spectrum in the United States, pandemic planning approaches that promote equity are critical if public officials are to develop effective adaptation, mitigation, response, and recovery plans that mobilize and serve diverse populations.

Conclusion

AA families continue to face a disproportionate burden of public health emergencies. This cultural exploration of AA familial experiences with the pandemic underscored the consequences of deep-rooted systemic racism in shaping these experiences and disparate adverse health outcomes. Although these families have inherent strengths through which they navigate and heal from public health crises, negative enablers create additional barriers to coping and building resilience. The expectation that families continue to lean into their cultural strengths to overcome crises without addressing external system-level factors not only perpetuates a sense of powerlessness but adds unnecessary stress to the system. Programs and policies that are cognizant of the inherent vulnerabilities of AA families and their cultural values are needed to elevate family-strengths while dismantling systemic barriers.

Acknowledgments

We acknowledge Verna Laboy and Judith Mutamba for their support with recruiting participants. We also acknowledge all those who shared their time reviewing the many iterations of this manuscript.

References

Adepoju, O. E., Han, D., Chae, M., Smith, K. L., Gilbert, L., Choudhury, S., & Woodard, L. (2021). Health disparities and climate change: The intersection of three disaster events on vulnerable communities in Houston, Texas. *International Journal of Environmental Research and Public Health, 19*(1), 35. https://doi.org/10.3390/ijerph19010035

Airhihenbuwa, C. O. (2007). *Healing our differences: The crisis of global health and the politics of identity.* Rowman & Littlefield.

Airhihenbuwa, C. O. (2020). Culture matters in communicating the global response to COVID-19. *Preventing Chronic Disease, 17.* https://doi.org/10.5888/pcd17.200245

Airhihenbuwa, C. O., Ford, C. L., & Iwelunmor, J. I. (2014). Why culture matters in health interventions: Lessons from HIV/AIDS stigma and NCDs. *Health Education & Behavior, 41*(1), 78–84.

Airhihenbuwa, C., Okoror, T., Shefer, T., Brown, D., Iwelunmor, J., Smith, E., Adam, M., Simbayi, L., Zungu, N., Dlakulu, R., & Shisana, O. (2009). Stigma, culture, and HIV and AIDS in the Western Cape, South Africa: An application of the PEN-3 cultural model for community-based research. *The Journal of Black Psychology, 35*(4), 407–432. https://doi.org/10.1177/0095798408329941

Anakwe, A., Majee, W., David, I., & BeLue, R. (2022). Unpreparedness and uncertainty: A qualitative study of African American experiences during COVID-19 pandemic. *Sociological Spectrum, 42*(3), 162–175

Anakwe, A., Majee, W., Noel-London, K., Zachary, I., & BeLue, R. (2021). Sink or swim: Virtual life challenges among African American families during COVID-19 lockdown. *International Journal of Environmental Research and Public Health, 18*(8), 4290.

Anderson, L. A. (2019). Rethinking resilience theory in African American families: Fostering positive adaptations and transformative social justice. *Journal of Family Theory & Review, 11*(3), 385–397. https://doi.org/10.1111/jftr.12343

Anderson, R. E. (2018). And still we rise: Parent–child relationships, resilience, and school readiness in low-income urban Black families. *Journal of Family Psychology, 32*(1), 60.

Andrasfay, T., & Goldman, N. (2020). Reductions in 2020 US life expectancy due to COVID-19 and the disproportionate impact on the Black and Latino populations. *Proceedings of the National Academy of Sciences*, 2021. **118**(5): pp. 1–6.

Artiga, S., B., Corallo, & Pham, O. (2020, August). *Racial disparities in COVID-19: Key findings from available data and analysis.* Kaiser Family Foundation. https:// www.kff.org/racial-equity-and-health-policy/issue-brief/racial-disparities-covid-19-key-findings- available-data-analysis/. - Google Search

Artiga, S., Garfield, R., & Orgera, K. (2020, April 7). Communities of Color at Higher Risk for Health and Economic Challenges due to COVID-19. *KFF.* https://www.kff.org/coronavirus-covid-19/issue-brief/communities-of-color-at-higher-risk-for-health-and-economic-challenges-due-to-covid-19/

Braun, V., & Clarke, V. (2006). Using thematic analysis in psychology. *Qualitative Research in Psychology, 3*(2), 77–101.

Bright, C. L. (2020). The two pandemics. *Oxford University Press, 44*(3), 139–142.

Centers for Disease Control and Prevention. (2020). *COVID-19 racial and ethnic health disparities: 1. Introduction.* https://stacks.cdc.gov/view/cdc/98554

Chaney, C. (2020). Family stress and coping among African Americans in the age of COVID-19. *Journal of Comparative Family Studies, 51*(3–4), 254–273. https://doi.org/10.3138/JCFS.51.3-4.003

Chang, J. E., Lai, A. Y., Gupta, A., Nguyen, A. M., Berry, C. A., & Shelley, D. R. (2021). Rapid transition to telehealth and the digital divide: Implications for primary care access and equity in a post-covid era. *The Milbank Quarterly, 99*(2), 340–368.

Conger, R. (2020). *Families in troubled times: Adapting to change in rural America.* Routledge.

Crable, M. (2021, March 19). The pandemic echoes a history of disruption for Black families, stretching back to slavery. *News and Events.* https://dornsife.usc.edu/news/stories/the-pandemic-echoes-a-history-of-disruption-for-black-families-stretching-back-to-slavery/

Davis, D. J., Chaney, C., & BeLue, R. (2020). Why "we can't breathe" during COVID-19. *Journal of Comparative Family Studies, 51*(3–4), 417–428.

Du Bois, W. E. B., & Eaton, I. (1996). *The Philadelphia Negro: A Social Study*. University of Pennsylvania Press.

Fairlie, R. W., Couch, K., & Xu, H. (2020). *The impacts of COVID-19 on minority unemployment: First evidence from April 2020 CPS microdata* (Working Paper 27246). National Bureau of Economic Research. https://doi.org/10.3386/w27246

Farrell, D., Greig, F., Wheat, C., Liebeskind, M., Ganong, P., Noel, P., & Jones, D. (2020). *Racial gaps in financial outcomes: Big Data Evidence* (SSRN Scholarly Paper 3582557). https://doi.org/10.2139/ssrn.3582557

Fothergill, A., Maestas, E. G., & Darlington, J. D. (1999). Race, ethnicity and disasters in the United States: A review of the literature. *Disasters, 23*(2), 156–1

George, C., & Toner, A. (2021). *Beyond 'food deserts': America needs a new approach to mapping food insecurity*. Brookings. https://www.brookings.edu/articles/beyond-food-deserts-america-needs-a-new-approach-to-mapping-food-insecurity/

Hill, R. B. (1999). *The strengths of African American families: Twenty-five years later*. ERIC.

Ismail, S. J., Tunis, M. C., Zhao, L., & Quach, C. (2021). Navigating inequities: A roadmap out of the pandemic. *BMJ Global Health, 6*(1), e004087. https://doi.org/10.1136/bmjgh-2020-004087

Iwelunmor, J., Newsome, V., & Airhihenbuwa, C. O. (2014). Framing the impact of culture on health: A systematic review of the PEN-3 cultural model and its application in public health research and interventions. *Ethnicity & Health, 19*(1), 20–46. https://doi.org/10.1080/13557858.2013.857768

Jackson II, R. L., Johnson, A. L., Hecht, M. L., & Ribeau, S. A. (2019). *African American communication: Examining the complexities of lived experiences*. Routledge.

Laditka, S. B., Murray, L. M., & Laditka, J. N. (2010). In the eye of the storm: Resilience and vulnerability among African American women in the wake of Hurricane Katrina. *Health Care for Women International, 31*(11), 1013–1027. https://doi.org/10.1080/07399332.2010.508294

Lee, E.-K. O., Shen, C., & Tran, T. V. (2009). Coping with Hurricane Katrina: Psychological distress and resilience among African American evacuees. *Journal of Black Psychology, 35*(1), 5–23. https://doi.org/10.1177/0095798408323354

Littlejohn-Blake, S. M., & Darling, C. A. (1993). Understanding the strengths of African American families. *Journal of Black Studies, 23*(4), 460–471. https://doi.org/10.1177/002193479302300402

Lopez, M. H., Rainie, L., & Budiman, A. (2020, May). Financial and health impacts of COVID-19 vary widely by race and ethnicity. *Pew Research Center*, 5.

Majee, W., Anakwe, A., Onyeaka, K., & Harvey, I. S. (2022). The past is so present: Understanding COVID-19 vaccine hesitancy among African American adults using qualitative data. *Journal of Racial and Ethnic Health Disparities, 10*(1), 462-474.

Masten, A. S., & Obradovic, J. (2008). Disaster preparation and recovery: Lessons from research on resilience in human development. *Ecology and Society, 13*(1), 9

McCoy, R. (2011). African American elders, cultural traditions, and the family reunion. *Generations, 35*(3), 16–21.

Moras, A., Shehan, C., & Berardo, F. M. (2018). African American families: Historical and contemporary forces shaping family life and studies. *Handbook of the Sociology of Racial and Ethnic Relations*, 91–107.

Morsy, L., & Rothstein, R. (2016). *Mass incarceration and children's outcomes: Criminal justice policy is education policy*. Washington DC

Nobles, W. W. (2007). African American family life. In *Black families, Harriette Pipes McAdoo (Ed.)*, (4th ed.). Sage.

Obinna, D. N. (2021). Essential and undervalued: Health disparities of African American women in the COVID-19 era. *Ethnicity & Health, 26*(1), 68–79.

Peterson, P. E. (2015). Government should subsidize, not tax, marriage: Social policies have influenced the rate of growth in single-parent families. *Education Next, 15*(2), 64–69.

Prime, H., Wade, M., & Browne, D. T. (2020). Risk and resilience in family well-being during the COVID-19 pandemic. *The American Psychologist, 75*(5), 631–643. https://doi.org/10.1037/amp0000660

Rossen, L. M. (2021). Disparities in excess mortality associated with COVID-19—United States, 2020. *MMWR. Morbidity and Mortality Weekly Report, 70*(33), 1114.

Ruggles, S. (1994). The origins of African-American family structure. *American Sociological Review*, 136–151.

Rushovich, T., Boulicault, M., Chen, J. T., Danielsen, A. C., Tarrant, A., Richardson, S. S., & Shattuck-Heidorn, H. (2021). Sex disparities in COVID-19 mortality vary across US racial groups. *Journal of General Internal Medicine, 36*(6), 1696–1701. https://doi.org/10.1007/s11606-021-06699-4

Sheridan, S. M., Sjuts, T. M., & Coutts, M. J. (2013). Understanding and promoting the development of resilience in families. *Handbook of Resilience in Children*, Sam Goldstein and Robert B. Brooks (Eds), Springer, 143–160.

Stelter, B. (2021, January 9). *Now it's sinking in: Wednesday's Capitol Hill riot was even more violent than it first appeared | CNN Business*. CNN. https://www.cnn.com/2021/01/09/media/reliable-sources-january-8/index.html

Thomas, A. (2017). Promoting culturally affirming parenting in African-American parents: Positive parenting in African American families. *CYF News, 1*.

van Dijk, J. A. G. M. (2006). Digital divide research, achievements and shortcomings. *Poetics, 34*(4), 221–235. https://doi.org/10.1016/j.poetic.2006.05.004

Walsh, F. (2015). *Strengthening family resilience*. Guilford publications.

6 Understanding How Disasters Worsen Disparities in Non-Communicable Diseases

Saria Hassan and Dabney P. Evans

Introduction

This chapter explores the intersection of non-communicable diseases (NCDs), disasters, and health disparities. NCDs are defined by the World Health Organization as conditions of long duration that are not passed from person to person but rather are a result of genetic, physiological, environmental, and behavioral factors. NCDs include diabetes, cardiovascular disease, respiratory conditions (asthma and chronic obstructive pulmonary disease), cancer, and mental health disorders (World Health Organization, 2021). Together, NCDs are the leading cause of death worldwide, contributing to 71% of all deaths globally. There are both modifiable behavioral risk factors as well as metabolic risk factors for NCDs. Behavioral risk factors include tobacco use, physical inactivity, excess salt/sodium intake, and tobacco use. Metabolic risk factors include elevated blood pressure, overweight/obesity, hyperglycemia, and hyperlipidemia. The world is seeing a rise in these risk factors driven by rapid urbanization, unhealthy lifestyles, and an aging population.

NCDs are managed by access to medication to treat chronic conditions, healthy lifestyle habits, and regular access to health professionals and the care they provide. Differential access to health care goods, facilities, and services has resulted in significant disparities in NCDs worldwide. Three-quarters of the 41 million deaths from NCDs worldwide occur in low- and middle-income countries (LMICs) (World Health Organization, 2021). Fifteen million people die prematurely—before age 70—from NCDs annually, with 85% of those deaths occurring in LMICs. Disparities in NCD prevalence and outcomes also occur within countries where structural and social determinants of health result in a higher prevalence of NCDs and worse NCD outcomes for historically oppressed populations, such as racial minorities, women, and poor people.

Unfortunately, these same populations are disproportionately affected by disasters. For our purposes, we understand disasters—including natural disasters, pandemics, and man-made crises—to be synonymous with complex humanitarian emergencies—"crises with consequences of such a vast magnitude and complexity that the human and societal needs far exceed the resources and capacity of the country or countries affected, often requiring a multinational or global response"(Evans et al., 2020). By the disruption these crises cause to social structures, government systems, and usual coping mechanisms, disasters disproportionately affect historically oppressed or otherwise vulnerable populations. In low-income nations with weaker healthcare infrastructure, the health of entire populations can be impacted. Within higher-income countries, structural and social determinants of health worsen the impact of disasters on low-income and otherwise disenfranchised individuals. Since management of NCDs relies heavily on a functioning health infrastructure and supply delivery system, disaster-induced disruptions can have significant implications on NCD-related outcomes in any setting.

DOI: 10.4324/9781003140245-6

Our objective is to describe how disasters disproportionately impact the lives of people living with NCDs. We then describe how disasters differentially impact vulnerable populations, leading to a worsening of underlying disparities in NCDs. We offer a framework to understand the mechanisms for these disparities, describing the intersection of disasters, NCDs, and structural and social determinants of health. We then utilize this framework in a case example proposing a formative approach to reducing NCD disparities resulting from disasters, strengthening resilience, and promoting health equity.

Disasters and Worsened NCD Outcomes

Information on the effect of disasters on NCD-related outcomes comes mainly from middle- and high-income countries. Most studies document mortality after a disaster and/or the reasons for hospitalization or emergency room visits after a disaster. This chapter relies on data from high-income settings, while acknowledging the need for additional research and data on NCDs and NCD-related disparities from low- and middle-income settings where disasters and crises disproportionately occur and where NCD prevalence is increasing.

The effects of disasters on NCD-related mortality are significant. Data from the United States has clearly documented that at least 35% of mortality after Hurricanes Irma and Maria were due to the exacerbation of preexisting medical conditions, including asthma and cardiovascular disease (Issa et al., 2018). In Puerto Rico, excess mortality estimates after Hurricanes Irma and Maria generated a great deal of controversy, given significantly higher deaths than officially reported; one-third of the estimated 4,645 excess deaths after Hurricane Maria were attributed to delayed or interrupted healthcare highlighting the importance of continued access to care for those with chronic diseases (Kishore et al., 2018). Similarly, one year after Hurricane Katrina, a 47% increase in mortality due to NCDs was observed (Ryan et al., 2015).

Health outcomes related to both diabetes and respiratory health have been shown to be negatively affected by disasters. In the aftermath of Hurricane Katrina, there was a documented increase in hemoglobin A1c levels in the 6–16 months following the storm (Satoh et al., 2019). Prior studies have shown an increase in diabetic foot infections after natural disasters (Saulnier et al., 2017). Respiratory conditions also worsen after disasters, with several studies documenting an increase in asthma exacerbations after disasters related to post-traumatic stress and poor air quality (Arcaya et al., 2014; Cowan et al., 2021).

Likewise, several studies have shown the adverse effects of disasters on cardiovascular health. A study in Louisiana, Georgia, in the United States looked at hospitalization for cardiovascular disease (CVD) after Hurricane Katrina and found a significant increase that was disproportionately found in low-income neighborhoods (Becquart et al., 2018). Another study looking at data in New Jersey after Hurricane Sandy showed that two weeks after the storm, there was an increase in the incidence of, and 30-day mortality from, myocardial infarction and stroke incidence (Swerdel et al., 2014). Data on earthquakes has shown their association with myocardial infarction, stress cardiomyopathy, heart failure, arrhythmias, and pulmonary embolism (Kloner, 2019; Leor et al., 1996).

In addition to physical health and disease, disasters pose major threats to mental health. Survivors of disasters show a wide range of mental health problems related to anxiety, depression, and post-traumatic stress disorder (Galea et al., 2005, 2008; Goenjian et al., 2000; Kumar et al., 2007; Masedu et al., 2014). This is precipitated by the increased levels of stress, disturbances in sleep, physical illness, and witnessing death and destruction. In addition to new-onset mental health problems, those with existing mental health problems are especially prone to the ill effects of disasters with exacerbations of underlying depression, anxiety, or psychotic disorders (Makwana, 2019).

Mechanisms to Explain How Disasters Worsen NCD Outcomes

There are several proposed mechanisms by which it is believed that disasters worsen NCD health outcomes. Here, we explore what evidence is available to support these theories: health service delivery disruption, stress-induced exacerbation of NCDs, limited access to healthy food, limited access to clean drinking water, and worsened air quality.

Between 2005 and 2020, natural disasters in the United States repeatedly caused significant destruction to healthcare infrastructure and the healthcare supply chain. Starting with Hurricane Katrina in 2006, severe levels of damage resulted in some hospitals shutting down permanently (Rodríguez & Aguirre, 2006). Hurricane Sandy not only destroyed hospitals, but studies documented the destruction of community pharmacies that are critical to care delivery. Hurricane Harvey similarly caused significant destruction to healthcare infrastructure, affecting healthcare utilization (Arya et al., 2016; Chambers et al., 2020; Sharpe & Clennon, 2020). This destruction is even more severe in LMICs. Cyclone Idai in 2019 resulted in damage to more than 50 health facilities across the Sofala Province of Mozambique (World Health Organization Africa, 2019). India sees severe flooding annually during the monsoon season, which leads to significant damage to hospital facilities and access to the hospitals (Phalkey et al., 2012).

In the same way that access to health care services is disrupted, disasters often result in disrupted access to food, especially fresh fruits and vegetables. In the aftermath of a disaster, there is a wide availability of unhealthy food items (soda, chips, fruit-flavored drinks), canned items with high salt content, and fewer fresh fruits and vegetables or frozen goods (Clay et al., 2021). Disasters lead to escalations in food insecurity levels in environments already suffering from significant malnutrition or undernutrition (UNICEF Mozambique, 2019).

Air quality, which directly affects chronic respiratory conditions and disasters, can impact environmental conditions affecting air quality. Flooding of homes results in significant mold build, triggering asthma exacerbations (Rath et al., 2011; Rao et al., 2007). In addition, wildfires result in smoke exposure that is harmful to those with respiratory conditions and those without these underlying conditions (Kiser et al., 2020).

Finally, strong evidence supports the association between negative mental health and other NCDs (Ali et al., 2020; Josiah et al., 2021; Rubio-Guerra et al., 2013; Schmitt et al., 2021). Data have shown that increasing anxiety and/or depression is/are associated with worse asthma outcomes, poor glycemic control, elevated blood pressure, and worse cardiovascular outcomes (Brunner et al., 2014; Landeo-Gutierrez & Celedón, 2020). Therefore, the increased mental health stressors caused by disasters will inevitably result in worsened control of other NCDs.

Framework to Understand How Disasters Contribute to Disparities in NCDs

Disasters do not impact everyone equally. Within the United States, communities of color, those living in low-income neighborhoods, the elderly, and those with disabilities bear a disproportionate burden of impact (Chakraborty et al., 2019; Kamo et al., 2011; Lane et al., 2013). Redlining policies and redistricting have resulted in low-income communities of color residing in flood-prone areas, environmental wastelands, and food desserts. In addition, these communities are more likely to live in substandard housing. These same groups are also less likely to evacuate in the setting of a pending storm or approaching disaster (Burger et al., 2017). Similarly, lower-income nations have limited capacity for disaster preparedness and response on the global stage, which results in disproportionate levels of damage, displacement, and health impacts than higher-income countries.

These same populations suffer a disproportionate burden of NCDs even before disasters. NCD disparities refer to the fact that historically oppressed populations in the United States have a higher prevalence of and worsened outcomes from common NCDs, including diabetes, cardiovascular disease, asthma, and mental health problems. Several studies have outlined the higher prevalence of diabetes among minority populations compared with their white counterparts: the risk of developing diabetes is 77% higher among African Americans than among non-Hispanic white Americans (National Center for Chronic Disease Prevention and Health Promotion, 2011); among Medicare beneficiaries, diabetes prevalence is 39% and 37% among Black non-Hispanic and Hispanic groups respectively compared with 24% in their white counterparts (Philip et al., 2021). Studies also show lower quality care and more complications of diabetes among minority populations. Similarly, the age-adjusted death rate from cardiovascular disease is 30% higher for African Americans than the overall U.S. population (CDC, 2022; Orimoloye et al., 2018). American Indian/Alaskan natives have a significantly higher prevalence of mental illness at 22% compared with 17% in their white counterparts (Whitesell et al., 2012); African Americans have a similar prevalence of mental illness than the general population but significantly lower rates of mental health service use (prescription medications and outpatient services) (SAMHSA, 2015). African American children are three times more likely to die of an asthma attack than their white counterparts (Asthma and Allergy Foundation of America, 2020). Disparities in the United States can also exist among socioeconomic status groups. Among women in the United States, obesity prevalence decreased with increased levels of income and educational attainment (Ogden et al., 2017). These significant disparities in NCDs in the United States depict the extent of health inequities. However, NCD disparities also refer to the fact that 77% of all NCD deaths occur in LMICs that bear the disproportionate burden of the effect of NCDs globally (World Health Organization, 2021).

These data show how historically underserved populations in the United States, as well as LMIC populations, suffer a disproportionate burden of NCDs and their consequences. These same populations suffer a disproportionate burden of disasters as outlined previously. There is, therefore, a cumulative effect that occurs when disasters disproportionately affect these populations – disasters will worsen NCDs and therefore exacerbate existing NCD disparities.

We offer a framework to address NCD disparities in disasters. The framework uses the Socio-Ecological Model to emphasize that individual, interpersonal, organizational, community, and policy factors contribute to existing disparities being worsened by disasters.

The Socio-Ecological Model

The Socio-Ecological Model (SEM) was developed initially in the 1970s to understand child development (Bronfenbrenner, 1977). It has since been formalized into a theory that depicts how the individual and their interactions and relationships with their surrounding environment can affect their behavior and health (Kilanowski, 2017). The SEM has been applied to health promotion, violence prevention, and chronic disease prevention (Centers for Disease Control and Prevention, 2021; Rimer & Glanz, 2005). Using the SEM provides a means to understand how factors shape behavior at the individual, interpersonal, community, societal, and policy levels. This model can also be applied to NCD disparities in disasters (Figure 6.1).

The individual level refers to the biological and personal history factors that influence behavior and health. These factors include race and ethnicity, income, educational level, and health insurance. These factors have been shown to underlay both NCD disparities and represent individual risk factors for populations most severely affected by disasters, including racial or ethnic minority, low-income, low educational attainment, and without health insurance. The interpersonal level refers to the individual's relationships and social networks that can influence their health and behaviors. These relationships play an essential role in the resilience of the individual and ability to overcome both NCD management challenges and the impact of disasters. The organizational level

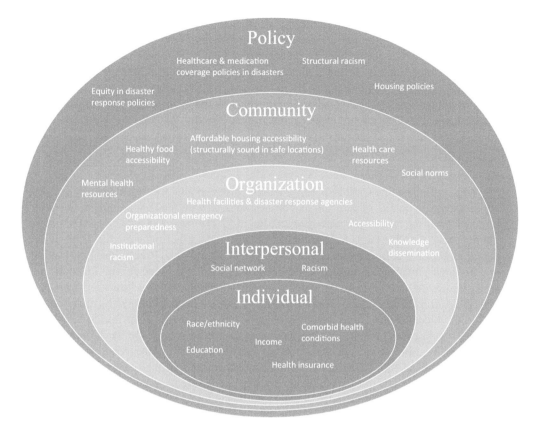

Figure 6.1 NCD Disparities in Disasters Framework: Causes of worsening disparities due to disasters using the Socio-Ecological Model.

refers to how individuals interface with entities related to their health. Here, we refer to the health care organizations and actors providing NCD-related care and the disaster management agencies providing disaster preparedness and protection measures. These organizations play an important role in preparing individuals for disasters, managing their chronic conditions during a disaster, and mitigating the impact of the disaster on vulnerable populations. Their effectiveness in achieving these goals is affected by a myriad of factors, including capacity, resources, knowledge, and institutional racism. The community level refers to structural factors that affect health as well as the social norms that influence individual behavior. Structural factors in this instance refer to access to safe, affordable housing, and access to fresh fruits and vegetables compared with access to fast food, and access to general health and mental health service centers. Social norms that impact acceptability of poor health habits such as unhealthy eating and smoking impact health behaviors. Lastly, the policy level refers to the local, state, and federal policies and laws that impact health behavior, access to care, and disease management. Here it refers to those regulations that impact community and organizational factors – for example, redlining policies, regulations/incentives for organizations and businesses in hard-to-reach places, and violence prevention allowing for safer walking environments. From a disaster perspective, regulations can affect access to preparedness material and equipment (e.g., insurance approval of advanced refills on chronic medication). It is imperative that policies enable access to health services, facilities, and personnel to not only address underlying disparities but reduce the impact of disasters disproportionately on different populations. General

Comment No. 14 (2000) on the right to the highest attainable standard of health (Article 12 of the International Covenant on Economic, Social and Cultural Rights) clearly articulates that the right to health includes "available, accessible, acceptable as well high-quality health care goods, facilities and services" (United Nations Human Rights Treaty Bodies, 2000). The International Convention on the Elimination of All Forms of Racial Discrimination—which has been ratified by many nations including the United States—also includes the right to health and other health-related rights (United Nations Human Rights Office of the High Commissioner, 1965).

Case Study

U.S. Virgin Islands in the Caribbean suffer a high burden of NCDs compounded by significant disparities in quality of care and outcomes compared with the U.S. mainland. In 2016, Puerto Rico had the highest prevalence of diabetes at 13.7% compared with other U.S. states with a median of 9.2%; the U.S. Virgin Islands with 11.7% was among the five states with the highest prevalence of diabetes (Centers for Disease Control and Prevention, 2020). With similarly high prevalence of hypertension (40% in Puerto Rico) and obesity (32% in the USVI), NCDs affect a vast proportion of the population of these two locations (Allende-Vigo, 2013; U.S. Virgin Islands Department of Health, 2020). Unfortunately, quality care and health outcomes have been documented to be worse in the U.S. territories compared with the U.S. mainland. When looking at performance measures for common chronic conditions among Medicare recipients, inhabitants of Puerto Rico fared worse (Rivera-Hernandez et al., 2016). When looking at hospital quality of care metrics, hospitals in the U.S. territories had higher 30-day mortality for common conditions requiring hospitalization (acute myocardial infarction, heart failure, pneumonia) (Nunez-Smith et al., 2011).

Unfortunately, these underlying NCD disparities are compounded by the higher exposure to disasters in the U.S. territories. The Caribbean in general has repeatedly experienced some of the world's most severe tropical storms. Puerto Rico was ranked as the location most severely affected by extreme weather events between 2000 and 2019 (Eckstein et al., 2021). With the high prevalence of underlying NCDs, NCD disparities, and vulnerability to extreme weather events, the U.S. territories of Puerto Rico and the U.S. Virgin Islands present an opportune context to develop interventions to reduce morbidity and mortality due to poorly managed NCDs after natural disasters.

In 2017, Puerto Rico and the U.S. Virgin Islands (USVI) were hit by Hurricanes Irma and Maria, two categories, five hurricanes. These back-to-back hurricanes resulted in over US$90 billion in infrastructure and crop damage leaving people without housing, food, water, and transportation. In addition, there was significant damage to health care infrastructure. Hurricane Irma completely destroyed the only hospital in St Thomas (USVI); twelve days later, Hurricane Maria destroyed 70% of the infrastructure on St. Croix (USVI), including the island's only hospital. Puerto Rico saw similar levels of damage resulting from both the hurricane-force winds and catastrophic flooding. Power and communications were wiped out leaving millions in Puerto Rico and the USVI in the dark for weeks. The estimated excess mortality from these storms is estimated at over 4,000 individuals. Much of this mortality was related to delayed or interrupted healthcare. This included inability to access medication, need for respiratory equipment requiring electricity, and closed medical facilities or absent doctors (Kishore et al., 2018). A study looking at the causes of excess mortality after Hurricane Maria in Puerto Rico found that the leading cause of death was cardiovascular disease (Cruz-Cano & Mead, 2019). Other causes included diabetes and Alzheimer's disease.

With the advent of climate change, it is projected that the Caribbean region will experience increasing severity of extreme weather events. To reduce future disaster-related morbidity and mortality after severe weather events, research is needed to help determine the best approaches for addressing the needs of people living with NCDs. We sought to address this gap by working with healthcare organizations that serve vulnerable populations in Puerto Rico and the USVI with a high prevalence of NCDs. Our objective was to develop sustainable approaches to reduce morbidity and mortality due to NCDs after disasters in Puerto Rico and the USVI. We partnered with federally qualified health centers (FQHCs) in these locations. FQHCs are community-based health care providers that receive funding from the U.S. Health Resources and Services Administration to provide primary care services in underserved areas. FQHCs are ideal partners because they work directly with the most vulnerable populations who suffer from a disproportionate burden of NCDs and effects of natural disasters. The work was done in close collaboration with a community and stakeholder advisory board. We applied the **NCD Disparities in Disasters Framework** to develop approaches at multiple levels of the SEM to reduce morbidity and mortality after disasters.

Our study used a sequential mixed-methods approach to understand the level of emergency preparedness at each of the FQHCs and the degree to which it addresses the needs of people living with NCDs. The study protocol and its components were reviewed and approved by the Emory University Institutional Review Board. The quantitative portion consists of a document review and a survey. The document review was conducted by a single researcher who reviewed all the emergency preparedness and response documentation for each FQHC to determine: (1) elements of the Centers for Medicare and Medicaid Services Emergency Preparedness Rule that were included and documented (Centers for Medicare & Medicaid Services, 2021); (2) How each plan specifically addressed the needs of people living with NCDs or could be modified to include items of importance to these populations. The survey was developed in collaboration with the stakeholder/community advisory board, FQHC leadership teams, and the FQHC disaster preparedness lead staff member. The purpose of the survey was to understand: (1) Prior experience with disasters while working at the FQHC; (2) The current level of familiarity with, and gaps in knowledge of, the center's emergency preparedness plan; (3) The level of importance attributed to PLNCDs in disasters; (4) Preferred ways in which the FQHC could better prepare its staff and patients for a disaster. The survey was piloted and translated into Spanish by a native speaker/by a speaker fluent in both Spanish and English. The survey was distributed via a staff listserv and during faculty/staff monthly meetings. Survey responses were anonymous. The qualitative portion of the study entailed in-depth interviews with staff who, based on the survey, were found to have either high or low levels of knowledge of the emergency preparedness plan and individuals with and without experience working during recent significant natural disasters. The interview guide explored experience providing care in the aftermath of a disaster and the degree to which the organization's emergency preparedness approach facilitated the ability to respond. The interview guide also explored how the organization was able to meet the needs of people living with NCDs and ways in which the emergency preparedness plan could better serve those needs.

Results of our mixed-methods analysis showed that of the staff (134) surveyed, only 25% felt mostly prepared for a disaster, and only 25% discussed disaster preparedness with their patients. Both those with high and low levels of knowledge of the center's emergency preparedness plan felt there was a need for more training and hands-on experience to better prepare for disasters. These individuals also shared a need for more resources to facilitate discussions with patients on preparedness. Individuals who had recently experienced disasters emphasized the continued mental health consequences and the importance of addressing mental health needs of patients and staff as part of the disaster response.

These results were directly translated into action at each of the centers using the NCD Disparities in Disasters Framework. At the individual level, we developed resources designed to empower individuals customized by NCD type to understand the best ways to prepare for a disaster given their chronic condition. Pamphlets and YouTube videos were created to provide tailored information for people at all education levels with the common chronic conditions of diabetes, hypertension, asthma, and existing mental health concerns. These pamphlets raised awareness on the best ways to prepare given their chronic health condition(s), the importance of community/family awareness and assistance, as well as the mental health impact of disasters. All pamphlets were reviewed by people living with chronic disease and edits/changes made accordingly. Pamphlets were then available in waiting rooms and distributed by providers. YouTube videos that summarized the pamphlet information was created for online streaming in FQHC waiting rooms allowing this content to reach the larger community and supporting the interpersonal level of the NCD Disparities in Disasters Framework to increase resilience among individuals with NCDs and their social network.

At the organizational level, a series of staff meetings were organized to review in detail the components of the center's emergency preparedness plans and answer any concerns that staff and providers had. These sessions emphasized the importance of familiarity with the plan and of sharing information with patients. We worked closely with leadership to refine the emergency preparedness plan to include activities specific to the needs of people living with NCDs. These included practices for sheltering in place including ensuring access to equipment and medication essential to people living with NCDs (nebulizers/inhalers, glucometers, blood pressure machine, and basic NCD medication), and providing nutrition access in the time of an emergency include options with low salt and sugar/carbohydrate content. In addition, access to emergency supplies for medication and equipment for people living with NCDs should be available to provide to patients in the aftermath of a natural disaster. There are now plans underway to organize a series of table-top exercises for each of the FQHCs to offer hands-on experience for staff/providers.

In the future, stakeholder meetings with community members and policymakers will examine measures to address housing, food, and healthcare access after a disaster. In collaboration with community-based organizations, we will develop approaches to reach out to the most vulnerable members of a disaster immediately before and after extreme weather events, provide food that is appropriate for people living with NCDs, clean water, and medication when needed. We will work with policymakers to address short-term approaches, including insurance coverage of early medication refill to help people stock up on supplies before an event, and comprehensive and easy-to-understand promotional campaigns to heighten awareness of the importance of preparation.

Through these activities, we will have addressed all levels of the NCDs Disparities in Disasters Framework to minimize the impact of natural disasters on worsening NCD disparities in the U.S. territories of Puerto Rico and the U.S. Virgin Islands.

Conclusion and Future Work

As we strive for health equity and eliminating health disparities, it is imperative to recognize the role of factors outside of our direct control such as disasters. Understanding how disasters worsen existing health disparities is critical to addressing health inequities in the United States and worldwide. We have outlined here how significant disparities in NCDs in the United States and worldwide are exacerbated by disasters. We have offered a framework to systematically think about the effect of disasters on NCD disparities and how to apply this framework to develop interventions to reduce that impact. Future work should develop methodologies to evaluate these interventions to understand their effect on health disparities but also ways of scaling up and scaling out these interventions to other contexts, including in low- and middle-income settings and among displaced and refugee populations.

References

Ali, M. K., Chwastiak, L., Poongothai, S., Emmert-Fees, K. M. F., Patel, S. A., Anjana, R. M., Sagar, R., Shankar, R., Sridhar, G. R., Kosuri, M., Sosale, A. R., Sosale, B., Rao, D., Tandon, N., Narayan, K. M. V., Mohan, V., & for the, I. S. G. (2020). Effect of a Collaborative Care Model on Depressive Symptoms and Glycated Hemoglobin, Blood Pressure, and Serum Cholesterol among Patients with Depression and Diabetes in India: The Independent Randomized Clinical Trial. *JAMA, 324*(7), 651–662. https://doi.org/10.1001/jama.2020.11747

Allende-Vigo, M. Z. (2013). Unequal Burden of Diabetes and Hypertension in the Adult Population of the San Juan Metropolitan Area of Puerto Rico. *Journal of Diabetes & Metabolism, 04*(04). https://doi.org/10.4172/2155-6156.1000261

Arcaya, M. C., Lowe, S. R., Rhodes, J. E., Waters, M. C., & Subramanian, S. V. (2014, 2014/12/01). Association of PTSD Symptoms with Asthma Attacks among Hurricane Katrina Survivors [https://doi.org/10.1002/jts.21976]. *Journal of Traumatic Stress, 27*(6), 725–729. https://doi.org/10.1002/jts.21976

Arya, V., Medina, E., Scaccia, A., Mathew, C., & Starr, D. (2016, Winter). Impact of Hurricane Sandy on Community Pharmacies in Severely Affected Areas of New York City: A Qualitative Assessment. *American Journal of Disaster Medicine, 11*(1), 21–30. https://doi.org/10.5055/ajdm.2016.0221

Asthma and Allergy Foundation of America. (2020). *Asthma Disparities in America: A Roadmap to Reducing Burden on Racial and Ethnic Minorities*. Retrieved from aafa.org/asthmadisparities

Becquart, N. A., Naumova, E. N., Singh, G., & Chui, K. K. H. (2018, Dec 28). Cardiovascular Disease Hospitalizations in Louisiana Parishes' Elderly before, during and after Hurricane Katrina. *International Journal of Environmental Research and Public Health, 16*(1). https://doi.org/10.3390/ijerph16010074

Bronfenbrenner, U. (1977). Toward an Experimental Ecology of Human Development. *American Psychologist, 32*(7), 513.

Brunner, W. M., Schreiner, P. J., Sood, A., & Jacobs, D. R., Jr. (2014). Depression and Risk of Incident Asthma in Adults: The CARDIA Study. *American Journal of Respiratory and Critical Care Medicine, 189*(9), 1044–1051. https://doi.org/10.1164/rccm.201307-1349OC

Burger, J., Gochfeld, M., Pittfield, T., & Jeitner, C. (2017, 2017/03/19). Responses of a Vulnerable Hispanic Population in New Jersey to Hurricane Sandy: Access to Care, Medical Needs, Concerns, and Ecological Ratings. *Journal of Toxicology and Environmental Health, Part A, 80*(6), 315–325. https://doi.org/10.1080/15287394.2017.1297275

CDC (2022). National Vital Statistics Report, Vol. 70, No. 8. Table 10. Retrieved from chrome-extension://efaidnbmnnnibpcajpcglclefindmkaj/https://www.cdc.gov/nchs/data/nvsr/nvsr70/nvsr70-08-508.pdf

Centers for Disease Control and Prevention (2020). Diabetes Report Card 2019. Atlanta, GA: Centers for Disease Control and Prevention, US Dept of Health and Human Services. Accessed online: www.cdc.gov/diabetes/library/reports/congress.html

Centers for Disease Control and Prevention. (2021). *The Social-Ecological Model: A Framework for Prevention*. Retrieved January 4 from https://www.cdc.gov/violenceprevention/about/social-ecologicalmodel.

html#:~:text=CDC%20uses%20a%20four%2Dlevel,%2C%20community%2C%20and%20societal%20 factors

Centers for Medicare & Medicaid Services. (2021). *Emergency Preparedness Rule*. CMS. Retrieved January 4 from https://www.cms.gov/medicare/health-safety-standards/quality-safety-oversight-emergency-preparedness/emergency-preparedness-rule

Chakraborty, J., Collins, T. W., & Grineski, S. E. (2019, Feb). Exploring the Environmental Justice Implications of Hurricane Harvey Flooding in Greater Houston, Texas. *American Journal of Public Health, 109*(2), 244–250. https://doi.org/10.2105/ajph.2018.304846

Chambers, K. A., Husain, I., Chathampally, Y., Vierling, A., Cardenas-Turanzas, M., Cardenas, F., Sharma, K., Prater, S., & Rogg, J. (2020). Impact of Hurricane Harvey on Healthcare Utilization and Emergency Department Operations. *The Western Journal of Emergency Medicine, 21*(3), 586–594. https://doi.org/10.5811/westjem.2020.1.41055

Clay, L. A., Slotter, R., Heath, B., Lange, V., & Colón-Ramos, U. (2021). Capturing Disruptions to Food Availability after Disasters: Assessing the Food Environment Following Hurricanes Florence and María. *Disaster Medicine and Public Health Preparedness*, 1–8. https://doi.org/10.1017/dmp.2021.145

Cowan, K. N., Pennington, A. F., Gregory, T., & Hsu, J. (2021, Feb 9). Impact of Hurricanes on Children with Asthma: A Systematic Literature Review. *Disaster Medicine and Public Health Preparedness, 16*(2), 778–782. https://doi.org/10.1017/dmp.2020.424

Cruz-Cano, R., & Mead, E. L. (2019, Jul 1). Causes of Excess Deaths in Puerto Rico after Hurricane Maria: A Time-Series Estimation. *American Journal of Public Health, 109*(7), 1050–1052. https://doi.org/10.2105/AJPH.2019.305015

Eckstein, David, Künzel, V., & Schafer, Laura (2021). *Global Climate Risk Index 2021: Who Suffers the most from Extreme Weather Events? Weather Related Loss Events in 2019 and 2000–2019*. GermanWatch.

Evans, Dabney P., Queen, E. L., & Martin, Lara S. (2020). Health and Human Rights in Conflict and Emergencies. In Lawrence O. Gostin, and Benjamin Mason Meier (eds), *Foundations of Global Health and Human Rights* (pp. 373–394). New York: Oxford Academic. https://doi.org/10.1093/oso/9780197528297.003.0018

Galea, S., Nandi, A., & Vlahov, D. (2005). The Epidemiology of Post-traumatic Stress Disorder after Disasters. *Epidemiological Review, 27*, 78–91. https://doi.org/10.1093/epirev/mxi003

Galea, S., Tracy, M., Norris, F., & Coffey, S. F. (2008, Aug). Financial and Social Circumstances and the Incidence and Course of PTSD in Mississippi during the First Two Years after Hurricane Katrina. *Journal of Traumatic Stress, 21*(4), 357–368. https://doi.org/10.1002/jts.20355

Goenjian, A. K., Steinberg, A. M., Najarian, L. M., Fairbanks, L. A., Tashjian, M., & Pynoos, R. S. (2000, Jun). Prospective Study of Post-traumatic Stress, Anxiety, and Depressive Reactions after Earthquake and Political Violence. *The American Journal of Psychiatry, 157*(6), 911–916. https://doi.org/10.1176/appi.ajp.157.6.911

Issa, Anindita, Ramadugu, K., Mulay, Prakash, Hamilton, Janet, Siegel, Vivi, Harrison, Chris, Campbell, Christine Mullarkey, Blackmore, Carina, Bayleyegn, Tesfaye, & Boehmer, Tegan (2018). Deaths Related to Hurricane Irma–Florida, Goergia, and North Carolina, Spetember 4–October 10, 2017. *Morbidity and Mortality Weekly Report (MMWR)*, 67.

Josiah, N., Starks, S., Wilson, P. R., Rodney, T., Arscott, J., Commodore-Mensah, Y., Turkson-Ocran, R. A., Mauney, K., Ogungbe, O., Akomah, J., & Baptiste, D. L. (2021, May). The Intersection of Depression, Anxiety, and Cardiovascular Disease among Black Populations Amid the COVID-19 Pandemic. *Journal of Clinical Nursing, 30*(9–10), e36–e40. https://doi.org/10.1111/jocn.15632

Kamo, Y., Henderson, T. L., & Roberto, K. A. (2011, 2011/10/01). Displaced Older Adults' Reactions to and Coping with the Aftermath of Hurricane Katrina. *Journal of Family Issues, 32*(10), 1346–1370. https://doi.org/10.1177/0192513X11412495

Kilanowski, J. F. (2017, 2017/10/02). Breadth of the Socio-Ecological Model. *Journal of Agromedicine, 22*(4), 295–297. https://doi.org/10.1080/1059924X.2017.1358971

Kiser, D., Metcalf, W. J., Elhanan, G., Schnieder, B., Schlauch, K., Joros, A., Petersen, C., & Grzymski, J. (2020, 2020/08/27). Particulate Matter and Emergency Visits for Asthma: A Time-series Study of Their Association in the Presence and Absence of Wildfire Smoke in Reno, Nevada, 2013–2018. *Environmental Health, 19*(1), 92. https://doi.org/10.1186/s12940-020-00646-2

Kishore, N., Marqués, D., Mahmud, A., Kiang, M. V., Rodriguez, I., Fuller, A., Ebner, P., Sorensen, C., Racy, F., Lemery, J., Maas, L., Leaning, J., Irizarry, R. A., Balsari, S., & Buckee, C. O. (2018). Mortality in Puerto Rico after Hurricane Maria. *New England Journal of Medicine, 379*(2), 162–170. https://doi.org/10.1056/NEJMsa1803972

Kloner, R. A. (2019, Sept). Lessons Learned about Stress and the Heart after Major Earthquakes. *American Heart Journal, 215*, 20–26. https://doi.org/10.1016/j.ahj.2019.05.017

Kumar, M. S., Murhekar, M. V., Hutin, Y., Subramanian, T., Ramachandran, V., & Gupte, M. D. (2007). Prevalence of Post-traumatic Stress Disorder in a Coastal Fishing Village in Tamil Nadu, India, after the December 2004 Tsunami. *American Journal of Public Health, 97*(1), 99–101. https://doi.org/10.2105/AJPH.2005.071167

Landeo-Gutierrez, J., & Celedón, J. C. (2020, Oct). Chronic Stress and Asthma in Adolescents. *Annals of Allergy, Asthma & Immunology, 125*(4), 393–398. https://doi.org/10.1016/j.anai.2020.07.001

Lane, K., Charles-Guzman, K., Wheeler, K., Abid, Z., Graber, N., & Matte, T. (2013). Health Effects of Coastal Storms and Flooding in Urban Areas: A Review and Vulnerability Assessment. *Journal of Environmental and Public Health, 2013*, 913064–913064. https://doi.org/10.1155/2013/913064

Leor, J., Poole, W. K., & Kloner, R. A. (1996, Feb 15). Sudden Cardiac Death Triggered by an Earthquake. *New England Journal of Medicine, 334*(7), 413–419. https://doi.org/10.1056/NEJM199602153340701

Makwana, N. (2019). Disaster and Its Impact on Mental Health: A Narrative Review. *Journal of Family Medicine and Primary Care, 8*(10), 3090–3095. https://doi.org/10.4103/jfmpc.jfmpc_893_19

Masedu, F., Mazza, M., Di Giovanni, C., Calvarese, A., Tiberti, S., Sconci, V., & Valenti, M. (2014). Facebook, Quality of Life, and Mental Health Outcomes in Post-disaster Urban Environments: The l'aquila Earthquake Experience. *Frontiers in Public Health, 2*, 286. https://doi.org/10.3389/fpubh.2014.00286

National Center for Chronic Disease Prevention and Health Promotion (U.S.), Division of Diabetes Translation. (2011). National Diabetes fact sheet, 2011. Retrieved from https://stacks.cdc.gov/view/cdc/13329

Nunez-Smith, M., Bradley, E. H., Herrin, J., Santana, C., Curry, L. A., Normand, S.-L. T., & Krumholz, H. M. (2011). Quality of Care in the U.S. Territories. *Archives of Internal Medicine, 171*(17), 1528–1540. https://doi.org/10.1001/archinternmed.2011.284

Ogden, C. L., Fakhouri, T. H., Carroll, M. D., Hales, C. M., Fryar, C. D., Li, X., & Freedman, D. S. (2017). Prevalence of Obesity among Adults, by Household Income and Education—United States, 2011–2014. *MMWR, 66*, 1369–1373.

Orimoloye, O. A., Budoff, M. J., Dardari, Z. A., Mirbolouk, M., Uddin, S. M. I., Berman, D. S., Rozanski, A., Shaw, L. J., Rumberger, J. A., Nasir, K., Miedema, M. D., Blumenthal, R. S., & Blaha, M. J. (2018, Oct 16). Race/Ethnicity and the Prognostic Implications of Coronary Artery Calcium for All-Cause and Cardiovascular Disease Mortality: The Coronary Artery Calcium Consortium. *Journal of the American Heart Association, 7*(20), e010471. https://doi.org/10.1161/JAHA.118.010471

Phalkey, R., Dash, S. R., Mukhopadhyay, A., Runge-Ranzinger, S., & Marx, M. (2012). Prepared to React? Assessing the Functional Capacity of the Primary Health Care System in Rural Orissa, India to Respond to the Devastating Flood of September 2008. *Global Health Action, 5*, 10.3402/gha.v3405i3400.10964. https://doi.org/10.3402/gha.v5i0.10964

Philip, S., Kelsy, K., Amy, S. I., Denys, L., Theresa, H. and Meagan, K. (2021). *Disparities in Diabetes Quality of Care and Potentially Preventable Utilization Among Medicare FFS Beneficiaries.* CMS OMH Data Highlight No. 25. Baltimore, MD: CMS Office of Minority Health.

Rao, C. Y., Riggs, M. A., Chew, G. L., Muilenberg, M. L., Thorne, P. S., Van Sickle, D., Dunn, K. H., & Brown, C. (2007). Characterization of Airborne Molds, Endotoxins, and Glucans in Homes in New Orleans after Hurricanes Katrina and Rita. *Applied and Environmental Microbiology, 73*(5), 1630–1634. https://doi.org/10.1128/AEM.01973-06

Rath, B., Young, E. A., Harris, A., Perrin, K., Bronfin, D. R., Ratard, R., Vandyke, R., Goldshore, M., & Magnus, M. (2011, Nov–Dec). Adverse Respiratory Symptoms and Environmental Exposures among Children and Adolescents Following Hurricane Katrina. *Public Health Reports (Washington, DC: 1974), 126*(6), 853–860.

Rivera-Hernandez, M., Leyva, B., Keohane, L. M., & Trivedi, A. N. (2016). Quality of Care for White and Hispanic Medicare Advantage Enrollees in the United States and Puerto Rico. *JAMA Internal Medicine, 176*(6), 787–794. https://doi.org/10.1001/jamainternmed.2016.0267

Rimer, Barbara K., & Glanz, K. (2005). *Theory at a Glance: A Guide for Health Promotion Practice.* U.S. Department of Health and Human Services, National Institutes of Health, National Cancer Institute

Rodríguez, H., & Aguirre, B. E. (2006, Fall). Hurricane Katrina and the Healthcare Infrastructure: A Focus on Disaster Preparedness, Response, and Resiliency. *Frontiers of Health Services Management, 23*(1), 13–23; discussion 25–30.

Rubio-Guerra, A. F., Rodriguez-Lopez, L., Vargas-Ayala, G., Huerta-Ramirez, S., Serna, D. C., & Lozano-Nuevo, J. J. (2013, Winter). Depression Increases the Risk for Uncontrolled Hypertension. *Experimental and Clinical Cardiology, 18*(1), 10–12. https://pubmed.ncbi.nlm.nih.gov/24294029; https://www.ncbi.nlm.nih.gov/pmc/articles/PMC3716493/

Ryan, B., Franklin, R. C., Burkle, F. M., Jr., Aitken, P., Smith, E., Watt, K., & Leggat, P. (2015). Identifying and Describing the Impact of Cyclone, Storm and Flood Related Disasters on Treatment Management, Care and Exacerbations of Non-communicable Diseases and the Implications for Public Health. *PLoS Currents, 7,* ecurrents.dis.62e9286d9152de04799644dcca04799647d04799288. https://doi.org/10.1371/currents.dis.62e9286d152de04799644dcca47d9288

SAMHSA. (2015). *Substance Abuse and Mental Health Services Administration, Racial/ Ethnic Differences in Mental Health Service Use among Adults.* HHS Publication No. SMA-15-4906. Rockville, MD: Substance Abuse and Mental Health Services Administration. http://www.samhsa.gov/data/.

Satoh, J., Yokono, K., Ando, R., Asakura, T., Hanzawa, K., Ishigaki, Y., Kadowaki, T., Kasuga, M., Katagiri, H., Kato, Y., Kurosawa, K., Miura, M., Nakamura, J., Nishitsuka, K., Ogawa, S., Okamoto, T., Sakuma, S., Sakurai, S., Satoh, H., Shimauchi, H., Shimokawa, H., Shoji, W., Sugiyama, T., Suwabe, A., Tachi, M., Takahashi, K., Takahashi, S., Terayama, Y., Tomita, H., Tsuchiya, Y., Waki, H., Watanabe, T., Yahata, K., & Yamashita, H. (2019). Diabetes Care Providers' Manual for Disaster Diabetes Care. *Journal of Diabetes Investigation, 10*(4), 1118–1142. https://doi.org/10.1111/jdi.13053

Saulnier, D. D., Brolin Ribacke, K., & von Schreeb, J. (2017, Oct). No Calm after the Storm: A Systematic Review of Human Health Following Flood and Storm Disasters. *Prehospital and Disaster Medicine, 32*(5), 568–579.

Schmitt, A., Bendig, E., Baumeister, H., Hermanns, N., & Kulzer, B. (2021, Feb). Associations of Depression and Diabetes Distress with Self-management Behavior and Glycemic Control. *Health Psychology, 40*(2), 113–124. https://doi.org/10.1037/hea0001037

Sharpe, J. D., & Clennon, J. A. (2020, Feb). Pharmacy Functionality during the Hurricane Florence Disaster. *Disaster Medicine and Public Health Preparedness, 14*(1), 93–102. https://doi.org/10.1017/dmp.2019.114

Swerdel, J. N., Janevic, T. M., Cosgrove, N. M., Kostis, J. B., & Myocardial Infarction Data Acquisition System Study, G. (2014). The Effect of Hurricane Sandy on Cardiovascular Events in New Jersey. *Journal of the American Heart Association, 3*(6), e001354–e001354. https://doi.org/10.1161/JAHA.114.001354

UNICEF Mozambique. (2019). *Mozambique: Children Living in Storm-affected Areas Face Worsening Food Insecurity and Nutrition Crisis Six Months after Cyclone Idai.* UNICEF. Retrieved January 4 from

United Nations Human Rights Office of the High Commissioner. (1965). *International Convention on the Elimination of All Forms of Racial Discrimination.*

United Nations Human Rights Treaty Bodies, E. a. S. C. (2000). *General Comment No. 14: The Right to the Highest Attainable Standard of Health* (article 12 of the International Covenant on Economic, Social and Cultural Rights). Geneva: UN. https://digitallibrary.un.org/record/425041

U.S. Virgin Islands Department of Health. (2020). *2020 United States Virgin Islands Community Health Assessment.* Christiansted: USVI.

Whitesell, N. R., Beals, J., Crow, C. B., Mitchell, C. M., & Novins, D. K. (2012). Epidemiology and Etiology of Substance Use among American Indians and Alaska Natives: Risk, Protection, and Implications for Prevention. *The American Journal of Drug and Alcohol Abuse, 38*(5), 376–382. https://doi.org/10.3109/00952990.2012.694527

World Health Organization. (2021). *Noncommunicable Diseases.* World Health Organization. Retrieved January 4th from https://www.who.int/news-room/fact-sheets/detail/noncommunicable-diseases

World Health Organization Africa. (2019). *Restoring Essential Health Services after Cyclone Idai in Mozambique.* Retrieved January 4 from https://www.afro.who.int/news/restoring-essential-health-services-after-cyclone-idai-mozambique#:~:text=More%20than%2050%20health%20facilities,System%20(known%20as%20HeRAMS)

7 Preparedness for Pandemic Disasters to Come

Mohamud Sheek-Hussein, Muhammad Abid, and Fikri Abu-Zidan

Background

In the history of pandemics, the coronavirus disease 2019 (COVID-19) pandemic ranks as the worst pandemic of the 21st century that public health officials have encountered. It is highly contagious and transmissible. The disease has a severe impact on vulnerable and disadvantaged members of the population, especially those who are already susceptible and marginalized within countries. Unfortunately, the pandemic is not over, with the development of new variants of concern and successive waves that are affecting many countries. COVID-19 was first detected in late December 2019 from a cluster of pneumonia of unknown etiology among people working in a seafood market in Wuhan, Hubei Province of China (Zhu et al., 2020). Since then, the world has changed dramatically. Data collected thus far from the Johns Hopkins "Global cases of COVID-19 Dashboard" on November 19, 2021, reveals that the total number of confirmed COVID-19 cases globally is 255,324,963, with 5,127,696 deaths; the total number of vaccinated individuals is 7,370,902,499 (JHU, 2021). The predicted endpoint for this COVID-19 pandemic and return to normalcy is still uncertain because of the appearance of new variants and lack of information on the effectiveness of COVID-19 vaccines to achieve an optimal level of herd immunity.

The appearance of new emerging infectious diseases has lately become unpredictable, which is regrettable given the scientific advances. In 2013, approximately 7 million deaths were reported globally from infectious diseases (Wang et al., 2016). Newly emerging infectious-disease epidemics and pandemics are rapidly increasing, and their control and prevention depend on a thorough understanding of the factors that determine the spread of the transmission. These factors include global interdependence, an increase in the proximity of humans and animals (zoonotic diseases), economic instability, and poverty. Inequality in nature and societal divide drive social tension, especially in the setting of a pandemic, as most societies are economically dominated by a small elite population that consequently results in a global disruption to human lives. Thus, it is predicted that the COVID-19 pandemic may stretch into 2022 and possibly beyond (Scheffer et al., 2017).

The COVID-19 pandemic has already claimed the lives of more Americans (approximately 736,000) than the Flu pandemic of 1918–1919 (675,000 deaths), which was considered the worst pandemic disease in human history (Johnson, 2021). The pandemic created significant disruptions to global healthcare services that became evidence of the international community's lack of preparedness. Furthermore, it amplified the already existing disparities in the health status of different social groups on both micro and macro levels (Valentine, 2020). The World Health Organization (WHO) reported concerns about systemic health inequities and their social, individual, communal, and economic impact on different populations. The global deaths have been disproportional, with the highest rates recorded among elderly people and ethnic minority groups in different countries, and even within countries, especially socioeconomically deprived populations and low-income

DOI: 10.4324/9781003140245-7

and low-wage laborers and migrant workers. This highlights the effect of globalization and interconnectedness among equity, inequity, and health outcomes, because during the COVID-19 pandemic that demanded dynamic systemic transformation even in the most developed western countries, there were socioeconomic inequalities, as reported by the European Union Statistics on Income and Living Condition that showed that socioeconomic inequalities in disability have increased in Europe over time since 2002 and 2017 (Rubio et al., 2021). This pandemic fundamentally has shown defiance and caused global disruption to healthcare systems (Shadmi et al., 2020). The effects of the pandemic have magnified the points where the systems are weakest. A review of COVID-19 in 28 selected countries' healthcare systems' resilience framework showed a failure of suitable health care delivery and fragmentation and suboptimal quality of care, which has resulted in an enormous cost to human and economic loss that requires changes to ensure better health care delivery (Haldane et al., 2021). With more than 5 million global deaths and persistent socioeconomic loss, there is a need for transformation of and investment in the improvement of resilience and preparedness. Resilience as defined by Thomas et al. (2020) highlights the "Ability to absorb, adapt and transform and learn from the shock of sudden extreme changes which will impact on the health system." Indeed, healthcare delivery resilience is the ability to manage and be prepared for eventual disasters and catastrophic events, such as the COVID-19 pandemic, which has caused enormous human and economic losses. Therefore, resilience should aim to identify and assess the consequence of human impact, such as psychological and physical results for the well-being of all people wherever they are, regardless of their sex, ethnicity, and religion (Khan et al., 2018). Accordingly, WHO guidelines (WHO, 2016) of the essential elements for a resilient public health emergency preparedness have been developed; the frameworks have described the complexity and impact on population's health in the short and long term. Thus, each country's public health plays a crucial role in reducing the risk for shortcoming emergency preparedness to ensure a timely, efficient, and effective response to any event at both local and national levels that concern communicable diseases that are potentially contagious and can cross borders. This chapter describes how each community/country can handle the challenges experienced in the COVID-19 pandemic and take this opportunity to be better prepared for similar future events.

Impact of COVID-19 on Health Inequalities

The COVID-19 pandemic has changed the life of each stratum in the community, different from any previously known epidemic or pandemic, such as plagues, smallpox, Spanish Flu, and SARS, Ebola in West Africa, Zika in South America, and Swine Flu, among the more recent ones. All these epidemics and pandemics have affected the environment and the economy by affecting agriculture, travel and tourism, livestock farming, factories, industry, and education (Siche, 2020). The mortality rate of the influenza pandemic of 1918–1920 was high and over 30-fold across different countries. Murray et al. predicted in 2006 that in a future pandemic, such deaths will mostly occur in poor countries where scarce health sources are already stretched by existing health priorities (Murray et al., 2006). Similarly, earlier studies (Sydenstricker, 1931) outlined that during the 1918 influenza epidemic, infection rates in America were significantly higher among the working class than in any other class. Owen et al. reported systemic inequities in access to the healthcare system in America upon comparing White American individuals with the African American people, concluding that African Americans have a higher rate of being uninsured and underinsured (Owen et al., 2020). Extensive research in international literature has shown that there was inequality in morbidity and mortality when comparing high- and low-income countries, e.g., a country like India with lower socioeconomic status had a 40 times higher mortality rate than Denmark. Mortality rates were also 20 times higher in South America than Europe (Murray et al., 2006). Williams et al. highlighted those racial differences in risk associated with COVID-19 on the health equity in the United States and defined a new kind of "herd immunity" (Williams & Cooper, 2020). This health disparity in the United States has failed to protect the most vulnerable people from COVID-19 infection, testing, detection, and immunizing; subsequently, those minorities might not have access to desirable screening practices and optimum treatment.

During this pandemic in the United States, the mortality rates for COVID-19 were particularly high in elderly subjects aged $\geq$90 years. Interestingly, more male than female subjects died in all age groups. However, the death rate in age-standardized male patients has reached almost 65.1 per 100,000 compared with 43.3 per 100,000 for female patients (Campbell & Caul, 2020). Furthermore, the death rate for Black men was 2.7 times higher than White men. Other reasons for this are speculated as being related to socioeconomic factors and underlying chronic diseases, which are disproportionately higher in the ethnic minority groups than the White population. The COVID-19 pandemic has shed light on the health inequalities in deprived communities, especially those from ethnic minority groups with a high rate of unemployment, and highlighted the existing barriers in accessing healthcare (Aldridge et al., 2020; Kirby, 2020). Similar scenarios have emerged from other countries like Germany and the United States (Huyser et al., 2021; Mishra et al., 2021; Wachtler et al., 2020).

Strategies recommended to improve equality and access to healthcare are legislative and require regulatory control to improve living conditions, availability of income support systems, job retention schemes, mortgage holidays, updated rules on eviction, increased housing benefits, reduction in price barriers to access preventive health services, provision of free school meals, local community support for vulnerable people, such as pregnant/postnatal women, and improving the overall accessibility of health services (WHO, 2021c).

Frontline Healthcare Workers (HCWs) against COVID-19 Pandemic

The COVID-19 pandemic has caused a massive burden on health services, especially among the HCWs worldwide. Per the WHO estimates (Patriti et al., 2020), COVID-19 has likely killed between 80,000 and 180,000 HCWs worldwide between January 2020 and May 2021, which is a tragic loss to society. Encouragingly, the reported rate of infections and deaths among healthcare staff has declined. Patriti et al.'s data illustrated that only two of five healthcare staff are fully vaccinated. The authors proposed appropriate actions such as the provision of personal protective equipment (PPE) and vaccination in all countries. HCWs had limited access to PPE in many countries, as witnessed in Italy. Several studies have shown that strategic plans to protect HCWs such as surgeons against COVID-19 were not optimal, contrary to the WHO standards in >70% of hospitals, while advanced PPE gear was used in all operations in <13% of all hospitals (Ruotsalainen et al., 2015).

Due to prolonged and direct exposure of HCWs to the COVID-19 infection, they are likely to suffer from psychological stress and mental ill-health. Public health physicians and nurses were more exposed to a highly contagious infection and uninterrupted long work hours, which has led to stress and work-related mental health issues, such as anxiety and burnout (Chirico et al., 2021; Koornneef et al., 2018). Particularly, HCWs are at a greater risk of mental and physical stress, anxiety, panic attacks, burnout, and post-traumatic stress disorders than others (Abdulrahman et al., 2018), and this has led to a negative impact not only on HCWs but also on the delivery of essential health care service and, consequently, decreasing the standard and quality due to staff shortages and increased costs (De Kock et al., 2021; Koornneef et al., 2018; Maslach et al., 1997). There are several contributory factors of burnout, including underlying organic illnesses, fear of infection and transmission to a family member, lack of PPE, lack of effective treatment, and the diversity and quantity of information (infodemic) (Dutour et al., 2021; Norful et al., 2021; Orrù et al., 2021). Evidently, recently published research data has shown the high prevalence of stress, anxiety, depression, and burnout in HCWs during COVID-19 in different hospital settings and countries (Barello et al., 2020; Çelmeçe & Menekay, 2020; Quintana-Domeque et al., 2021). Quintana-Dominique et al. (2021) reported that medical doctors in the United Kingdom and Italy have shown high prevalence of anxiety and depression in the first and second waves of the COVID-19 pandemic (Pappa et al., 2020). Twelve cross-sectional studies in China and Singapore reported a prevalence of 23.2% and 22.8% for anxiety and depression in HCWs, respectively (Lewnard & Lo, 2020).

Mental Health and the COVID-19 Pandemic

Stress, anxiety, worry, and fear are perceived as normal responses to real threats; however, the social impact of the COVID-19 pandemic and the public health authority response, such as social distancing measures, lockdown, and quarantine, can lead to psychiatric consequences (Asmundson & Taylor, 2020; Brooks et al., 2020). Both the infected and non-infected population may be susceptible as a result of certain experiences such as widespread anxiety (42) and social isolation (Asmundson & Taylor, 2020), hence, extra stress among HCWs and other essential supplementary workers were reported. Unemployment and insufficient earnings and income were additional stressors. The negative dimension of hidden mental disorder has magnified the COVID-19 pandemic effects indirectly through individual experiences and subjective fear of being infected with the virus, loss of job, stigmatization (Jones et al., 1998), and amnesia or traumatic memories of severe illness (Rogers et al., 2020). Mental disorders and their sequelae of brain damage could arise either through direct or indirect effects of CNS infection via immune response (Taquet et al., 2021a). Systematic and meta-analyses have shown that large populations have not experienced a psychiatric disorder following COVID-19 infection; thus, there is not much data to support that neuropsychiatric complications outside of short-term delirium were prevalent in COVID-19-affected individuals. A study by Taquet et al. showed that patients who survived COVID-19 have an increased risk of psychiatric sequelae independent of known physical factors (Gostin et al., 2021; Taquet et al., 2021b).

COVID-19 Pandemic: Unprecedented Public Health Challenges

This unprecedented COVID-19 pandemic has been challenging for all countries at national and international capacities to prepare and respond swiftly. On the global level, the healthcare system is under severe pressure to contain and mitigate the spread of COVID-19. It has revealed the vulnerabilities, limitations, and gaps in the health care services at the global and local levels not only in poorer developing countries but also in western developed countries. The most urgent of these limitations are shortages in bed capacity and medical supply in intensive-care units (ICU), qualified, professional frontline HCWs, and sufficient PPE to protect against COVID-19. Overcoming these challenges is fundamental to ensuring accessible and affordable health for all equitably; therefore, strengthening a swift and effective response to the pandemic is a holistic approach to realizing the One Health One-World concept. As zoonotic diseases continue to cross the species barrier to humans, the COVID-19 pandemic may not be the last one facing the world. Another significant challenge is the lack and insufficient exchange of international scientific knowledge with the public health workforce, information and data systems, integrity and ethics availability of public health laboratories, effective and genuine global cooperation, and impartial distribution of vaccine and medical resources (Etienne et al., 2020; Godlee, 2021).

COVID-19 Pandemic Health Systems Resilience

Universally, the COVID-19 pandemic is considered the most challenging public health emergency at all levels, including national, regional, and international capacities for preparedness and response (Haldane et al., 2021). The success of such plans in each country is dependent on the organization of the existing healthcare system infrastructure, financing, and organization across all levels in a coordinated manner (el Bcheraoui et al., 2020). This pandemic has shed light on the limitations of many healthcare services that were previously considered as high-performing and resilient (HOC, 2021).

As Godlee (Godlee, 2021) summarized, the entire world has dealt poorly with COVID-19, with no country being well prepared. Even the United Kingdom's pandemic response was inadequate in its planning and preparedness. They failed to learn lessons from previous pandemics and showed suboptimal performance, United Kingdom performed less than other European countries (Coccolini et al., 2021). This report highlights the gaps in the areas of pandemic preparedness, lockdown and social distancing, testing and contact tracing, social care, at-risk communities, and vaccines. The pandemic exposed the vulnerability of the country to whole-system emergencies. It was believed that most high-income countries have resilient healthcare services; in fact, in this crucial time, they lacked the capability and capacity to deal with many patients and protect frontline health care workers in the early phase of the COVID-19 pandemic. Therefore, one of the critical elements of pandemic preparedness is better emergency preparedness in healthcare systems when responding to any novel healthcare crisis (Kapiriri et al., 2021). A comparative analysis of 18 African countries of their COVID-19 pandemic plans showed some aspects of the expected priority settings and processes, but none of the national plans addressed all quality parameters (CDC, 2021).

Last year, the WHO produced timely guidelines and a training framework to strengthen the health systems recovery by setting the standards for the post-emergency recovery of health systems that can be adopted in different settings (WHO, 2020).

COVID-19 Pandemic Mitigation and Prevention

COVID-19 mitigation is intended to be used by individuals and social and community organizations for governments to implement effective strategies to reduce COVID-19 transmission and its rapid spread in the community. The initial prevention of COVID-19 infection was a non-pharmaceutical intervention, such as mandatory facial mask covering, emphasis on individual and social distancing, personal hygiene, education awareness, lockdown campaigns, and stay-at-home orders, eventually contributing to the controlling of the pandemic in certain areas. The interventions included COVID-19 testing, case and close contact tracing, self-isolation, quarantine, active surveillance in the community, mitigation measures to prevent and control further transmission in the community, particularly for susceptible and vulnerable people, pregnant women, people with chronic diseases and comorbidities, and for those with severe illnesses and complications. The objective of effective mitigation strategies in all countries regardless of whether they are rich or poor countries was to curb transmission of COVID-19 infection in the community, aiming to minimize the overall rate of transmission, by implementing proper isolation of those infected with the virus, quarantine those suspected to be exposed to the virus, limiting public congregate settings (Wu & McGoogan, 2020).

COVID-19 Pandemic and Critical Care Management

Intensive-care management in severe cases of COVID-19: The overall case-fatality rate from different parts of the world ranged between 0.25% and 3% (Khan et al., 2020; Wilson et al., 2020). Severe COVID-19 infection is more common in the elderly and those who have underlying chronic comorbidities, such as obesity, diabetes, hypertension, cardiac conditions, and chronic obstructive pulmonary disease (Roche, 2021). The management of critically ill patients is an important part of the response to this pandemic, including coordinating different medical teams, containing the infection, treating patients, and protecting healthcare professionals and their staff. Despite the wide use of empirical antibiotics and antivirals, no effective treatments are available. More recently, the efficacy of a few treatments are emerging from clinical trials, such as the use of dexamethasone in those who need supplemental oxygen, use of monoclonal antibody treatment (Ronapreve: a combination of casirivimab and imdevimab) to reduce hospital admission or death by 70% in high-risk non-hospitalized patients (NICE, 2021), tocilizumab in hospitalized patients with severe COVID-19 pneumonia who have either completed a course of dexamethasone or not received another interleukin-6 inhibitor during admission (Greenwood, 2014). Furthermore, in clinical trials, antivirals such as molnupiravir and ritonavir, taken orally, have shown promise in reducing the risk of death and hospitalization in mild and moderate cases. These drugs are recommended as soon as possible after a positive COVID-19 test, and within five days of symptom onset. Increased availability of these drugs in low- and middle-income countries will be advantageous for the worldwide control of this pandemic.

COVID-19 Vaccinations

Immunization has enormously contributed to reducing infectious diseases globally and is the most successful public health achievement (Zhu et al., 2020). The major success in public health is the eradication of smallpox, the world's first deadly and disfiguring disease finally eradicated in 1979 (JHU, 2021). Out of the three wildtype polioviruses, namely type 1, type 2, and type 3, the polio vaccine has eradicated types 2 and 3 and only type 1 poliovirus remains (CDC, 2020). Vaccine development has always been very challenging, requiring extensive experimental and clinical trials, and its efficacy and immunogenicity need rigorous testing before approval by regulatory bodies, such as the Food and Drug Administration in the United States (Scheffer et al., 2017).

During this crucial COVID-19 pandemic, there has been an overwhelming need for safe, effective, and long-standing high immunogenic COVID-19 vaccines. As no country was prepared for this pandemic, the WHO started working tirelessly with partners to develop, manufacture, and deploy safe and effective vaccines (WHO, 2019). Earlier in the COVID-19 pandemic, only non-pharmacological public health measures were implemented at individual and community levels to prevent its transmission, such as wearing a facemask, social distancing, lockdowns, and frequent handwashing. Soon after, the race for vaccine development started for COVID-19 (WHO, 2020). A few months later, different COVID-19 vaccines were developed, tested, and found to offer varying levels of protection to control this pandemic. The current vaccines have been shown to decrease the number of hospitalizations, admissions to ICUs, and deaths. Fortunately, those vaccinated produced high titers of antibodies because some people do not produce, or produce low levels of, protective antibodies due to genetic predisposition, immunosuppression, or other disorders. It was also observed that immunity produced by the vaccines might be waning slowly over time and booster doses may be required to increase immunity to a protective level (Sheek-Hussein & Abu-Zidan, 2020).

The WHO COVID-19 Dashboard display on November 19, 2021 showed that a total of 7,370,902,499 vaccine doses had been administered (JHU, 2021). There is no transparent and equitable allocation of the available vaccine supply for developing countries; therefore, there is an urgent need for affordable and accessible vaccines against SARS-CoV-2 not only for developing countries but also for those underserved minorities within countries.

Since the availability of effective vaccines, the first users were those who were able to afford the cost of vaccines in high-income countries. Developing countries in the African continent accounted for just 2.6% of the globally administered doses, and many regions of low-income countries did not receive enough vaccine supply. The United Nations and WHO sponsored and supported the global program COVAX that was responsible to distribute vaccines to all countries and was able to obtain and ensure a fair distribution of vaccines to both rich and poor countries (WHO, 2021a,b).

Although COVID-19 vaccines are a vital tool in the global fight against coronavirus, these alone will not end the COVID-19 pandemic. A cohort study by Singanayagam et al. in October 2021 has shown that vaccinations reduce the risk of the delta variant infection and accelerate its clearance (Singanayagam et al., 2021). Hence, basic public health and disease control measures, such as "Testing, isolating, treating, and contact tracing," should continue (Lovelace, 2021).

Vaccine mistrust, anti-vaccine propaganda, and vaccine hesitancy are increasing on a global scale, which has a potential impact on accepting COVID-19 vaccines (Greenwood & MacDonald, 2021). This could drive further expansion of the epidemic.

COVID-19 Pandemic, Findings, Insights, and Solutions

Currently, Europe is going through the fourth wave of the ongoing COVID-19 pandemic, which will cause more deaths during the winter. There are many reasons for this increase, such as insufficient vaccine uptake; relaxation of public health measures, such as wearing face masks in public places and individual and social distancing; and the belief of some individuals that the pandemic is over. Furthermore, there is a massive and growing anti-vaccination campaign worldwide. We describe our lessons from this ongoing pandemic to build a more resilient health system.

Resilient health systems and early-warning surveillance systems are crucial for the rapid detection of any public health event of international concerns; additionally, assessment, contact tracing, reporting, and managing the cases and outbreaks is equally critical. Even rich high-income countries with vigorous healthcare services have struggled to manage this pandemic. They have often been short of public health professionals, such as doctors and nurses, and have not had enough capabilities and capacity to treat a large number of infected cases with COVID-19 and protect their HCWs in the early stage of the outbreak. Some of the screening tools used for COVID-19 testing were developed in January 2020, but despite all those efforts, they failed to translate into an effective, reliable test protocol in 2020. In the later stages of the pandemic, most resources from the prevention and chronic disease treatment plan programs were directed and shifted, which resulted in compromising the care of other patients with chronic diseases. This has affected lower-income countries to the point of the collapse of their precarious healthcare and economic systems. All such future plans should be more explicit and monitor surge capacity in its long-term organization and funding. There should be protocols and standard care for infection control and prevention to cover unexpected staffing issues, HCWs, bed capacity, and physical infrastructure.

Clearly, this pandemic has taken a massive toll on social care, particularly on the aging population, who have been at the greatest risk of death from severe COVID-19 infection. Planning for future pandemics should include improvement in the social care sector to address issues like funding, staff shortages, lack of sensitive and specific testing, difficulty in obtaining PPE, and improvement of infection control in such settings.

Inconsistencies exist across the world regarding how deaths are reported. For example, in the United Kingdom, COVID-19 deaths have been reported as those who died within 28 days of a positive real-time polymerase chain reaction (RT-PCR) test result. It offered statistics on daily deaths with COVID-19 on the death certificate. There is a need to agree on international standards of reporting COVID-19 deaths such as that recognized by the International Classification of Diseases.

Uptake COVID-19 Vaccination

Vaccines are crucial as they aim to increase population immunity on a global scale and are one of the most cost-effective tools in terms of public health interventions. Nevertheless, although nearly 8 billion doses of COVID-19 vaccines have been administered globally, the vaccine uptake has been variable due to limited vaccine availability in many countries, especially low-income countries, or refusal to take the vaccine especially in high-income countries. Distribution of the vaccines through the COVAX program needs strengthening to benefit low-income and low- to middle-income countries. As HCWs work in the frontline in high-risk areas, some countries consider making these vaccines mandatory to improve their uptake. Communication about the benefits of vaccination, their production, funding, and the results of research trials should be shared transparently in public campaigns to increase awareness. Engagement of local religious communities should be considered along with other stakeholders' involvement. Use of social media and traditional media is crucial, especially to control misinformation and the spread of fake news. Unfortunately, anti-vaccine propaganda has become stronger in recent times and led to misinformation around the globe. As a result, many people are hesitant and indecisive about accepting the COVID-19 vaccine, which is a growing public health concern and requires a long-standing public trust in vaccines to be established (Dhama et al., 2021).

Ethics and Scientific Integrity

Since the start of the pandemic, there has been an explosion of information in the media regarding the source, nature of the virus, and its behavior, different tests used to identify the infection, public health measures, effective vaccines, and other treatments. The medical and academic community has responded very promptly to produce research-based information. There was also a lack of coordination and ethics that disguised the true scientific information. There has also been a lack of international coordination to evaluate and assess conflicts of interest and of commercial revenue and organizational matters seen in the areas of vaccines/drugs experimentation, production, and their distribution. Over the years, there have been high expectations from modern medicine and the human spirit, and faith in science has substantially grown with communities generally becoming more self-educated and empowered to access health information. During this pandemic, there has been an increased request for proper and reliable information both from professionals and politicians alike. There should be clarity in the messages to people regarding what is known at present, what we can achieve, and what is unknown or out of our control and comprehension. This approach will build trust; otherwise, the response will create misunderstanding, disappointment, and confusion. Health advice and hotlines should be accessed and available for diversified people in a wide range of different languages as well as outreach planning programs that reflect the most effective strategic technique with respect to cultural diversity context of different communities, different beliefs, and values in all countries.

Global Equity and Equality

This unprecedented COVID-19 pandemic has had an uneven impact across the global population, with certain strata in each section of society suffering significantly higher illness, distress, and deaths than the nation as a whole. This pandemic has highlighted the pre-existing social disparities and inequities with respect to income, financial status, and healthcare access; people who earn less, are less educated, and belong to ethnic minorities are disproportionately affected by higher rates of severe COVID-19 infection because of the lack of facilities in accessing the needed healthcare.

There is a real need for plan of care for those who require it; such plans of action should be prepared in advance to reduce and minimize these disparities and increase the affordability and accessibilities to healthcare facilities for the entire population in the community, starting from prevention, health education, and awareness to enable them to access the healthcare that they deserve.

Health Care from a Global Perspective

With globalization and the spread of infections across the globe, there is a need to share the actual distribution of healthcare assistance across the world. The emerging and re-emerging infectious diseases are unpredictable; therefore, mass vaccination and stronger immunity-building will protect and prevent the spread and transmissibility of new infections. The unequal distribution of the vaccine doses has been observed even within the high-income countries. There is a need for much wider sharing of health system tools, facilities, and development of infrastructure to reduce such discrepancies.

"One Globe One Health Approach"

The One Health, One-World concept is based on a holistic approach to addressing that humans and animals share and live in one environment; therefore, it is important to strengthen the foundation to better understand sociocultural practices, ecosystems, and the health of humans and animals, and plants. There is a need to understand the connectivity between humans and animals to be better prepared for any future pandemics.

Digital Technologies in the Public Health Care System

During this pandemic, there has been an impact due to globalization on health everywhere in all communities' acceptance and use of digital health technologies, which requires the development of infrastructure for such technologies and sharing its distribution globally. Modern advanced medical technologies, when incorporated into medical practice, could likely reduce the pressure on the hospital infrastructure and resources by preventing unnecessary visits.

Vulnerabilities of HCWs

Many health systems were unable to protect their HCWs resulting in them being infected and/ or dying. Availability of appropriate PPE, proper triage, and standard precaution and infection control measures were major challenges at the beginning of the pandemic. There is a real need for a strategic plan to provide and secure a sufficient supply of PPE for all HCWs in the future. In some specialized disciplines, the workforce was strengthened by recruiting new leavers or retirees that increased their risk of acquiring this infection. Support for the overworked HCWs and those who were possibly experiencing burnout was also missing, resulting in their low performance and further compromised health and safety (Greenberg et.al., 2020).

Summary

The global lack of preparedness for infectious epidemics and pandemics, as demonstrated by the COVID-19, put on full display the vulnerable nature of our current systems that promote health. The pandemic's disruption of healthcare services revealed a lack of preparedness and inequities in healthcare access in different areas, with greater fatality rates among the elderly, minorities, and low-income groups. Healthcare system failures resulted in more than 5 million deaths worldwide and enormous social and economic costs. In comparison to the 1918–1920 influenza mortality, the current COVID-19 pandemic mortality was as high as 30-fold across several countries, with per-head income accounting for a major portion of this variation. This health inequality was evident in the United States, which revealed a failure to protect the most vulnerable population from COVID-19 infection during the stages of testing, detection, and immunization; as a result, those minorities may not have had access to the screening and treatment that they require. Additionally, age has played a significant factor in COVID-19 mortality. During this pandemic in the United Kingdom, the mortality rates for COVID-19 were particularly higher in elderly patients aged ≥90 years. More male than female patients died in all age groups. However, the death rate in age-standardized analysis for males reached almost 65.1 per 100,000 as compared with 43.3 per 100,000 in females. Patients who survived COVID-19 have an increased risk of psychiatric sequelae, independent of known physical factors.

This pandemic will function as a catalyst for change and strategic and worthwhile investment in more resilient healthcare services. This chapter describes and illustrates the obstacles faced by many communities worldwide during the current response to this pandemic, and the lessons learned that could apply in the future. In the case of a pandemic, there should be mechanisms in place for multilevel strategies to tackle infection prevention and control; complete pandemic preparedness; and rapid response, including adequate medical staff, bed capacity, and physical infrastructure; vaccine availability; overcoming anti-vaccine propaganda; and imparting education and awareness regarding vaccine hesitancy and spread of misinformation. These approaches must address inequality to ensure adequate and equal health care to those most vulnerable and in need; moreover, these approaches must be inclusive in terms of research and technology and accessible globally.

References

Abdulrahman, M., Farooq, M., al Kharmiri, A., al Marzooqi, F., & Carrick, F. (2018). Burnout and depression among medical residents in the United Arab Emirates: a multicenter study. *Journal of Family Medicine and Primary Care, 7*(2). https://doi.org/10.4103/jfmpc.jfmpc_199_17

Aldridge, R. W., Lewer, D., Katikireddi, S. V., Mathur, R., Pathak, N., Burns, R., Fragaszy, E. B., Johnson, A. M., Devakumar, D., Abubakar, I., & Hayward, A. (2020). Black, Asian and minority ethnic groups in England are at increased risk of death from COVID-19: indirect standardisation of NHS mortality data. *Wellcome Open Research, 5*. https://doi.org/10.12688/wellcomeopenres.15922.1

Asmundson, G. J. G., & Taylor, S. (2020). Coronaphobia: fear and the 2019-nCoV outbreak. *Journal of Anxiety Disorders, 70*. https://doi.org/10.1016/j.janxdis.2020.102196

Barello, S., Palamenghi, L., & Graffigna, G. (2020). Burnout and somatic symptoms among frontline healthcare professionals at the peak of the Italian COVID-19 pandemic. *Psychiatry Research, 290*. https://doi.org/10.1016/j.psychres.2020.113129

Brooks, S. K., Webster, R. K., Smith, L. E., Woodland, L., Wessely, S., Greenberg, N., & Rubin, G. J. (2020). The psychological impact of quarantine and how to reduce it: rapid review of the evidence. *The Lancet, 395*(10117). https://doi.org/10.1016/S0140-6736(20)30460-8

Campbell, A., & Caul, S. (2020). Deaths involving COVID-19, England and Wales: deaths occurring in May 2020. Office for National Statistics. https://www.ons.gov.uk/peoplepopulationandcommunity/birthsdeathsandmarriages/deaths/bulletins/deathsinvolvingcovid19englandandwales/deathsoccurringinjune2020

Çelmeçe, N., & Menekay, M. (2020). The effect of stress, anxiety and burnout levels of healthcare professionals caring for COVID-19 patients on their quality of life. *Frontiers in Psychology, 11*. https://doi.org/10.3389/fpsyg.2020.597624

Center for Disease Control and Prevention. (2020). Polio disease and poliovirus. *Center for Disease Control and Prevention.* https://www.cdc.gov/cpr/polioviruscontainment/diseaseandvirus.htm.

Center for Disease Control and Prevention. (2021). Framework for implementation of COVID-19 community mitigation measures for lower-resource countries. *Center for Disease Control and Prevention.* https://www.cdc.gov/coronavirus/2019-ncov/global-covid-19/index.html

Chirico, F., Nucera, G., & Magnavita, N. (2021). Protecting the mental health of healthcare workers during the COVID-19 emergency. *BJPsych International, 18*(1). https://doi.org/10.1192/bji.2020.39

Coccolini, F., Cicuttin, E., Cremonini, C., Tartaglia, D., Viaggi, B., Kuriyama, A., Picetti, E., Ball, C., Abu-Zidan, F., Ceresoli, M., Turri, B., Jain, S., Palombo, C., Guirao, X., Rodrigues, G., Gachabayov, M., Machado, F., Eftychios, L., Kanj, S. S., ... Sartelli, M. (2021). A pandemic recap: lessons we have learned. *World Journal of Emergency Surgery, 16*(1). https://doi.org/10.1186/s13017-021-00393-w

de Kock, J. H., Latham, H. A., Leslie, S. J., Grindle, M., Munoz, S. A., Ellis, L., Polson, R., & O'Malley, C. M. (2021). A rapid review of the impact of COVID-19 on the mental health of healthcare workers: implications for supporting psychological well-being. *BMC Public Health, 21*(1). https://doi.org/10.1186/s12889-020-10070-3

Dhama, K., Sharun, K., Tiwari, R., Dhawan, M., Emran, T. bin, Rabaan, A. A., & Alhumaid, S. (2021). COVID-19 vaccine hesitancy - reasons and solutions to achieve a successful global vaccination campaign to tackle the ongoing pandemic. *Human Vaccines & Immunotherapeutics, 17*(10). https://doi.org/10.1080/21645515.2021.1926183

Dutour, M., Kirchhoff, A., Janssen, C., Meleze, S., Chevalier, H., Levy-Amon, S., Detrez, M. A., Piet, E., & Delory, T. (2021). Family medicine practitioners' stress during the COVID-19 pandemic: a cross-sectional survey. *BMC Family Practice, 22*(1). https://doi.org/10.1186/s12875-021-01382-3

el Bcheraoui, C., Weishaar, H., Pozo-Martin, F., & Hanefeld, J. (2020). Assessing COVID-19 through the lens of health systems' preparedness: time for a change. *Globalization and Health, 16*(1). https://doi.org/10.1186/s12992-020-00645-5

Etienne, C. F., Fitzgerald, J., Almeida, G., Birmingham, M. E., Brana, M., Bascolo, E., Cid, C., & Pescetto, C. (2020). COVID-19: Transformative actions for more equitable, resilient, sustainable societies and health systems in the Americas. *BMJ Global Health, 5*(8). https://doi.org/10.1136/bmjgh-2020-003509

Godlee, F. (2021). Covid 19: why we need a global pandemic treaty. *BMJ.* https://doi.org/10.1136/bmj.n2963

Gostin, L. O., Halabi, S. F., & Klock, K. A. (2021). An international agreement on pandemic prevention and preparedness. *Journal of the American Medical Association, 326*(13). https://doi.org/10.1001/jama.2021.16104

Greenberg, N., Docherty, M., Gnanapragasam, S., & Wessely, S. (2020). Managing mental health challenges faced by healthcare workers during covid-19 pandemic. *The BMJ, 368.* https://doi.org/10.1136/bmj.m1211

Greenwood, B. (2014). The contribution of vaccination to global health: past, present and future. *Philosophical Transactions of the Royal Society B: Biological Sciences, 369*(1645). https://doi.org/10.1098/rstb.2013.0433

Greenwood, M., & MacDonald, N. (2021). Vaccine mistrust: a legacy of colonialism. *Royal Society of Canada.* https://rsc-src.ca/en/voices/vaccine-mistrust-legacy-colonialism

Haldane, V., de Foo, C., Abdalla, S. M., Jung, A. S., Tan, M., Wu, S., Chua, A., Verma, M., Shrestha, P., Singh, S., Perez, T., Tan, S. M., Bartos, M., Mabuchi, S., Bonk, M., McNab, C., Werner, G. K., Panjabi, R., Nordström, A., & Legido-Quigley, H. (2021). Health systems resilience in managing the COVID-19 pandemic: lessons from 28 countries. *Nature Medicine, 27*(6). https://doi.org/10.1038/s41591-021-01381-y

House of Commons Health and Social Care and Science and Technology Committees. (2021). Coronavirus: lessons learned to date. *U.K. Parliament.* https://committees.parliament.uk/work/657/coronavirus-lessons-learnt/publications/

Huyser, K. R., Yang, T. C., & Yellow Horse, A. J. (2021). Indigenous peoples, concentrated disadvantage, and income inequality in New Mexico: a ZIP code-level investigation of spatially varying associations between socioeconomic disadvantages and confirmed COVID-19 cases. *Journal of Epidemiology and Community Health.* https://doi.org/10.1136/jech-2020-215055

Johns Hopkins University. (2021). *COVID-19 dashboard.* Johns Hopkins University.

Johnson, C. K. (2021). COVID has killed about as many Americans as the 1918–19 flu. *A.P. News.* https://apnews.com/article/science-health-pandemics-united-states-coronavirus-pandemic-c15d5c6dd7ece-88d0832993f11279fbb

Jones, C., Humphris, G. M., & Griffiths, R. D. (1998). Psychological morbidity following critical illness – The rationale for care after intensive care. *Clinical Intensive Care, 9*. https://doi.org/10.1080/714029095

Kapiriri, L., Kiwanuka, S., Biemba, G., Velez, C., Razavi, S. D., Abelson, J., Essue, B. M., Danis, M., Goold, S., Noorulhuda, M., Nouvet, E., Sandman, L., & Williams, I. (2021). Priority setting and equity in COVID-19 pandemic plans: a comparative analysis of 18 African countries. *Health Policy and Planning.* https://doi.org/10.1093/heapol/czab113

Khan, Y., O'Sullivan, T., Brown, A., Tracey, S., Gibson, J., Généreux, M., Henry, B., & Schwartz, B. (2018). Public health emergency preparedness: a framework to promote resilience. *BMC Public Health, 18*(1). https://doi.org/10.1186/s12889-018-6250-7

Khan, G., Sheek-Hussein, M., al Suwaidi, A., Idris, K., & Abu-Zidan, F. (2020). Novel coronavirus pandemic: a global health threat. *Turkish Journal of Emergency Medicine, 20*(2). https://doi.org/10.4103/2452-2473.285016

Kirby, T. (2020). Evidence mounts on the disproportionate effect of COVID-19 on ethnic minorities. *The Lancet. Respiratory Medicine, 8*(6). https://doi.org/10.1016/S2213-2600(20)30228-9

Koornneef, E. J., Dariel, A., Elbarazi, I., Alsuwaidi, A. R., Robben, P. B. M., & Nikiforakis, N. (2018). Surveillance cues do not enhance altruistic behavior among anonymous strangers in the field. *PLoS One, 13*(8). https://doi.org/10.1371/journal.pone.0197959

Lewnard, J. A., & Lo, N. C. (2020). Scientific and ethical basis for social-distancing interventions against COVID-19. *The Lancet Infectious Diseases, 20*(6). https://doi.org/10.1016/S1473-3099(20)30190-0

Lovelace, B. (2021). WHO warns coronavirus vaccine alone won't end pandemic: 'we cannot go back to the way things were.' *CNBC.*

Maslach, C., Jackson, S. E., & Leiter, M. P. (1997). Maslach Burnout Inventory: Third edition. In C. P. Zalaquett & R. J. Wood (Eds.), *Evaluating stress: A book of resources* (pp. 191–218). Scarecrow Education.

Mishra, V., Seyedzenouzi, G., Almohtadi, A., Chowdhury, T., Khashkhusha, A., Axiaq, A., Wong, W. Y. E., & Harky, A. (2021). Health inequalities during COVID-19 and their effects on morbidity and mortality. *Journal of Healthcare Leadership, 13*. https://doi.org/10.2147/JHL.S270175

Murray, C. J., Lopez, A. D., Chin, B., Feehan, D., & Hill, K. H. (2006). Estimation of potential global pandemic influenza mortality on the basis of vital registry data from the 1918–20 pandemic: a quantitative analysis. *Lancet, 368*(9554). https://doi.org/10.1016/S0140-6736(06)69895-4

Norful, A. A., Rosenfeld, A., Schroeder, K., Travers, J. L., & Aliyu, S. (2021). Primary drivers and psychological manifestations of stress in frontline healthcare workforce during the initial COVID-19 outbreak in the United States. *General Hospital Psychiatry, 69*. https://doi.org/10.1016/j.genhosppsych.2021.01.001

Orrù, G., Marzetti, F., Conversano, C., Vagheggini, G., Miccoli, M., Ciacchini, R., Panait, E., & Gemignani, A. (2021). Secondary traumatic stress and burnout in healthcare workers during COVID-19 outbreak. *International Journal of Environmental Research and Public Health, 18*(1). https://doi.org/10.3390/ijerph18010337

Owen, W. F., Carmona, R., & Pomeroy, C. (2020). Failing another national stress test on health disparities. *JAMA - Journal of the American Medical Association, 323*(19). https://doi.org/10.1001/jama.2020.6547

Pappa, S., Ntella, V., Giannakas, T., Giannakoulis, V. G., Papoutsi, E., & Katsaounou, P. (2020). Prevalence of depression, anxiety, and insomnia among healthcare workers during the COVID-19 pandemic: a systematic review and meta-analysis. *Brain, Behavior, and Immunity, 88*. https://doi.org/10.1016/j.bbi.2020.05.026

Patriti, A., Baiocchi, G. L., Catena, F., Marini, P., Catarci, M., Beatrice, D. V., Massimo, S. P. N., Walter, S., Mario, S., Roberto, P., Fortunato, A. M., Marco, S., Antonio, G., Dario, M., Andrea, R., Stefano, B., Giuseppe, C., Alessandro, C., Felice, B., … Mario, I. S. (2020). Emergency general surgery in Italy during the COVID-19 outbreak: first survey from the real life. *World Journal of Emergency Surgery, 15*(1). https://doi.org/10.1186/s13017-020-00314-3

Quintana-Domeque, C., Lee, I., Zhang, A., Proto, E., Battisti, M., & Ho, A. (2021). Anxiety and depression among medical doctors in Catalonia, Italy, and the U.K. during the COVID-19 pandemic. *PloS One, 16*(11), e0259213.

Roche. (2021). Japan becomes first country to approve Ronapreve (casirivimab and imdevimab) for the treatment of mild to moderate COVID-19. *Roche.* https://www.roche.com/media/releases/med-cor-2021-07-20.htm

Rogers, J. P., Chesney, E., Oliver, D., Pollak, T. A., McGuire, P., Fusar-Poli, P., Zandi, M. S., Lewis, G., & David, A. S. (2020). Psychiatric and neuropsychiatric presentations associated with severe coronavirus infections: a systematic review and meta-analysis with comparison to the COVID-19 pandemic. *The Lancet Psychiatry*, *7*(7). https://doi.org/10.1016/S2215-0366(20)30203-0

Rubio Valverde, J. R., Mackenbach, J. P., & Nusselder, W. J. (2021). Trends in inequalities in disability in Europe between 2002 and 2017. *Journal of Epidemiology and Community Health*, *75*(8). https://doi.org/10.1136/jech-2020-216141

Ruotsalainen, J., Verbeek, J., Mariné, A., & Serra, C. (2015). Preventing occupational stress in healthcare workers. *Cochrane Database of Systematic Reviews*, *4*. www.cochranelibrary.com.

Scheffer, M., van Bavel, B., van de Leemput, I. A., & van Nes, E. H. (2017). Inequality in nature and society. *Proceedings of the National Academy of Sciences of the United States of America*, *114*(50). https://doi.org/10.1073/pnas.1706412114

Shadmi, E., Chen, Y., Dourado, I., Faran-Perach, I., Furler, J., Hangoma, P., Hanvoravongchai, P., Obando, C., Petrosyan, V., Rao, K. D., Ruano, A. L., Shi, L., de Souza, L. E., Spitzer-Shohat, S., Sturgiss, E., Suphanchaimat, R., Uribe, M. V., & Willems, S. (2020). Health equity and COVID-19: global perspectives. *International Journal for Equity in Health*, *19*(1). https://doi.org/10.1186/s12939-020-01218-z

Shah, W., Hillman, T., Playford, E. D., & Hishmeh, L. (2021). Managing the long term effects of covid-19: summary of NICE, SIGN, and RCGP rapid guideline. bmj, 372.

Sheek-Hussein, M., & Abu-Zidan, F. M. (2020). Invited editorial. Covid-19 vaccine: hope and reality. *African Health Sciences*, *20*(4). https://doi.org/10.4314/ahs.v20i4.3

Siche, R. (2020). What is the impact of COVID-19 disease on agriculture? *Scientia Agropecuaria*, *11*(1). https://doi.org/10.17268/sci.agropecu.2020.01.00

Singanayagam, A., Hakki, S., Dunning, J., Madon, K. J., Crone, M., Koycheva, A., Derqui-Fernandez, N., Barnett, J. L., Whitfield, M. G., Varro, R., Charlett, A., Kundu, R., Fenn, J., Badhan, A., Dustan, S., Tejpal, C., Vetkar, A., Cutajar, J., Quinn, V., … Lalvani, A. (2021). Community transmission and viral load kinetics of SARS-CoV-2 Delta (B.1.617.2) variant in vaccinated and unvaccinated individuals. *SSRN Electronic Journal*. https://doi.org/10.2139/ssrn.3918287

Siu, Y. M. J. (2008). The sars-associated stigma of SARS victims in the post-sars era of Hong Kong. *Qualitative Health Research*, *18*(6), 729–738. https://doi.org/10.1177/1049732308318372

Sydenstricker, E. (1931). The incidence of influenza among persons of different economic status during the epidemic of 1918. *Public Health Reports (Washington, DC: 1974)*, *121*. https://doi.org/10.2307/4579923

Taquet, M., Dercon, Q., Luciano, S., Geddes, J. R., Husain, M., & Harrison, P. J. (2021a). Incidence, co-occurrence, and evolution of long-COVID features: a 6-month retrospective cohort study of 273,618 survivors of COVID-19. *PLoS Medicine*, *18*(9). https://doi.org/10.1371/journal.pmed.1003773

Taquet, M., Luciano, S., Geddes, J. R., & Harrison, P. J. (2021b). Bidirectional associations between COVID-19 and psychiatric disorder: retrospective cohort studies of 62 354 COVID-19 cases in the USA. *The Lancet Psychiatry*, *8*(2). https://doi.org/10.1016/S2215-0366(20)30462-4

Thomas, S., Sagan, A., Larkin, J., Cylus, J., Figueras, J., & Karanikolos, M. (2020). *Strengthening health systems resilience: key concepts and strategies*. World Health Organization.

Valentine, N. (2020). Extent, scope and impacts of COVID-19 on health inequities: the evidence. *World Health Organization*. https://www.who.int/docs/default-source/documents/social-determinants-of-health/overview---covid-19-impacts-(nicole-valentine).pdf

Wachtler, B., Michalski, N., Nowossadeck, E., Diercke, M., Wahrendorf, M., Santos-Hövener, C., Lampert, T., & Hoebel, J. (2020). Socioeconomic inequalities in the risk of SARS-CoV-2 infection – first results from an analysis of surveillance data from Germany. *Journal of Health Monitoring*, *5*(7), 18.

Wang, H., Naghavi, M., Allen, C., Barber, R. M., Carter, A., Casey, D. C., Charlson, F. J., Chen, A. Z., Coates, M. M., Coggeshall, M., Dandona, L., Dicker, D. J., Erskine, H. E., Haagsma, J. A., Fitzmaurice, C., Foreman, K., Forouzanfar, M. H., Fraser, M. S., Fullman, N., … Zuhlke, L. J. (2016). Global, regional, and national life expectancy, all-cause mortality, and cause-specific mortality for 249 causes of death, 1980–2015: a systematic analysis for the global burden of disease study 2015. *The Lancet*, *388*(10053), 1459–1544.

Williams, D. R., & Cooper, L. A. (2020). COVID-19 and health equity - a new kind of "herd immunity." *JAMA - Journal of the American Medical Association, 323*(24). https://doi.org/10.1001/jama.2020.8051

Wilson, N., Kvalsvig, A., Barnard, L. T., & Baker, M. G. (2020). Case-fatality risk estimates for COVID-19 calculated by using a lag time for fatality. *Emerging Infectious Diseases, 26*(6). https://doi.org/10.3201/EID2606.200320

World Health Organization. (2016). *A strategic framework for emergency preparedness.* https://iris.who.int/bitstream/handle/10665/254883/9789241511827-eng.pdf

WHO. (2019). https://www.who.int/news/item/24-08-2020-172-countries-and-multiple-candidate-vaccines-engaged-in-covid-19-vaccine-global-access-facility

World Health Organization. (2021a). Health and care worker deaths during COVID-19. https://www.who.int/news/item/20-10-2021-health-and-care-worker-deaths-during-covid-19

World Health Organization. (2021b). Vaccine equity. https://www.who.int/campaigns/vaccine-equity

World Health Organization. (2021c). Policies, regulations and legislation promoting healthy housing: a review. https://www.who.int/publications/i/item/9789240011298

World Health Organization. Regional Office for the Eastern Mediterranean. (2020). *Implementation guide for health systems recovery in emergencies: transforming challenges into opportunities.* World Health Organization. Regional Office for the Eastern Mediterranean. https://apps.who.int/iris/handle/10665/336472.

Wu, Z., & McGoogan, J. M. (2020). Characteristics of and important lessons from the coronavirus disease 2019 (COVID-19) outbreak in China: summary of a report of 72 314 cases from the Chinese center for disease control and Prevention. *Jama, 323*(13), 1239–1242.

Zhu, N., Zhang, D., Wang, W., Li, X., Yang, B., Song, J., Zhao, X., Huang, B., Shi, W., Lu, R., Niu, P., Zhan, F., Ma, X., Wang, D., Xu, W., Wu, G., Gao, G. F., & Tan, W. (2020). A novel coronavirus from patients with pneumonia in China, 2019. *New England Journal of Medicine, 382*(8). https://doi.org/10.1056/nejmoa2001017

8 Cross-National Newspaper Coverage of Climate Change

Community Structure Theory and "Buffered" Health and Female Privilege

John C. Pollock, Faris El Akbani, Avantika D. Butani, Robert Robinson, and Miranda Crowley

Introduction

Climate change is one of the greatest threats to human civilization generating effects, such as extreme weather events, rising sea levels, and threats to the food supply (United Nations, 2019, para 1). One of the main causes of climate change is the release of carbon dioxide and other greenhouse gases into the atmosphere from human activity (United Nations, 2019, para 3). In 2015, the United Nations (UN) Climate Change Conference negotiated a global agreement, referred to as the "Paris Agreement," to reduce global emissions to prevent the average global temperature from rising above 2°Celsius from pre-industrial levels (Denchak, 2018, para. 4).

Media framing of global issues, such as climate change, is a dimension of media impact that can influence public opinion. Framing "signifies the structuring power of context … in which people produce and exchange messages" (D'Angelo, 2018, p. 23). Two major media frames will be used in this study. The first frame posits that a country's domestic "government" is primarily responsible for addressing climate change and mitigating its effects. The other climate change frame posits that "society" is responsible for addressing climate change through private, non-profit, and other non-governmental organizations (NGO) as well as foreign aid. It is assumed that the framing of responsibility for climate change in newspapers can vary by country.

Newspapers will be used to examine cross-national coverage of climate change. Newspapers are a reliable source of information because they are read by the well-educated and by political and economic elites (Singer, 2013). In addition, newspapers are prominent intermedia agenda-setters for other platforms, such as radio, television, and the internet. Newspapers are also easily accessible to the public and serve as community forums for the exchange of views.

Expecting that demographics and characteristics of countries have a great influence on how media report on social and political change, our study will use community structure theory, to examine media coverage of climate change worldwide. The community structure approach is defined as "a form of quantitative content analysis that focuses on the ways in which key characteristics of communities … are related to the content coverage of newspapers in those communities" (Pollock 2007, p. 23). Two critical questions guide this study: How much variation exists in cross-national news coverage of climate change? Then, how much does that variation in coverage connect to demographic differences among countries?

Community Structure Theory

In order to complete a thorough analysis of climate change in cross-national coverage, scholarly literature in communication studies was compared with that in biology, sociology, and political

DOI: 10.4324/9781003140245-8

science from 2015 onward, yielding substantial results in other fields, but only a few in communication studies. Community structure theory is a subset of media sociology, which foregrounds questions about history, power, inequality, control, institutions, autonomy, and human agency (Waisbord, 2014, p. 17), integrating into the study of media sociological questions about identity, class, and collective action (Waisbord, 2014, p. 5; see also Benson, 2013; Schudson, 2008; Tumber, 2000; Zelizer, 2004). Community structure theory focuses on the ways community characteristics help shape media coverage (Pollock, 2007, p. 23).

Community structure theory provides a bottom-up lens to understand how newspapers frame narratives. Funk and McCombs (2017) define community structure theory as the "conceptual inverse" of agenda-setting. The theory focuses on demographic characteristics of communities as "bottom-up" shapers of news instead of "top-down" national news leaders as "intermedia agenda-setters" (McCombs, 2004) and drivers of public perception. Consequently, community structure theory is a "central pillar of modern communication research" (Funk & McCombs, 2017, p. 845), providing a powerful framework for analyzing society's influence on media coverage.

U.S. precursors to the community structure model originated in the early 20th century by sociologist and communication scholar Robert Park (1922) and later by Morris Janowitz (1952), both of the University of Chicago, who challenged the traditional belief that media mainly influence society by arguing that society also influences media, Janowitz arguing that press coverage could serve as an index of the social structure and values of distinct communities. Later in the 20th century, University of Minnesota scholars Tichenor, Donohue and Olien introduced "structural pluralism," finding that compared with newspapers in small homogeneous cities, newspapers in large cities reflected the "structural" or demographic "pluralism" found in varied, diverse social systems (1973, 1980). Eventually, these scholars developed a "guard dog" hypothesis (Donohue, Tichenor, & Olien, 1995), which argues that media typically reflect political and economic elite interests more than the interests of the general public.

Despite the Minnesota scholars' predictions, their intellectual offspring reached somewhat different conclusions, arguing that media may accommodate social change, aligning with the views of dominant ethnic groups (Hindman, 1999) or sizable protest groups (Mcleod & Hertog, 1992, 1999), accommodating social change (Demers & Viswanath, 1999, p. 34). Other significant community structure contributions were made by Nah and Armstrong (2013), Yamamoto (2013), Watson and Riffe (2013), and Pollock and Storey (2012).

Three additional contributions were added by Pollock and colleagues to what they call "community structure theory." First, they conducted the first studies using cities nationwide and cross-national samples to link multiple city and national-level structural characteristics to variations in newspaper coverage of critical events. Second, they combined measurements of both article "content" and article "prominence" to create a single composite score called a "Media Vector." Third, Pollock et al.'s studies confirm that media can mirror the interests of society's most "vulnerable" citizens (Pollock, 2007, 2013a, 2013b, 2015), contrary to Donohue, Tichenor, and Olien suggesting that media usually serve as "guard dogs" for political and economic elites (1995). It is informative that using a systematic empirical study, scholars have found that "bottom up" community structure predictions compared favorably with those made by "top-down" agenda-setting theory (Funk & McCombs, 2017).

Hypotheses

Based on previous community structure theory studies, two umbrella hypotheses were constructed to analyze cross-national media coverage of climate change: buffer and vulnerability (Pollock, 2007).

Buffer Hypothesis

Privilege. The buffer hypothesis suggests that privileged individuals or groups in a community who are "relatively buffered" from conditions of poverty and uncertainty, and newspapers in such communities, have proved broadly supportive of human rights claims (Pollock, 2007, pp. 61–100), specifically addressing health care access, female empowerment, communication access, and resource access. Overall privilege can be measured cross-nationally through various characteristics, including but not limited to, gross domestic product (GDP), GDP per capita, and life expectancy rates in particular countries, all of which can be examined in connection with newspaper reporting on climate change.

The buffer hypothesis is supported by numerous U.S. and cross-national studies. In U.S. studies, for example, the higher the percent of college-educated people in a city, the greater the media support for Anita Hill's testimony to the 1991 Clarence Thomas Senate Judiciary Committee hearings, for physician-assisted suicide for seniors, and for research on embryonic stem cells, helping those suffering from multiple types of intransigent conditions and diseases (Pollock, 2007, pp. 61–100). In cross-national studies, the higher the GDP in a nation, the more favorable the coverage of the United Nations (Gratale, et al., 2005) and of NGOs' efforts to fight AIDS (Eisenberg et al., 2006), and higher GDP per capita is linked to media emphasis on government responsibility for human trafficking (Alexandre, et al., 2014) and for COVID-19 interventions, with positive media coverage also linked to higher female and male life expectancy at birth as well as literacy rates (Fleischman, et al., 2021). Buffered, privileged groups are likely linked to coverage more favorable to (or emphasizing more government responsibility for) human rights claims. Since climate change has become a prevalent human rights issue, it is reasonable to expect that privileged groups will be linked to greater media emphasis on government responsibility for climate change, a progressive position. Therefore:

H1a: *The higher a nation's GDP, the more media emphasis on government responsibility to address climate change (Central Intelligence Agency (CIA, 2020).*

H1b: *The higher a nation's GDP per capita, the more media emphasis on government responsibility to address climate change (CIA, 2020).*

H1c: *The higher a nation's life expectancy at birth, the more media emphasis on government responsibility to address climate change (CIA, 2020).*

Health care access. A strong indicator of privilege in any community is access to health care. Cross-national health care access can be measured by calculating the number of physicians, hospital beds, and midwives per 100,000 citizens, all three of which are strongly associated with media emphasis on government responsibility for COVID-19 (Fleischman, et al., 2021). One cross-national study on climate change found that the greater the number of hospital beds and physicians per 100,000, the greater the media support for the government to address climate change (Pollock, Reda et al., 2010). A similar study found physicians/100,000 associated with media emphasis on government responsibility to halt human trafficking (Purandare et al., 2021) and hospital beds/100,000 associated with media emphasis on government responsibility for mental health access (Yasin et al., 2020). A country that portrays abundant concern for the health of its residents may display coverage emphasizing more government responsibility to reduce the effects of climate change. Therefore:

H1e: *The greater the number of physicians per 100,000 citizens in a country, the more media emphasis on government responsibility to address climate change (United Nations Statistics Division, 2020).*

H1f: *The greater the number of hospital beds per 100,000 citizens in a country, the more media emphasis on government responsibility to address climate change (United Nations Statistics Division, 2020).*

H1g: *The greater the number of midwives per 100,000 citizens in a country, the more media emphasis on government responsibility to address climate change (United Nations Statistics Division, 2020).*

Female empowerment/privilege. Female empowerment is vital to the coverage of climate change because of the issues of climate-related child hunger and mortality rate among infants, which affect mothers greatly. Female empowerment variables—such as female life expectancy, female school life expectancy, female literacy rate, and percent female enrollment in secondary school, all significantly linked with media emphasis on government responsibility for COVID-19 (Fleischman, et al., 2021)—produce significant results when analyzing human rights issues (Pollock, 2015). A cross-national study on the 1995 Beijing conference efforts to promote women's rights found that the higher a country's level of female life expectancy at birth, the more favorable the coverage of women's rights broadly, such as the rights of children and the right to protest (Hammer, Mitchell, Shields, & Pollock, 2006). Female life expectancy at birth was also associated with media emphasis on government responsibility for rape and rape culture (Johnson, et al., 2021). Similarly, the greater the female school life expectancy in a nation, the more media emphasis on government responsibility for human trafficking (Alexandre, et al., 2014) and (along with female enrollment in secondary school) for addressing rape and rape culture (Johnson, et al., 2021).

Female workplace presence is one index of the relative economic and political influence and authority of women in a community. The higher the percent of females in the workforce, the more media emphasis on government responsibility for HIV/AIDS (Etheridge, et al., 2014) and for transit migration (Pollock, O'Brien et al., 2019) and the more favorable the coverage of transgender rights (Pollock, Buonaro, Gomez et al., 2017, p. 18). Regarding climate change, it is likely that media would support the interests of advantaged female stakeholders because they are generally associated with "buffered," privileged groups. As a result:

H2a: *The higher a nation's female life expectancy, the more media emphasis on government responsibility to address climate change (CIA, 2020).*

H2b: *The higher a nation's female labor force participation rate, the more media emphasis on government responsibility to address climate change (CIA, 2020).*

H2c: *The higher a nation's female school life expectancy, the more media emphasis on government responsibility to address climate change (CIA, 2020).*

H2d: *The higher a nation's female literacy rate, the more media emphasis on government responsibility to address climate change (CIA, 2020).*

H2e: *The higher a nation's female enrollment in secondary school, the more media emphasis on government responsibility to address climate change (CIA, 2020).*

Communication privilege and penetration. Media access is another indicator of privilege, therefore suggesting that nations with greater media access will support government responsibility to reduce climate change. Studies have found positive correlations between media access and emphasis on government responsibility. More broadband subscriptions per 100 in a country have been linked to media emphasis on government responsibility for human trafficking (Alexandre, et al., 2014), and broadband subscriptions and literacy rates have been connected to media emphasis on government responsibility for mental health access (Yasin et al., 2020) and for COVID-19 (Fleischman, et al., 2021). Because media access and penetration are indicators of "buffered" privilege, news coverage in these circumstances is expected to support government responsibility for climate change. Therefore:

H3a: *The higher the percent covered with a mobile phone network in a nation, the more media emphasis on government responsibility to address climate change (Organisation for Economic Co-Operation and Development, 2020).*

H3b: *The higher the number of broadband subscriptions per 100 residents in a nation, the more media emphasis on government responsibility to address climate change (Organisation for Economic Co-Operation and Development, 2020).*

H3c: *The higher a nation's literacy rate, the more media emphasis on government responsibility to address climate change (CIA, 2020).*

Resource privilege: Energy production/consumption, infrastructure, and sub-economy stakeholders. Privileged stakeholder groups in nations that have high "resource privilege" (e.g., energy production and consumption rates, along with abundant roads and industrial production) were associated generally with media support for substantial government activity on climate change. The greater the natural gas production and natural gas consumption in a nation, the greater the media emphasis on government activity addressing climate change (Pollock, Reda et al., 2010) and COVID-19, coverage of which is also associated with electricity and oil consumption (Fleischman et al., 2021). Similarly, higher levels of coal production and consumption are linked to greater media emphasis on government responsibility for halting human trafficking (Purandare, et al., 2021) and for providing food security for a nation's population (Govindarajan, et al., 2021). In addition, the greater the presence of relatively "modern" forms of energy production (electricity) and consumption (electricity and gas), the greater the media emphasis on government responsibility for women's reproductive rights (Pollock, Buonauro, Gomez, et. al., 2017).

Tested measures included gas, electrical, coal, and oil production and consumption, along with the length of road network and industrial production growth rate. Almost none of the correlations between these measures of resource privilege and coverage emphasizing government responsibility for climate change was significant at all, with the exception of industrial production growth rate (see Table 8.4: Pearson correlations).

Vulnerability Hypothesis

The vulnerability hypothesis, also referred to as the "unbuffered" hypothesis, posits connections between vulnerable populations and coverage. Although vulnerable groups do not typically have strong affiliations with "maximum newspaper readership," the vulnerability hypothesis assumes that media coverage will usually mirror the ideas and concerns associated with the vulnerable in a community, whether city or nation state (Pollock, 2007, pp. 137–170). The vulnerability hypothesis challenges the "guard dog" hypothesis of Donohue, Tichenor, and Olien (1995), finding that media often reflect the interests not of elites but of vulnerable populations, regarding such issues as capital punishment, abortion, the "Occupy" movement, universal health care, physician-assisted suicide, immigration reform, genetically modified foods—GMOs and COVID-19 government interventions (respectively, Pollock, 2007, pp. 138–146; Pollock, et al., 1978; Pollock, 2013a, pp. 1–30; Kiernicki et al., 2013a; Pollock & Yulis, 2004; Pollock, Gratale, Teta et al., 2014; Pollock, Peitz, et al., 2017; and Pollock, et al., 2021).

Cross-national studies have discovered that several measures of vulnerability often correspond to media emphasis on government assistance. The higher the percentage of a nation's population younger than 15, the greater the media emphasis on government responsibility to reduce child labor (Kohn & Pollock, 2014). More media coverage emphasizing government responsibility for

GMOs (Pollock, Peitz, et al., 2017) is also linked to higher fertility rates. Since vulnerable populations suffer disproportionately higher health and livelihood risks from climate change, coverage in less advantaged countries is expected to be more supportive of government responsibility for addressing climate change. Therefore:

H4a: *The higher a nation's poverty level, the more media emphasis on government responsibility to address climate change (United Nations Statistics Division, 2020).*

H4b: *The higher a nation's fertility rate, the more media emphasis on government responsibility to address climate change (United Nations Statistics Division, 2020).*

H4c: *The higher the percentage of a nation's population younger than 15, the more media emphasis on government responsibility to address climate change (United Nations Statistics Division, 2020).*

Health vulnerability. Health indicators such as infant mortality rates, malnutrition, and deaths per 100,000 due to cholera can reveal which populations have limited access to medical resources. One cross-national study found that the higher the percent without improved water services, and the higher the infant mortality rate, the more media emphasis on government responsibility for water handling (Wissel, et al., 2014). Also, higher infant mortality rates are connected to media emphasis on government responsibility for child labor (Kohn & Pollock, 2014), and the higher percent undernourished in a country, the more media emphasis on government responsibility for HIV/AIDS (Etheridge, et al., 2014). Since connections are expected between measures of health vulnerability and more media emphasis on government responsibility for climate change, a profound issue connected to a wide range of cultural values and traditions, the following is predicted:

H6a: *The higher a nation's infant mortality rate, the more media emphasis on government responsibility to address climate change (United Nations Statistics Division, 2020).*

H6b: *The higher the percentage of undernourished in a nation, the more media emphasis on government responsibility to address climate change (United Nations Statistics Division, 2020).*

H6c: *The greater the percent of people without access to improved water services, the more media emphasis on government responsibility to address climate change (CIA, 2020).*

H6d: *The greater the prevalence of adult HIV per 100,000 in a nation, the more media emphasis on government responsibility to address climate change (CIA, 2020).*

Political vulnerability. National strategic context (Pollock & Guidette, 1980) and political instability can play a role in reporting on political and social change, including climate change. Political instability (measured, inversely, by a sophisticated "Global Peace Index") is likely to generate supplications for government assistance, likely reflected in media coverage emphasizing government responsibility for efforts to stabilize or normalize human relations and environmental conditions of all kinds, including climate change. (A nation's Global Peace Index/instability score is a composite score combining 23 indicators that examine relative peace or instability in a country: Institute for Economics and Peace, 2020).[1] One study found that the greater the political instability in a country, the more media emphasis on government responsibility for food security (Sparano, et al., 2020). Accordingly, for climate change:

H7a: *The higher a nation's Global Peace Index (the less peaceful a country), the more media emphasis on government responsibility to address climate change (Institute for Economics and Peace, 2020).*

Agricultural dependence. The proportion of a country's land and other resources that are used for agricultural purposes is known as agricultural dependence. If a nation focuses more on agriculture, we can assume the less developed and industrialized that country will be, manifesting an increase in vulnerability. Previous studies found that the more agricultural land in a given country, the more favorable the media coverage of GMO usage (Pollock, Peitz et al., 2017), and the more media emphasis on government responsibility for transit migration (Pollock, O'Brien et al., 2019), food security (Sparano, et al., 2020), drug trafficking, and condom promotion (Pollock, 2020). Therefore:

H8a: The higher a nation's percentage of agricultural land, the more media emphasis on government responsibility to address climate change (World Bank, 2020).

H8b: The greater the value added to a nation's GDP from agriculture, the more media emphasis on government responsibility to address climate change (World Bank, 2020).

H8c: The greater the crop production index score in a nation, the more media emphasis on government responsibility to address climate change (World Bank, 2020).

H8d: The greater the food production index in a nation, the more media emphasis on government responsibility to address climate change (World Bank, 2020).

Methodology

To investigate coverage of climate change, a cross-national sample of 21 major newspapers/news services was extracted from NewsBank and AllAfrica databases using search terms "climate change," "global warming," and "policies.*" Sampling all news or feature articles of 250 words or more in the specified time frame, excluding editorials and letters to the editor, and utilizing any of the search terms in the headline or first paragraph yielded a total of 454 articles. The compilation of publications included articles from the following: *Agence France Presse*, *Anadolu Agency* (Turkey), *The Bangkok Post* (Thailand), *China Daily*, *The Daily Nation* (Kenya), *Daily News Egypt*, Deutsche Press Agentur (Germany), *El Mercurio* (Chile), *El Universal* (Mexico), *The Japan Times*, *La Nación* (Argentina), *The Namibian*, *The Nation* (Pakistan), *New Strait Times* (Malaysia), *The New Times* (Rwanda), *New Vision* (Uganda), *The New York Times* (United States), *The Sydney Morning Herald* (Australia), *The Times* (United Kingdom), *The Times of India*, and *The Toronto Star* (Canada). A larger sample of newspapers was drawn initially, but some newspapers in the larger sample were ultimately not included either because of language limitations of researchers or because so few articles (less than 10) were encountered in the sample period for a given newspaper.

The inception point of data collection was December 12, 2015, the day that the global community adopted the "Paris Agreement" at the UN Framework Convention on Climate Change. The "Paris Agreement" is the most ambitious global agreement to address climate change because all nations were committed to "[combat] climate change and [adapt] to its impacts" (Denchak, 2018, para 4). The sample period ended on September 27, 2020, the last day of Climate Week NYC 2020, a summit hosted by the United Nations that brought international leaders together to discuss climate change issues (Climate Week NYC, 2020, para 1).

Article Prominence

Each article was assessed through two different measures: prominence and direction. The first measure determines the "prominence" of each article, based on the editors' judgments on its significance. A score ranging from 3 to 16 was attributed to each article based on four elements: article

Table 8.1 Prominence Score (For Coding Database)*

Dimension	4	3	2	1
Placement	Front page first section	Front page inside section	Inside page first section	Other
Headline size (# of words)	10+	9-8	7-6	5 or fewer
Article length (# of words)	1000 +	750–999	500–749	250–499
Photos/graphics	2 or more	1		

* Prominence Score copyright John C. Pollock, 1994–2023.

placement, headline size, article length, and photos/graphics. Articles with a higher number of points received a greater attention score. The prominence score is outlined below.

Article Direction

After receiving a prominence score, an article was assigned a "direction" category based on the content of the frames it used. "Direction" indicated whether an article primarily focused on "government" or "society" responsibility to address climate change, or whether it was "balanced/neutral." The articles were coded for these directions based on the following criteria:

(0) Articles emphasizing government responsibility, in particular increased government efforts, for addressing climate change were coded as "government." (b) Articles interpreted emphasizing society responsibility—individuals, non-government agencies, charities, or foreign aid—in particular increased societal efforts, for addressing climate change were coded as "societal responsibility." (c) Articles perceived to be nonpartisan regarding action on climate change, or covering both sides of this issue in approximately equal measure, were classified as "balanced/neutral," as were articles that simply offered current events, data, or statistics.

Coefficient of Intercoder Reliability. Precisely 276 of 454 articles, or approximately 61%, were double-coded for content direction, yielding a Scott's Pi coefficient of intercoder reliability of 0.7204.

Calculating Media Vectors

0.0. The Janis-Fadner Coefficient of Imbalance was applied to calculate a "Media Vector" after analyzing 21 newspapers from nations worldwide. The Media Vector was calculated by combining prominence and directional scores to measure article "projection" onto audiences (Pollock, 2007, p. 49). The "magnitude" of the Media Vector was measured by the article's prominence. The "direction" was defined by the article's emphasis on either government or society responsibility in addressing climate change. Media Vector scores range from +1.00 and −Coverage emphasizing government efforts to address climate change yielded a score between 0 and +1.00, while coverage emphasizing societal efforts to address climate change yielded scores between 0 and −1.00. This formula is depicted in Table 8.2.

Results

In evaluating newspaper coverage on addressing climate change, this study compared Media Vectors from 21 different countries from December 12, 2015 to September 27, 2020. All Media

Table 8.2 Media Vector Formula*

g = sum of the prominence scores coded "government responsibility" s = sum of the prominence scores coded "societal responsibility"

n = sum of the prominence scores coded "balanced/neutral" r = g + s + n

If g > s (the sum of the government prominence scores is greater than the sum of the societal prominence scores), the following formula is used:

Government Media Vector:

$$GMV = \frac{(g2 - gs)}{r2} \quad \left(\text{Answer lies between } 0 \text{ and } +1.00 \right)$$

If g < s (the sum of the societal prominence scores is greater than the sum of the government scores), the following formula is used:

Societal Media Vector:

$$SMV = \frac{(gs - s2)}{r2} \quad \left(\text{Answer lies between } 0 \text{ and } +1.00 \right)$$

* Media Vector copyright John C. Pollock, 2000-2023

Table 8.3 Media Vectors

Nation	Newspaper	Media Vector
France	*Agence France Presse*	0.4777
Chile	*El Mercurio*	0.4160
Australia	*Sydney Morning Herald*	0.4103
Germany	*Deutsche Press Agentur*	0.3880
United Kingdom	*The Times*	0.2614
India	*The Times of India*	0.2354
Malaysia	*The New Strait Times*	0.2175
Argentina	*La Nación*	0.2132
United States	*The New York Times*	0.2112
Canada	*The Toronto Star*	0.2030
Uganda	*New Vision*	0.1534
Mexico	*El Universal*	0.1449
China	*China Daily*	0.1246
Japan	*Japan Times*	0.0963
Kenya	*Daily Nation*	0.0671
Pakistan	*The Nation*	0.0425
Thailand	*The Bangkok Post*	0.0290
Rwanda	*The New Times*	0.0244
Egypt	*Daily News Egypt*	0.0193
Namibia	*The Namibian*	0.0142
Turkey	*Anadolu Agency*	0.0130

Vectors emphasized governmental responsibility for addressing climate change. The highest Media Vector was 0.4777 (*Agence France Presse*), the lowest, 0.0130 (*Anadolu Agency*), and range was 0.4647. Table 8.3 offers a complete list of the Media Vector scores found in this study, listed from most positive to most negative.

Pearson correlations were calculated by using SPSS to search for connections between country characteristics and variation in newspaper coverage (Table 8.4).

Table 8.4 Pearson Correlation

Country Characteristic	Pearson Correlation	Significance
Greater number of midwives per 100,000	0.718	0.000**
Broadband subscriptions per 100 people in a nation	0.640	0.001**
Female school life expectancy	0.608	0.002**
GDP per capita	0.600	0.002**
Male life expectancy at birth	0.593	0.002**
Physicians per 100,000	0.584	0.003**
Female life expectancy at birth	0.563	0.004**
Global Peace Index	−0.553	0.005**
Percentage of female enrollment in secondary school	0.542	0.007**
Literacy rate	0.528	0.007**
Percentage of population Younger than 15	−0.508	0.009**
Infant mortality rate	−0.501	0.009*
Value added to GDP from agriculture	−0.537	0.009*
Female literacy rate	0.499	0.011*
Percentage undernourished	−0.446	0.021*
Adult HIV cases per 100,000	−0.501	0.024*
Fertility rate	−0.418	0.030*
Percent of the nation's population without access to improved water services	−0.401	0.036*
Food production index	−0.377	0.046*
Poverty level	−0.378	0.050*
Nation's industrial production growth rate	−0.368	0.050*
Crop production index score	−0.324	0.076
Stock of direct foreign investment at home (CIA)	0.317	0.081
Hospital beds per 100,000	0.274	0.122
Oil production	−0.240	0.147
Daily newspapers per 1000 people	0.199	0.207
Electricity production	0.143	0.268
Percentage of population covered by a mobile phone network	0.142	0.269
Length nation's road network (km)	0.126	0.294
Natural gas consumption	0.126	0.294
GDP	0.113	0.313
Electricity consumption	0.093	0.345
Percentage females in the Workforce	0.070	0.381
Coal consumption	−0.064	0.397
Oil consumption	−0.066	0.408
Length of paved roads (km)	0.055	0.411
Percentage of permanent cropland in a nation	0.018	0.469
Percent agricultural land in a nation	0.017	0.470
Natural gas production	−0.013	0.481

Discussion of Significant Findings: "Buffer" Hypothesis Confirmed

This cross-national study yielded significant findings regarding numerous measures of privilege. It is striking that the "buffered" health privilege measure of midwives and other health privilege indicators were the most significant findings, while measures of energy production and consumption, often connected to climate change, were statistically unrelated to media coverage.

Health (especially Female) Privilege Robustly Associated with Coverage Emphasizing Government Responsibility for Addressing Climate Change.

As predicted, the greater the number of midwives per 100,000 residents in a country ($r = 0.718$, $p = 0.000$), the more media emphasis on government responsibility to address climate change. Three other measures of health access privilege were also strongly linked to coverage emphasizing government responsibility for climate change, including: male life expectancy at birth ($r = 0.593$, $p = 0.002$); greater number of physicians per 100,000 citizens in a country ($r = 0.584$, $p = 0.003$); and female life expectancy at birth ($r = 0.563$, $p = 0.004$). It is noteworthy that two measures of female health access privilege, midwives/100,000 residents and female life expectancy at birth, are strongly associated with coverage supporting government responsibility for climate change.

Female, Economic, and Communication Privilege Also Associated with Media Emphasis on Government Responsibility for Climate Change.

Two broad indicators of privilege, one of female advantage—female school life expectancy ($r = 0.608$, $p = 0.002$), the other of economic advantage—higher levels of GDP/capita ($r = 0.600$, $p = 0.002$). were also associated strongly with coverage emphasizing government responsibility for climate change, as were two indicators of communication resource privilege: higher numbers of broadband subscriptions per 100 citizens in a nation ($r = 0.640$, $p = 0.001$) and higher literacy rates ($r = 0.0528$, $p = 0.007$).

Almost all Indicators of "Vulnerability" Were Associated with Coverage Emphasizing "Less" Government Responsibility for Climate Change

By contrast, media emphasis on government responsibility for climate change was significantly and negatively associated with many indicators of vulnerability, including: Global Peace Index—measuring political instability ($r = -0.553$, $p = 0.005$); percent population under 15 years old ($r = -0.508$, $p = 0.009$); infant mortality rate ($r = -0.501$, $p = 0.009$); value added to GDP from agriculture ($r = -0.537$, $p = 0.009$); percent undernourished ($r = -0.446$, $p = 0.021$); adult HIV cases/100,000 ($r = -0.501$, $p = 0.024$); fertility rates ($r = -0.418$, $p = 0.030$); percent population without access to improved water services ($r = -0.401$, $p = 0.036$); food production index ($r = -0.377$, $p = 0.046$); and poverty level ($r = -0.378$; $p = 0.050$).

Regression Analysis

A regression analysis identified midwives (46.7% of the variance), physicians/100,000 (4.9%), and GDP per capita (5.2%) collectively accounting for 56.9% of the variance associated with coverage emphasizing government responsibility for climate change (Table 8.5).

Conclusion

Despite geographic, economic, and social diversity in all 21 sampled nations, media coverage everywhere emphasized government responsibility for addressing climate change. Overall, the "buffer" hypothesis associating privilege with sympathetic coverage of human rights claims was confirmed. Countries with higher levels of healthcare privilege, as measured by midwives per

Table 8.5 Regression Analysis for Cross-national Coverage of Climate Change

Model (Predictors)	R	R^2 Cumulative	R^2 Change	F Change	Sig, F Change
Midwives	0.684	0.467	0.467	14.91	0.001
Midwives, physician/100,000	0.719	0.516	0.049	1.629	0.220
Midwives, physician/100,000, GDP per capita	0.754	0.569	0.052	1.822	0.197

100,000 residents, were robustly linked with significant media emphasis on government responsibility for addressing climate change (accounting for 46.7% of the variance), as were other measures of health or female privilege, including physicians/100,000 (another 4.9% of variance), male and female life expectancy at birth, and female school life expectancy, along with indicators of economic and communication privilege, including GDP/capita (5.2% pf variance), broadband subscriptions/100, and higher literacy rates.

How do the roles that midwives play—less prestigious with typically less training than other healthcare professionals, often local, and requiring high amounts of interpersonal contact—become closely connected with variations in national coverage of climate change across the globe? That question deserves exploration in future research, along with questions about the curious absence of almost any significant connections between levels of resource privilege (high levels of electricity, gas, coal, and oil production and consumption) and media emphasis on government responsibility for climate change. Only industrial production growth rate was significantly (negatively) associated with the Media Vector ($r = -0.367$, $p = 0.050$).

Empirically, media coverage of climate change can be associated with multiple indicators of "buffered" health and female privilege linked to coverage emphasizing government responsibility for the issue. Methodologically, the composite Media Vectors sensitively portrayed combinations of measures of "prominence" and "direction" to reflect different levels of media support for government responsibility to address climate change. Theoretically, by emphasizing the influence of national demographics, community structure theory complements agenda-setting theory at the national level, highlighting, as found empirically by prominent agenda-setting scholars (Funk & McCombs, 2017), the way demographics and prominent newspapers can both affect coverage of important issues, including climate change.

Note

1 The Global Peace Index composite score looks at: the level of perceived criminality in society, the number of internal security officers and police per 100,000 people, number of homicides per 100,000 people, number of jailed population per 100,000 people, ease of access to small arms and light weapons, intensity of organized internal conflict, level of violent crime, likelihood of violent demonstrations, political instability, political terror scale, volume of transfers of major conventional weapons (imports) per 100,000 people, impact of terrorism, number of deaths from internal organized conflict, the number and duration of internal conflicts, military expenditure as a percentage of GDP, the number of armed services personnel per 100,000 people, financial contribution to UN peacekeeping missions, nuclear and heavy weapons capabilities, number of refugees and internally displaced people as a percentage of the population, volume of transfers of major conventional weapons as exports per 100,000 people, relations with neighboring countries, the number, duration, and role in external conflicts, and the number of deaths from organized external conflict (Institute for Economics and Peace, 2020).

References

Alexandre, K., Sha, C., Pollock, J.C., Baier, K., & Johnson, J. (2014). Cross-national coverage of human trafficking: A community structure approach. *Atlantic Journal of Communication, 22*(3/4), 160–174.

Benson, R. (2013). *Shaping immigration news: A French-American comparison.* Cambridge, UK: Cambridge University Press.

Buonauro, B., Pollock, J.C., Gomez, O., Galfo, A., Salmon, M., & Hart-McGonigle, T. (2017, April). *Cross-national newspaper coverage of women's reproductive rights 2011- 2015: A community structure approach* [Paper presentation]. Biannual conference of the DC Health Communication Conference, Fairfax, VA.Central Intelligence Agency (CIA). (2020). *The world factbook 2020–2021.* https://www.cia.gov/library/publications/resources/the-world-factbook/

Climate Week NYC. (2020, September). Climate week NYC 2020. *Climate Week NYC*. Retrieved from https://www.climateweeknyc.org/climate-week-nyc-2020

D'Angelo, P. (Ed.) (2018). *Doing news framing analysis II: Empirical and theoretical perspectives.* London: Routledge.

Demers, D.P., & Viswanath, K. (Eds.) (1999). *Mass media, social control, and social change: A macrosocial perspective.* Ames, IA: Iowa State University Press.

Denchak, M. (2018, December 12). Paris climate agreement: Everything you need to know. *Natural Resources Defense Council.* Retrieved from https://www.nrdc.org/stories/paris- climate-agreement-everything-you-need-know

Donohue, G.A., Tichenor, P.J., & Olien, C. (1995). A guard dog perspective on the role of media. *Journal of Communication, 45*, 115–132.

Eisenberg, D., Kester, A., Caputo, L., Sierra, J., & Pollock, J.C. (2006, November). *Cross-national coverage of NGO's efforts to fight AIDS: A community structure approach* [Paper presentation. Annual conference of the National Communication Association, San Antonio, TX.

Etheridge, J., Zinck, K., Pollock, J.C., Santiago, C., Halicki, K., & Badalamenti, A. (2014). Cross-national coverage of HIV/AIDS: A community structure approach. *Atlantic Journal of Communication, 22*(3/4), 175–192.

Fleischman, J., Sacco, C., Sippy, S., Uhl, A., Pollock, J.C., & Crowley, M. (2021, April). *Cross- national news coverage of government responses to COVID-19: Community structure theory and privileged health access (especially for women).* Paper presented at the DC Health Communication Conference, Fairfax, VA.

Funk, M.J., & McCombs, M. (2017). Strangers on a theoretical train: Inter-media agenda setting, community structure, and local news coverage. *Journalism Studies, 18*(7), 845–865.

Govindarajan, S., Natalicchio, A., Rodriguez, M., Bialoblocki, S., Pollock, J.C., & Crowley, M. (2021, April). *Cross-national coverage of food security: Community structure theory and privileged resources.* Paper presented at the DC Health Communication Conference, Fairfax, VA.

Gratale, S., Hagert, J., Dey, L., Pollock, J., D'Angelo, P., Braddock, P., Montgomery, A. (2005, May). *International coverage of United Nations efforts to combat AIDS: A structural approach* [Paper presentation]. Annual conference of the International Communication Association, New York, NY.

Hammer, B., Mitchell, E., Shields, A., & Pollock, J.C. (2006, November). *Cross-national coverage of "Beijing Plus Ten": Women's rights in the ten years after the 1995 Beijing Conference* [Paper presentation]. Annual conference of the National Communication Association, San Antonio, TX.

Hindman, D.B. (1999). Social control, social change and local mass media. In D. Demers & K. Viswanath (Eds.), *Mass media, social control, and social change: A macrosocial perspective* (pp. 99–116). Ames, IA: Iowa State University Press.

Institute for Economics and Peace (2020). *Global peace index 2020.* https://www.visionofhumanity.org/wp-content/uploads/2020/10/GPI_2020_web.pdf

Janowitz, M. (1952). *The community press in an urban setting.* Glencoe, Il: The Free Press.

Johnson, L.-A., Hines, M., Villanueva, V., Lipsey, D., Pollock, J.C., & Marta, A. (2021, April). *Cross-national media coverage of rape and rape culture: Community structure theory and "buffered" female privilege.* Paper presented at the DC Health Communication Conference, Fairfax, VA.

Kiernicki, K., Pollock, J.C., & Lavery, P. (2013a). Nationwide newspaper coverage of universal health care: A community structure approach. In J.C. Pollock (Ed.), *Media and social inequality: Innovations in community structure research* (pp. 116–134). London: Routledge.

Kohn, J.G., & Pollock, J.C. (2014, July). Cross-national coverage of child labor: A community structure approach. *Atlantic Journal of Communication, 22*(3/4), 211–228.

McCombs, M. (2004). *Setting the agenda: The mass media and public opinion.* Malden, MA: Blackwell Publishing.

McLeod, D.M., & Hertog, J.K. (1992). The manufacture of public opinion by reporters: Informal cues for public perceptions of protest groups. *Discourse and Society, 3*, 259–275.

McLeod, D.M., & Hertog, J.K. (1999). Social control, social change and the mass media's role in the regulation of protest groups. In D. Demers & K. Viswanath (Eds.), *Mass media, social control, and social change: A macrosocial perspective* (pp. 305–331). Ames, IA: Iowa State University Press.

Nah, S., & Armstrong, C. (2013). Structural pluralism in journalism and media studies: A concept explica-
tion and theory construction. In J.C. Pollock (Ed.), *Media and social inequality: Innovations in community
structure research* (pp. 31–52). Routledge.

Organisation for Economic Co-operation and Development (OECD). (2020). *Statistics from a to z.* http://
www.oecd.org/statistics/

Park, R. (1922). *The immigrant press and its control.* New York, NY: Harcourt.

Pollock, J.C. (2007). *Tilted mirrors: Media alignment with political and social change- A community structure approach.* Cresskill, NJ: Hampton Press.

Pollock, J.C. (Ed.) (2013a). *Media and social inequality: Innovations in community structure research.* London: Routledge.

Pollock, J.C. (2013b). Community structure research. In P. Moy (Ed.), *Oxford bibliographies online.* Oxford,
UK: Oxford University Press.

Pollock, J.C. (Ed.) (2015). *Journalism and human rights: How demographics drive media coverage.* London:
Routledge.

Pollock, J.C. (2020). Empowering the vulnerable: Using community structure theory to analyze relationships
between demographics and health communication. *International Journal of Nursing Sciences 7,* 516–518.
doi: https://doi.org/10.1016/j.ijnss.2020.05.007.

Pollock, J.C., Buonauro, B., Hosonitz, A., Kordomenos, C., Phelan, C., & Salmon, M. (2017). *Nationwide
newspaper coverage of transgender rights: A community structure approach* [Paper presentation]. Conference of the International Communication Association, San Diego, CA.

Pollock, J.C., Crowley, M., Govindarajan, S., Lewis, A., Marta, A., Purandare, R., & Sparano, J.N. (2021). US
nationwide coronavirus newspaper coverage of state and local government responses: Community structure theory and community "vulnerability". In J.C Pollock & D. Kovach (Eds.), *COVID-19 in international
media: Global pandemic responses.* New York and London: Routledge.

Pollock, J.C., Gratale, S., Anas, A., Kaithern, E., & Johnson, K. (2014). Nationwide newspaper coverage
of posttraumatic stress: A community structure approach. *Atlantic Journal of Communication, 22*(3/4),
275–291.

Pollock, J.C., Gratale, S., Teta, K., Bauer, K., & Hoekstra, E. (2014). Nationwide newspaper coverage of immigration reform: A community structure approach. *Atlantic Journal of Communication, 22*(3/4), 259–274.

Pollock, J.C., & Guidette, C. (1980). Mass media, crisis, and political change: A community structure approach. In Dan Nimme (Ed.), *Communication yearbook IV* (pp. 309–324). New Brunswick, NJ: Transac-
tion Books.

Pollock, J.C., O'Brien, K., Ouelette, M., Gottfried, M., Kovacs, P., Hart-McGonigle, T., Longo, L., & Cook,
J.P. (2019b). Cross-national newspaper coverage of transit migration: Community structure theory and
national vulnerability. *International Communication Research Journal, 54*(1), 34–67.

Pollock, J.C., Peitz, K., Watson, E., Esposito, C., Nichilo, P., Etheridge, J., Morgan, M., & Hart-McGonigle,
T. (2017b, June). Comparing cross-national coverage of genetically modified organisms: A community
structure approach. *Journalism & Mass Communication Quarterly, 94*(2), 571–596.

Pollock, J.C., Reda, E., Bosland, A., Hindi, M., & Zhu, D. (2010, June). *Cross-national coverage of climate
change: A community structure approach* [Paper presentation]. Annual conference of the International
Communication Association, Singapore.

Pollock, J.C., Robinson, J.L., & Murray, M.C. (1978). Media agendas and human rights: The Supreme Court
decision on abortion. *Journalism Quarterly, 53*(3), 545–548, 561.

Pollock, J.C., & Storey, D. (2012). Comparing health communication. In F. Esser & T. Hanitzsch (Eds.),
Handbook of comparative communication research (pp. 161–184). New York, NY: Routledge.

Pollock, J.C., & Yulis, S.G. (2004). Nationwide newspaper coverage of physician assisted suicide: A community structure approach. *Journal of Health Communication, 9*(4), 281–307.

Purandare, R., Griffith, T., Ochoa, M., Muniappan, D., Pollock, J.C., & Marta, A. (2021, April). *Cross-
national coverage of human trafficking: Community structure theory, health vulnerability, and resource
privilege.* Paper presented at the DC Health Communication Conference, Fairfax, VA.

Schudson, M. (2008). *Why democracies need an unlovable press.* Cambridge, UK: Polity.

Singer, J.B. (2013). The ethical implications of an elite press. *Journal of Mass Media Ethics, 28*(3), 203–216.

Sparano, J.N., Adams, A., Mazzullo, J., Rainero, R., Pollock, J.C., & Crowley, M. (2020, April). *Cross-national media coverage of food insecurity: Community structure theory and national vulnerability.* Paper presented at the annual conference of the New Jersey Communication Association, New Brunswick, NJ.

Tichenor, P.J., Donohue, G., & Olien, C. (1973). Mass communication research: Evolution of a structural model. *Journalism Quarterly, 50*(3), 419–425.

Tichenor, P.J., Donohue, G., & Olien, C. (1980). *Community conflict and the press.* Thousand Oaks, CA: Sage.

Tumber, H. (2000). Introduction: Academic at work. In H. Tumber (ed.), *Media power, professionals, and policies* (pp. 1–12). London: Routledge.

United Nations. (2019). *Climate change.* United Nations. Retrieved from https://www.un.org/en/sections/issues-depth/climate-change/index.html

UNICEF. https://www.unicef.org/publications/index_96412.html

United Nations Statistics Division. (2020). *UNSD statistical databases*, NY United Nations. https://unstats.un.org/databases.htm

Waisbord, S. (Ed.) (2014). *Media sociology: A reappraisal.* Cambridge, UK: Polity Press.

Watson, B., & Riffe, D. (2013). Structural determinants of local public affairs place blogging: Structural pluralism and community stress. In J.C. Pollock (Ed.), *Media and social inequality: Innovations in community structure research* (pp. 91–116). London: Routledge.

Wissel, D., Ward, K., Pollock, J.C., Hipper, A., Klein, L., & Gratale, S. (2014). Cross-national coverage of water handling: A community structure approach. *Atlantic Journal of Communication, 22*(3/4), 193–210.

World Bank (2020). *World development indicators 2020.* World Bank — 2020 – elibrary.worldbank.org

Yamamoto, M. (2013). Mass media as a macrolevel source of social control: A new direction in the community structure model. In J.C. Pollock (Ed.), *Media and social inequality: Innovations in community structure research* (pp. 53–70). London: Routledge.

Yasin, S., Khan, S., Lanfranchi, V., Natarajan, S., Pollock, J.C., & Crowley, M. (2020, April). *Cross-national coverage of access to mental health services: Community structure theory and "buffered" privilege.* Paper presented at the biannual University of Kentucky Health Communication Conference, Lexington, KY.

Zelizer, B. (2004). *Taking journalism seriously: News and the academy.* Thousand Oaks, CA: Sage.

9   Disaster Response Inclusiveness to Persons with Disabilities and the Elderly in the Philippines

*Joseph Christian Obnial, Jacqueline Veronica Velasco,
Hillary Kay Ang, Paulene Miriel Viacrusis,
and Don Eliseo Lucero-Prisno III*

Introduction

The Philippines is one of the most disaster-stricken nations in the world. Across countries with the highest disaster risk globally, the Philippines ranked the third with at least 60% of its total land area being exposed to numerous hazards and 74% of its total population having been considered vulnerable to the impact of these hazards (UN Office for Disaster Risk Reduction, 2019). This vulnerability to disasters can be partly explained by the Philippines' location along the "Pacific Ring of Fire", presenting a serious risk to the safety of the population in the face of events like volcanic eruptions and earthquakes (UN Office for Disaster Risk Reduction, 2019). It experiences 20 typhoons on a yearly average and ranks in the top three countries in terms of exposures, to tropical storms (European Commission Disaster Risk Management Knowledge Centre, 2021). Flooding in low-lying areas due to the annual monsoon is another problem, contributing up to 80% of natural disasters in the Philippines (Bolletino et al., 2018). In addition, the occurrence of droughts and landslides contribute to the vulnerability of the population considering that major sources of livelihood depend on the state of the environment (UN Office for Disaster Risk Reduction, 2019). Worsened by high concentrations of people and a shift in economic activities of industrial mining, these factors threaten to lower protective shields against natural disasters (Jha et al., 2018; UNDRR, 2019).

Damages and losses due to natural disasters deal a huge socioeconomic blow in this low to middle income country, especially as they traverse its poorest areas (Bolletino et al., 2018; Jha et al., 2018). In the past three decades, the economic toll of storms alone has cost the country at least USD20 billion (ADB, 2021). In response, the country has invested heavily in disaster risk management infrastructure. Despite these efforts, the country still finds it difficult to provide adequate disaster risk mitigation (Jha et al., 2018). One such example is the government's shortcomings in response to Typhoon Haiyan. Generally considered one of the worst disasters in the history of the world, the typhoon struck the country in 2013, leaving thousands of people, including the elderly and persons with disabilities (PWDs), desolate and out of their homes.

Vulnerabilities, Risks, and Disasters

A disaster is defined as 'a sudden, calamitous event that seriously disrupts the functioning of a community or society, eventually causing human, material, economic or environmental losses that exceed the community or society's ability to cope using its own resources' (The International Federation of Red Cross, n.d.). Disasters massively impact aspects of humanity and result in the loss of human lives, property, agriculture, and economic livelihood.

Risks and vulnerabilities are concepts central to the discussions of disasters. Risk is defined as 'the interaction of a hazard's consequences with its probability or likelihood' (Coppola, 2011).

DOI: 10.4324/9781003140245-9

Vulnerability, in contrast, is the likelihood of being affected by an event that varies across different populations (United Nations Office for Disaster Risk Reduction, 2019). From an epidemiologic perspective, the focus has now shifted from risk to a focus on vulnerability. This is true particularly in public health due to limitations when using the former concept. Risk focuses on individual acts while vulnerability emphasizes understanding of the shared characteristics of a group of people within the society that lead to bad outcomes such as disasters (Frohlich and Potvin, 2008). Thus, in the current public health domain, there is now an emphasis on 'vulnerable populations' which this study will highlight.

Persons with Disabilities and the Elderly as Vulnerable Populations

A vulnerable population is broadly defined by the Iowa Public Health Preparedness Program (as cited by Nick et al., 2009) as "any individual, group, or community whose circumstances create barriers to obtaining or understanding information, or the ability to react as the general population". Some of the circumstances that create barriers include age, socioeconomic level, religion, ethnicity, language, citizenship, culture, and geography. The physical, mental, emotional, and cognitive states are also known determinants of vulnerability.

Such a population group may include the ill and disabled, the elderly (Shi & Stevens, 2021), young children, the poor, and other so-called marginalized groups. These groups have a shared characteristic leading them to more insecure situations when disasters strike. Minimizing vulnerability in the context of disasters, considered acute public health events, improves the collective health of vulnerable populations and all populations in general (Stephenson et al., 2013).

In particular, the elderly and PWD populations are commonly overlooked during disaster responses, where access and mobility are limited because of their pre-existing conditions. This was seen in Typhoon Haiyan where two-fifths of the population's mortality belonged to the elderly (CHRP, 2021). High dependence on families is very critical to get away from hazards and to acquire easy access to community resources (Maltais, 2019). Post-disaster, financial difficulties arise and hinder disaster rehabilitation and recovery. Following suspension of economic activities, incurring loans, and selling personal items are inevitable in order to sustain their financial needs, such as medicines for their pre-existing illnesses. Furthermore, reluctance in expressing their needs leads to local response prioritizing the younger population (Maltais, 2019). With the fast turnover of government officials every election, advocates tend to lean on the indifference of local governments, including the PWDs and the elderly (Bolte et al., 2014). Evacuation centers are insufficient for all community residents leading to the elderly prioritizing younger family members before them. As a result, the elderly and PWDs are significantly more vulnerable during disasters and post-disaster. An inclusive disaster risk management is needed to consider the increased needs of the elderly and PWDs.

Basics of Disaster Risk Management

Disaster risk management (DRM) refers to the creation of systems and the organization and direction of resources to reduce vulnerability and reinforce resilience (Bolte et al., 2014). It encompasses four stages that can be called the DRM Cycle (Figure 9.1): prevention/mitigation, preparedness, response, and rehabilitation and reconstruction (Asian Disaster Reduction Center, 2009). The first two stages happen prior to the disaster, while the last two stages happen after the disaster. Prevention/mitigation refers to efforts that reduce or mitigate damage (Asian Disaster Reduction Center, 2009). Examples of these are construction of dams or flood reservoirs and retrofitting of vulnerable buildings. Preparedness refers to activities and measures to ensure effective response to disasters. They do not aim to avert the occurrence of a disaster (Asian Disaster Reduction Center, 2009).

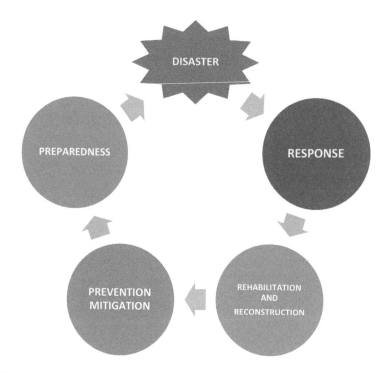

Figure 9.1 Disaster risk management cycle.

Examples of these are emergency drills, early-warning systems, and stockpiling of resources. Response refers to the immediate actions taken after disaster strikes (Asian Disaster Reduction Center, 2009). These include evacuation and rescue efforts, relocation to evacuation sites, and administration of first aid. Finally, rehabilitation and reconstruction refer to measures made for the affected population to return to normal or a new normal (Asian Disaster Reduction Center, 2009). These can range from immediate measures, such as restoring essential services like food and water, to more long-term measures, such as livelihood support programs, disaster resistant reconstruction, and land planning.

The cycle emphasizes the fact that DRM is a continuous process that always has to be taken note of. In order to truly reduce vulnerability, preparations must be made even before there is an immediate threat of disaster. DRM efforts must be all-encompassing and must be able to protect all members of its community regardless of age, gender, disability, or other factors (Bolte et al., 2014).

The Call for Disaster Justice

DRM undoubtedly has a social aspect. It is not confined to solely managing physical exposure, but also mitigating social vulnerability. As discussed in the previous sections, the elderly and PWDs are included among the most vulnerable due to several perpetuating factors. It is during calamities that these vulnerabilities are further magnified (Lukasiewicz & Dovers, 2018). According to the United Nations (2015), it is largely the responsibility of the government to ensure justice in the wake of disasters. Thus, it must be called to the attention of such disaster management actors to ensure that all members of the community including the vulnerable minority are delivered with just preparedness, response, and recovery protocols. Fighting injustice is a step forward to increasing community resilience during disasters and calamities. Continuing to view such inadequate attempts to address social vulnerability as a misfortune rather than injustice, disaster justice will remain as a concept often overlooked for proper action (Verchick, 2012).

Objectives

This chapter aims to assess the disaster response and impact of typhoons in the Philippines on the elderly and PWDs and identify the points of improvement for disaster response organizations in hopes that ultimately disaster justice is duly delivered to the people of the nation. Possible solutions on the way forward will also be discussed to ensure a culture of preparedness and resilience in light of future catastrophic events.

Methods

This study conducted a narrative review regarding the state of PWDs and the elderly in the Philippines. Literature included newspaper articles, journal articles, policy documents, and gray literature to acquire data on the experiences of PWDs and the elderly in the context of disasters and natural calamities. Search terms include "disaster preparedness", "disasters", "evacuation", "typhoons", "earthquakes", "PWDs", "persons with disabilities", "elderly", and "senior citizens". Eligibility criteria included content in either English, Tagalog, or any Filipino language and must include a mention of PWDs and the elderly in the aftermath of a disaster. Relevant policy documents were also qualitatively analyzed to acquire data on the policies and laws that are currently being implemented to ensure DRM-inclusiveness of PWDs and the elderly. Data was gathered using PubMed, Google Scholar, and Google. Articles were obtained from local and national news outlets, as well as non-governmental and governmental organizations reporting on the matter.

The state of PWDs and the elderly and the current policies implemented to address their inclusion to DRM were analyzed together. This is to obtain information on the current status of PWDs and the elderly during disasters and review the adequacy of government policies in ensuring DRM-inclusiveness in these populations. The analytical process used to frame the analysis is shown in Figure 9.2.

Results

A total of 25 documents (Table 9.1) from the Philippines were reviewed and analyzed. Fourteen online articles and two news clips comprising interviews and news articles regarding PWDs and

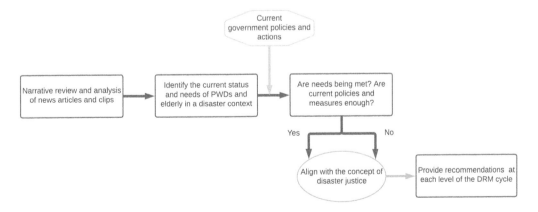

Figure 9.2 Conceptual framework for analysis.

Table 9.1 Newspaper Articles, Government Documents, and Policy Papers Included in the Study

No.	Document	Source
1	Online article: Typhoon leaves elderly more vulnerable	https://www.thenewhumanitarian.org/news/2013/11/18/typhoon-leaves-elderly-more-vulnerable
2	Online article: Catanduanes 70-year-old, PWD rescued from Ulysses flooding	https://www.gmanetwork.com/news/topstories/regions/764036/catanduanes-70-year-old-pwd-rescued-from-ulysses-flooding/story/
3	Online article: Older people disproportionately affected by Typhoon Haiyan	https://www.helpage.org/newsroom/latest-news/older-people-disproportionately-affected-by-typhoon-haiyan/
4	Online article: Where are PWDs during disasters?	https://www.rappler.com/moveph/86256-persons-with-disability-disasters-cebu/
5	Online article: For Filipinos with disabilities, climate change and natural disasters are a dangerous mix	https://theworld.org/stories/2018-07-13/disabled-community-coastal-philippine-city-feels-forgotten
6	Online article: Philippines: Earthquakes injure Hundreds	https://www.hi-us.org/news_earthquakes_in_the_philippines_humanity_inclusion_responds_to_the_needs_of_the_most_vulnerable
7	Online article: PCG saves two PWDs accidentally left behind during evacuation	https://www.untvweb.com/news/pcg-saves-two-pwds-accidentally-left-behind-during-evacuation/
8	Online article: Philippines: Task force launched to support older people in emergencies. HelpAge International	https://www.helpage.org/newsroom/latest-news/philippines-task-force-launched-to-support-older-people-in-humanitarian-responses/
9	Online article: Typhoon Haiyan one year on: Older people key to rebuilding communities	https://www.helpage.org/newsroom/latest-news/typhoon-haiyan-one-year-on-older-people-key-to-rebuilding-communities/
10	Online article: Disability Inclusiveness Vital to Risk Reduction in the Philippines	https://www.preventionweb.net/blog/disability-inclusiveness-vital-risk-reduction-philippines
11	Online article: One year after Haiyan: feeling safer and better prepared	https://ageingasia.org/haiyan-salud/
12	Online article: PWDs emphasize need to involve in disaster risk reduction programs	https://cebudailynews.inquirer.net/150751/pwds-emphasize-need-involve-disaster-risk-reduction-programs#ixzz7X81irxwJ
13	Online article: PWDs left behind in Marikina's disaster preparedness efforts	https://news.abs-cbn.com/focus/09/29/17/evacuation-centers-relief-goods-not-pwd-inclusive
14	Online article: Why the Deaf and Blind are vulnerable during disasters	https://www.rappler.com/moveph/98514-deaf-blind-challenges-disasters/
15	News clip: Faces of Resilience – Philippines	https://www.youtube.com/watch?v=OJeA3SMVySc
16	News clip: Thousands of Yolanda survivors yet to benefit from government housing program	https://www.youtube.com/watch?v=bHfCPTKJG9o
17	Government Data: Senior Citizen Comprised 6% of the Population	https://psa.gov.ph/content/senior-citizen-comprised-six-percent-population

18	Republic Act 10524: An Act Expanding The Positions Reserved For Persons With Disability	https://www.ncda.gov.ph/disability-laws/republic-acts/republic-act-no-10524-an-act-expanding-the-positions-reserved-for-persons-with-disability-amending-for-the-purpose-republic-act-no-7277-as-amended-otherwise-known-as-the-magna-carta-for-persons/
19	Republic Act 7277: Magna Carta for Disabled Persons	https://pcw.gov.ph/republic-act-7277-magna-carta-for-disabled-persons/#:~:text=AN%20ACT%20PROVIDING%20FOR%20THE,SOCIETY%20AND%20FOR%20OTHER%20PURPOSES.
20	Republic Act 10121: Philippine Disaster Risk Reduction and Management Act of 2010	https://pcw.gov.ph/republic-act-10121-philippine-disaster-risk-reduction-and-management-act-of-2010/
21	House Bill No. 10472: An Act Establishing Evacuation Centers in Every Barangay and Appropriating Funds Therefor	https://hrep-website.s3.ap-southeast-1.amazonaws.com/legisdocs/basic_18/HB10472.pdf
22	Policy Document: Making the Invisible Visible! The Significance of an Integrated Data Management System for Persons with Disabilities at National Level. Philippine Statistics Authority	https://psa.gov.ph/sites/default/files/8.3.3%20Making%20the%20Invisible%20Visible%21%20The%20Significance%20of%20an%20Integrated%20Data%20Management%20System%20for%20Persons%20with%20Disabilities%20.pdf
23	Policy Document: Disaster Preparedness and Local Governance in the Philippines	https://pidswebs.pids.gov.ph/CDN/PUBLICATIONS/pidsdps1852.pdf
24	Policy Document: Operational Framework of Disability Inclusive Development	http://www.ncda.gov.ph/wp-content/uploads//2017/01/DID_Operational-Framework-2.pdf
25	Policy Document: National Disaster Risk Reduction and Management Plan 2020–2030	https://ndrrmc.gov.ph/attachments/article/4147/NDRRMP-Pre-Publication-Copy-v2.pdf

the elderly in relation to disasters was included in the review to document the states of these populations during disasters. Nine documents comprising national laws, government data, policy papers, and government memoranda were reviewed to elicit the current status of Philippine policies regarding DRM and the elderly and PWDs.

State of the Elderly during Disasters

The Philippines holds the 24th ranking in magnitude and 121st in percentage share of the elderly senior citizens (Reyes et al., 2019). According to the 2015 Census of Population and Housing, 7.5% (7,548,769) of the total population are senior citizens (Reyes et al., 2019). Data gathered showed the region that houses the greatest number of elderly populations based on statistics is the National Capital Region (Reyes et al., 2019). The 2005 Philippine Statistics Authority census states that 2.5 million households were headed by senior citizens (Philippine Statistics Authority, 2005). A projection of 11.4% increase by 2030 and of 15.9% increase by 2045 shows a steady increase in the elderly population. This indicates that in the decades to come, a significant number of the population in the Philippines may be extremely vulnerable during a disaster or natural crisis.

The increase in the vulnerability of the elderlies is pronounced during disaster emergencies. This is linked with poverty and isolation (HelpAge International, n.d.). For HelpAge International, the spiral of problems caused by poverty affects their basic needs, mobility, access to services, and social, economic, and legal status. Poverty is the result of a lower labor force and less access to pensions of the elderlies (Reyes et al., 2019). It is also stated that most of the elderlies are less economically active than younger individuals, and the elderlies are tasked to take care of the younger children in the family. During Typhoon Ulysses 2020, a 70-year-old woman taking care of her daughter, who herself was a PWD, were not evacuated upon arrival of the storm. They were trapped during severe flooding and were unable to hear their rescuers due to heavy rain and the rushing floodwaters (Casilao, 2020). In the case of Typhoon Haiyan, challenges in mobility and lack of assistance are disproportionately accounted for (Kulcsar, 2013). These pose a threat to elderlies who live alone because they can be easily displaced to unfamiliar surroundings and often risk separation from their family. This leads to isolation and oftentimes would lead to them having been left alone to fend for themselves (HelpAge International, n.d.). In addition to the current issues, there is a need to require more healthcare services due to the growing population of elderlies who suffer from various medical diseases and comorbidities (Reyes et al., 2019).

Despite the safety at evacuation centers, the elderly are at a disadvantage. Interviews with the elderly show that they have shown difficulty adapting to these environments (The New Humanitarian, 2013). There is also a lack of accessibility at the evacuation centers for these populations. It is harder for the elderly to queue for food and the makeshift areas have not been modified enough to ensure mobility for the elderly as a consequence of the rapidity with which these centers have been created (The New Humanitarian, 2013).

Beyond the disaster, the elderly faced difficulties with recovery and rehabilitation, with many not being included in cash-for-work programs (Gillam, 2014). Most notably, six years after Haiyan, rehabilitation for many survivors has still been incomplete, as some are unable to fully benefit from housing programs of the government (CNN, 2019). On the other hand, some have been experiencing difficulties rebuilding their sources of incomes because coconut and fruit trees were toppled by typhoons (HelpAge International, n.d.). Some elderly individuals have partial disabilities as well, rendering them unable to stray far from their homes, a potential vulnerability for future calamities (HelpAge International, n.d.).

State of PWDs during Disasters

Meanwhile, PWDs have also shown to be extremely vulnerable in the face of calamities. Republic Act (RA) 10524 of the Philippines consider PWDs as "those individuals who suffer long-term physical, mental, intellectual or sensory impairments, which, upon interaction with various barriers, may hinder their full and effective participation in society on an equal basis with others" (Republic Act 10524, 2013). People with disabilities comprise 1.57% of the total Philippine population (De Luna-Narido & Tacadao, 2021). According to the 2010 Census of Population and Housing, among the 1.443 million Filipinos with disabilities, 50.9% are male and the remaining 49.1% are female. Cases of disabilities were highest among 5–19 years old and 45–64 years old, a majority of which are in the working age group (De Luna-Narido & Tacadao, 2021).

PWDs in the Philippines often feel forgotten when it comes to DRM initiatives (Imperial & Morales, 2017; Luardo, 2017). Some PWDs even find it difficult to ask for aid during disasters themselves and have a hard time knowing where to go (UN Office for Disaster Risk Reduction, 2021). For the deaf and blind, in particular, there are no DRM guidelines that cater to their specific needs (Deaf Disaster Assistance Team-DRR, 2015). PWD groups state the need for their inclusion in the DRM planning process. In addition, some stress the importance of capacity-building for PWDs, such as through training in the basics of disaster rescue that could prove invaluable in assisting their family members during calamities (Imperial & Morales, 2017).

PWDs may be dependent on abled persons and their caregivers for quick evacuation, leaving them vulnerable in times of disaster. During super Typhoon Haiyan in 2013, several family members testified having to carry their disabled relative to evacuation centers through long distances, sometimes even taking several trips at a time (UNDRR, 2013). On the other hand, there are also instances wherein the disabled relative was left behind in small confinements while the other family members evacuated during the onslaught of the super typhoon (Serafica, 2015). The disabled member has been unable to secure themselves in the absence of assistance, posing great risks during emergencies. Other issues include the difficulty of transferring these PWDs to higher areas, especially to escape flooding. A report during Typhoon Haiyan stated how some PWDs could only stay on the ground floor due to being wheelchair-bound (Strother, 2018). This keeps them trapped should there be massive flooding inside the home. A PWD even stated that the flood actually went in and went as far up as her waist, and she could not do anything about it due to her spinal cord injury (Strother, 2018). There are also concerns of accidentally leaving behind PWDs during evacuation activities (Cerrudo, 2020). The Philippine Coast Guard (PCG) reports rescuing PWDs with mental illnesses who have been left behind after their families have evacuated. Although the PCG allayed concerns of them being intentionally left behind (Cerrudo, 2020), this further reveals another issue. Due to lockdowns and closing off of disaster-prone areas during evacuation, it is difficult for families to come back and retrieve their PWD family members.

The challenges faced by PWDs do not end upon reaching evacuation centers. Safety, protection, and access to basic needs are still areas of concern. Limited resources and remote accessibility hamper PWDs from reaching distribution sites in earthquake evacuation centers (Humanity and Inclusion, n.d.). Lack of inclusiveness in DRM planning results not only in difficulty to evacuate but PWDs also find that the evacuation facilities themselves are inaccessible to their needs (Clarin, 2021; Imperial & Morales, 2017). Public schools are usually used for emergency evacuations and non-enforcement of PWD-inclusive regulations make it difficult for affected individuals to navigate through the facilities (i.e., difficult to traverse areas due to lack of ramps, insufficient door widths). Finally, nutrition of those with special needs is not prioritized, evidenced by the lack of suitable relief goods for those who have difficulty swallowing or for children with special dietary restrictions (Imperial & Morales, 2017).

Philippine Policies on PWDs and the Elderly

Domingo and Manejar (2018) discuss the local government efforts on disaster preparedness and local governance of the Philippines. For the elderly, these involve building contingency plans and evacuation areas and conducting surveys and training on the elderly population for the improvement of disaster preparedness among local communities. Monitoring and evaluation are conducted to track the progress of planning. Canham (2014) states that the difficulties for the elderlies during Typhoon Haiyan paved the way for non-government organizations to step-up, such as the Coalition of Services of the Elderly (COSE). COSE partnered with HelpAge International to launch the Aging and Disability Task Force in the Philippines. Advocacy to include the elderlies in the assessment of disaster emergencies have also been given importance, in addition to emphasizing the crucial roles they play within their families and communities during emergency responses (Canham, 2014; HelpAge International, n.d.). Moreover, wider policymaking and full implementation of laws and rights of the elderlies have been points of focus by this task force. Lastly, efforts have been made by the group to ensure that all government relief and recovery strategies include affected elderlies (Canham, 2014).

For the disabled, major laws include the Magna Carta for Persons with Disabilities, or RA 7277 and its amendment RA 10524. These discuss the rights and privileges of PWDs. Supplements to this law further elaborate on accessibility regulations and programs and services for PWDs. The Philippine Disaster Risk Reduction Management Act of 2010 also has sections that focus on increasing resilience in the face of disaster and reducing vulnerabilities. However, these laws do not have specific sections on how to be PWD-inclusive when it comes to disaster management. These are all general laws with no specific details on how to deal with vulnerable PWDs and their clear inclusion in the disaster response.

Recently, however, there have been attempts to improve disability and elderly inclusivity in disaster management. In 2017, the National Council on Disability Affairs created an Operational Framework on Disability Inclusive Development that includes the establishment of disability inclusive DRM in their outcomes (National Council on Disability Affairs, 2017). However, no report as to the success of this outcome has yet been published. The National Disaster Risk Reduction and Management Plan (NDRRMP) 2020–2030 also emphasized the inclusion of PWDs, older age groups, and other marginalized groups in DRM planning. The NDRRMP also highlighted the importance of PWD-inclusive early-warning signs by including it in one of its outcomes (National Disaster Risk Reduction and Management Council, 2020). Meanwhile, House Bill 10472, a proposed bill to erect evacuation centers in every *barangay*, also has provisions to ensure all centers will adhere to accessibility laws (Banas-Nograles, 2021). Lastly, the 2021 Senate Finance Committee approved a budget for disability-friendly infrastructure. This includes the budget for building handrails, tactile paving, toilets, and paved walkways in public areas, particularly in schools. However, there is still a lack of simple ramps, non-skid flooring, signages, toilet and washrooms, and parking slots in several buildings and establishments, despite having laws for such basic requirements. There is still a long way to go for PWD and elderly inclusivity in many aspects of society. Endeavors to promote disability inclusion and to lift barriers that hinder PWDs from opportunities are still advocated (Luna, 2020).

Discussion

Understanding Disaster Justice in the Context of PWDs and the Elderly

'Disaster justice' pertains to the concept that the state has the legal responsibility and moral obligation to safeguard its people from the ravages of disasters (Bankoff, 2018). When the government fails to protect its people, this becomes a form of injustice and a violation of the contract of the democratic principles agreed upon as part of the duties of the state to its people (Verchick, 2012). It is mandated that the state has the duty and obligation to protect and shield its people from hazards and physical harm through policies and laws and to provide more equitable attention to those who are marginalized (Clarinval and Hunt, 2014). In the context of a disaster, Alessandra Jerolleman (2019) argues that 'there can be no resilience if there is no justice, and that recovery cannot truly occur if it is not just.'

Since justice is the concept of fairness, this concept needs to be applied to several circumstances, not just in disaster situations. Social justice is the manifestation of fairness within the society. This means equal rights, treatment, and opportunities for all ("What Is Social Justice?", 2016). On the other hand, health justice is the just and fair opportunity to be healthier by removing obstacles to health, such as poverty and discrimination, and by providing access to essential needs, such as a good job with fair pay, quality education, housing, and of course, healthcare ("Health Justice: Empowering Public Health and Advancing Health Equity – Network for Public Health Law", 2018). Through discussion of the different kinds of justice, it is impossible to isolate each variable as they all play intersectoral roles. In a pre-disaster setting, in order for the state to optimally deliver one type of justice, it would also require the other. This is even more evident in post-disaster settings, wherein the concept of disaster justice comes to intermix with social and health justice.

As stated by Michael Mendez,

> While disasters themselves may not discriminate, they are a product of human decision-making that often disproportionately impacts low-income communities…due to existing structural inequalities in society. Every part of a disaster — including vulnerabilities, preparedness, response, and rebuilding — is to some extent a social calculus. Therefore, the question of whose lives get priority before, during, and after a disaster is critically important.
>
> ("Seeking social justice in disaster", 2021)

Going beyond this, the same can be applied to marginalized groups such as PWDs and the elderly. Since these two groups are without a doubt more vulnerable than the average population, when disaster hits, the importance of delivering social, health, and disaster justice is even more pronounced.

Applying justice in the context of disasters has its roots in the study of environmental justice. "An environmental injustice occurs when an individual or a group bears disproportionate risks, has unequal access to environmental goods, or has less opportunity to participate in environmental decision-making" (Shrader-Frechette, 2002 cited in Jerolleman, 2019). Environmental justice carries with it the notion of "a more equitable distribution of goods and bads, along with more public participation in the process of distribution and evaluation" (Shrader-Frechette, 2002 cited in Jerolleman, 2019). The idea of justice as an equitable or fair distribution, however, has further evolved to encompass full and informed participation as equally integral components (Jerolleman, 2019).

Post-disaster inequality has always been observed in many global occurrences of disasters. For example, Kammerbauer and Wamsler (2017) noted that the marginalization of some social groups often become evident in recovery efforts that ensue from the occurrence of disasters that thus impede the attainment of sustainable goals. For instance, case studies in the districts of Fischerdorf and Natternberg of the German city of Deggendorf, following the 2013 floods in Europe, reveal that insured homeowners did not receive funding from the state for the reason that they were not qualified for government funding. While uninsured homeowners received government assistance, inequalities among low-income tenants were augmented due to post-flood rent increases. Thus, the magnitude of inequality can be dichotomized among those who are insured and uninsured in the 2013 flooding in Europe.

When looking at injustice through system failures, experts attribute this to the governing class. In an article by Ireni-Saban (2012), she aptly mentioned a major reflection of current management and governance issues: 'recent studies on disaster resilience policies focus on government and administrative shortcomings that prevent communities from improving their life circumstances.' Related to it are failures due to logistics and lack of funds. Many governments have limited budgets to address the risks the country faces. Policymakers would channel funds to risks that pose the biggest threat to society (Coppola, 2011), thereby resulting in some hazards mitigated, while the rest are neglected. An example is climate change. This hazard is not a priority in many countries and is not easily felt and appreciated. Other failures are due to the lack of use of evidence. The need to implement best practices in disaster management should be anchored on evidence (Lee, 2016).

In the occurrence of disasters in the Philippines, vulnerable populations such as PWDs and the elderly are often left out. In relation to the elderly, evidence has shown that they are often overlooked in emergency relief systems as they fail to consider the different needs and challenges faced by the elderly (Adams et al., 2011). This aggravates the present vulnerability they already have and worsens their ability to respond and adapt to disasters. Application of the concept of disaster justice here would therefore entail the creation of systems that are able to account for the specific needs of the elderly in all aspects of emergency response, both from preparedness to response and recovery. This would include the provision of plans and designs of emergency response that are appropriate for the elderly, training of necessary skills, and provision of equipment to aid not just the elderly but the first responders as well, and to provide nutritional, medical, and psychosocial support (Adams et al., 2011). The state will then be able to lessen the disproportionate impact of disaster on this special population.

The same applies to PWDs who also have additional specific needs and different capabilities that are overlooked during emergency response. An example of this is that PWDs have limited access to early-warning information and if they do, they are less likely to be able to respond adequately to it as they are limited by their disability (i.e., being unable to walk and being hard of hearing) (Ton & Adamson, 2020). Post-disaster, PWDs continue to be vulnerable as under-resourced PWDs are unable to access basic needs and services (Ton & Adamson, 2020). Therefore, in order to deliver disaster justice to these individuals, it is important to understand and address the social inequities hampering them. This would include maximizing the environment of PWDs for them to be able to respond better to disaster situations. Examples of this include implementation of additional early-warning communication channels to reach people with hearing and cognitive disabilities and modification of the built environment to make it more accessible to those with mobility disabilities (Ton & Adamson, 2020). Provision of social services and support to aid these individuals during a crisis is also essential. Through these efforts, PWDs can also become more resilient to disasters.

Addressing PWD and Elderly Inclusiveness in Disaster Responses in the Philippines According to the DRM Stages

Prevention and Mitigation

Prevention and mitigation measures for disasters will mostly be non-specific to PWDs and the elderly but will be beneficial for all as they limit the impact of disasters and reduce the amount of area affected by these events. In the Philippines, more focus is given to disaster preparedness and response as opposed to prevention (UN Office for Disaster Risk Reduction, 2019). As one of the most disaster-prone countries, the government must heavily invest in disaster prevention and mitigation efforts through strengthening infrastructure and increasing their ability to withstand hazards (United Nations, 2015). Reforestation efforts must be revisited to reduce the intensity of typhoons and tide walls can also be studied as to their feasibility in the country, as is the construction of erosion control dams. Overhauling drainage systems in the urban areas can also aid in reducing the incidence of massive flooding. Research and development on seismic design and construction of earthquake-proof facilities must also be explored.

Preparedness

PWDs and the elderly must be actively involved in the planning and implementation of inclusive disaster responses. Local government units must contact local PWD groups and elderly associations to enable them to participate in planning activities (Bolte et al., 2014). Committees must also identify issues with which these stakeholders may not be able to participate (Bolte et al., 2014). These barriers must be removed, and committees must make sure that these stakeholders are present in any consultative meetings. Caretakers and their family must also be included in these discussions to get their opinions.

Local PWD organizations have also been mobilizing to train their constituents in disaster management. As such, government arms, such as the NDRRMC and the Department of Social Welfare and Development, must engage and partner up with these organizations. This has already been reported in some areas of the Philippines (Bolte et al., 2014) and must be applied nationwide. These organizations are willing to aid the government but must also be tapped through formal partnerships. These efforts must be brought to the national scale through partnerships with different regional interest groups.

Bolstering emergency measures is crucial for any inclusive DRM to succeed. Information collected during the stakeholder meetings and data gathering must be implemented at all levels of government. Organizational structures must be inclusive to PWDs and the elderly (International Institute of Rural Reconstruction & Give2Asia, 2018). This may include a sectoral group for the elderly and PWDs that can cater to their issues in the event of emergencies. Drills that include the PWD and elderly must be conducted regularly so that family members and caretakers have adequate knowledge and practice of how to evacuate with their more vulnerable members. The smallest government unit in the Philippines, the *barangay*, must conduct regular home visits to identify beneficiaries and identify issues that can be prepared for (International Institute of Rural Reconstruction & Give2Asia, 2018). Finally, regulations regarding inclusive early-warning systems (National Disaster Risk Reduction and Management Council, 2020) must be monitored up until their fulfillment nationwide.

Response

During calamities, evacuation centers and shelters offer solace and protection to everyone displaced by these events. These shelters must be adequately modified to meet the needs of PWDs and the elderly. Proper queueing and prioritization during meals, adequate dietary modification, and compliance with accessibility requirements as stated by law must be established in these areas. These include the inclusion of PWD restrooms and bath areas, inclusion of guardrails and ramps, and proper lighting to ensure a safe environment for these populations. In addition, adequate manning of these facilities must be enforced. Medical professionals that have proper experience in the care of the elderly and PWDs must be available. This may include physical therapists, nurses, caregivers, and social workers (Benson & Aldrich, 2007).

In emergency situations, these are difficult to prepare. As such, it is imperative that these be planned by the national government organizations in cooperation with the local government units so that these are included in the creation of shelters. A common blueprint for these DRM-inclusive shelters should be provided so to ensure ease and standardization of their construction. Because of the regular use of public schools as evacuation centers in the Philippines, proper enforcement of PWD-inclusive building regulations must be ensured to properly accommodate these populations. Temporary PWD-friendly facilities may be added to these schools to accommodate evacuees should outright renovation of the public-school facilities be impossible.

Recovery, Rehabilitation, and Reconstruction

Livelihood and financial support must be ensured to PWDs and the elderly in the aftermath of calamities. These groups are more vulnerable when it comes to rebuilding their livelihoods compared with able-bodied individuals especially considering their increased financial requirement because of their medical conditions. As such, these groups must be prioritized in any assistance programs and cash-for-work systems. HelpAge International, with COSE has pioneered an assistance program for the elderly with the help of local organizations after Haiyan (Gillam, 2014). This may serve as a blueprint for the local and national government in its livelihood support to these vulnerable groups. Pension packages for the elderly must also be reconsidered to provide financial stability to those who can no longer work.

Further reconstruction of communities must also have the elderly and PWDs in mind. New housing should comply with accessibility laws to ensure adequate living conditions for these special groups. This should also be the case in rebuilding disaster-affected infrastructure. Buildings and facilities must be accessible to wheelchairs and assistive devices and include ramps to enable PWDs to escape through the higher floors should they be trapped by heavy flooding. Regular visits must also be made to assess the status of these individuals and offer special assistance for their needs (MDC, n.d.).

Conclusion

The Philippines is still far from being disability and elderly inclusive with regard to disasters. Despite the yearly onslaught of natural disasters in the country, the government is still not ready to assist these populations when these calamities happen. It is therefore imperative to focus on these populations and include them in all plans from evacuation to rehabilitation.

Further laws must be passed to ensure that these issues are brought to light and legal instruments are provided to encourage local government units and the national government to give due consideration for the plights of these vulnerable populations. Dialogues must be initiated with their representative groups, and they must be included in any discussions on DRM. As one of the most disaster-stricken nations of the world, it is the responsibility of the nation and its government to ensure equity and justice in these vulnerable populations, especially in times of disasters.

A culture of preparedness and resilience cannot be done overnight. It entails years of planning, execution, and constant evaluation to cultivate such culture. The private citizens and NGOs have paved the way toward this path and the government must meet them halfway and lend their support to these populations as dictated by disaster justice. Only then can a perpetual state of readiness be realized not just for the average citizen, but for the marginalized citizenry as well.

References

Adams, V., Kaufman, S., van Hattum, T., & Moody, S. (2011). Aging Disaster: Mortality, Vulnerability, and Long-Term Recovery among Katrina Survivors. *Medical Anthropology*, *30*(3), 247–270. https://doi.org/1 0.1080/01459740.2011.560777

Asian Development Bank. (2021, July). *Disaster Resilience in Asia: A Special Supplement of Asia's Journey to Prosperity: Policy, Market, and Technology Over 50 Years*. https://www.adb.org/publications/disaster-resilience-asia

Asian Disaster Reduction Center. (2009). *Total Disaster Risk Management – Good Practices 2009*. https://www.adrc.asia/publications/TDRM2005/TDRM_Good_Practices/GP2009_e.html

Banas-Nograles, S. L. (2021, November 15). *House Bill No. 10472: An Act Establishing Evacuation Centers in Every Barangay and Appropriating Funds Therefor.* Republic of the Philippines House of Representatives. From https://www.congress.gov.ph/members/search.php?id=banas

Bankoff, G. (2018). Blame, Responsibility and Agency: "Disaster Justice" and the State in the Philippines. *Environment and Planning E: Nature and Space, 1*(3), 363–381. https://doi.org/10.1177/2514848618789381

Benson, W. F., & Aldrich, N. (2007). CDC's Disaster Planning Goal: Protect Vulnerable Older Adults. *CDC Health Aging Program*. https://www.cdc.gov/aging/pdf/disaster_planning_goal.pdf

Bolletino, V., Alcayna, T., Enriquez, K., & Vinck, P. (2018, June). *Perceptions of Disaster Resilience and Preparedness in the Philippines*. Harvard Humanitarian Initiative. https://hhi.harvard.edu/publications/perceptions-disaster-resilience-and-preparedness-philippines

Bolte, P., Marr, S., & Sitompul, D. (2014). *Empowerment and Participation Good Practices from South & South-East Asia in Disability Inclusive Disaster Risk Management*. Handicap International. https://www.preventionweb.net/files/38358_38358hiempowermentandparticipationi.pdf

Canham, C. (2014, May 29). *Philippines: Task Force Launched to Support Older People in Emergencies*. HelpAge International. https://www.helpage.org/newsroom/latest-news/philippines-task-force-launched-to-support-older-people-in-humanitarian-responses/

Casilao, J. L. (2020, November 13). *Catanduanes 70-year-old, PWD Rescued from Ulysses Flooding | News |*. GMA News Online. Retrieved November 11, 2021, from https://www.gmanetwork.com/news/topstories/regions/764036/catanduanes-70-year-old-pwd-rescued-from-ulysses-flooding/story/

Cerrudo, A. (2020, January 20). PCG Saves Two PWDs Accidentally Left behind during Evacuation. *UNTV News*. https://www.untvweb.com/news/pcg-saves-two-pwds-accidentally-left-behind-during-evacuation/

CHRP. (2021, January). *Call for Inputs in Relation to the Human Rights Council Resolution A/Hrc/Res/44/7 on Human Rights and Climate Change*. Commission on Human Rights of the Philippines. https://www.ohchr.org/Documents/Issues/ClimateChange/RightsOlderPersons/ chrphilippines-submission.docx

Clarin, C. B. (2021, July 15). *Disability Inclusiveness Vital to Risk Reduction in the Philippines*. PreventionWeb. Retrieved February 4, 2022, from https://www.preventionweb.net/blog/disability-inclusiveness-vital-risk-reduction-philippines

CNN. (2019, November 7). Thousands of Yolanda Survivors Yet to Benefit from Government Housing Program [Video]. YouTube. https://www.youtube.com/watch?v=bHfCPTKJG9o

Coppola, D. P. (2011). *Introduction to International Disaster Management* [E-book] (2nd ed.). Elsevier Gezondheidszorg.

De Luna-Narido, S., & Tacadao, M. (2021). *A Study on Employment Profile of Persons with Disabilities (PWDs) in Selected Regions in the Philippines*. Institute for Labor Studies, Department of Labor and Employment (Philippines). https://ils.dole.gov.ph/downloads/file/171-a-study-on-employment-profile-of-persons-with-disabilities-pwds-in-selected-regions-in-the-philippines

Deaf Disaster Assistance Team - DRR. (2015, July 6). *Why the Deaf and Blind Are Vulnerable during Disasters*. RAPPLER. Retrieved January 3, 2022, from https://www.rappler.com/moveph/98514-deaf-blind-challenges-disasters/

Domingo, S., & Manejar, A. (2018, December). *Disaster Preparedness and Local Governance in the Philippines*. Philippine Institute for Development Studies. https://pidswebs.pids.gov.ph/CDN/PUBLICATIONS/pidsdps1852.pdf

European Commission Disaster Risk Management Knowledge Centre. (2021). *INFORM Risk Country Risk Profile*. DRMKC - Disaster Risk Management Knowledge Centre. Retrieved October 29, 2021, from https://drmkc.jrc.ec.europa.eu/inform-index/INFORM-Risk/Country-Risk-Profile/moduleId/1767/id/419/controller/Admin/action/CountryProfile

Frohlich, K. L., & Potvin, L. (2008). Frohlich and Potvin Respond. *American Journal of Public Health, 98*(8), 1352. https://doi.org/10.2105/AJPH.2008.141309

Gillam, S. (2014, August 11). *Typhoon Haiyan One Year On: Older People Key to Rebuilding Communities.* HelpAge International. Retrieved January 21, 2022, from https://www.helpage.org/newsroom /latest-news/typhoon-haiyan-one-year-on-older-people-key-to-rebuilding-communities/

Health Justice: Empowering Public Health and Advancing Health Equity - Network for Public Health Law. Network for Public Health Law. (2018). Retrieved 29 January 2022, from https://www.networkfor phl.org/news-insights/health-justice-empowering-public-health-and-advancing-health-equity/.

HelpAge International. (n.d.). *Older People in Disasters and Humanitarian Crises: Guidelines for Best Practice.* https://www.helpage.org/silo/files/older-people-in-disasters-and-humanitairan-crises-guidelines-for-best-practice.pdf

Humanity and Inclusion. (n.d.). *Philippines: Earthquakes Injure Hundreds.* Retrieved January 29, 2022, from https://www.hi-us.org/news_earthquakes_in_the_philippines_humanity_inclusion_responds _to_ the_ needs_of_the_most_vulnerable

Clarinval, C., & Hunt, M. R. (2014). Disaster, Displacement and Justice: Powers and Faden's Theory of Social Justice and the Obligations of Non-governmental Organizations Towards Internally Displaced Persons. *Bioethica Forum.* https://doi.org/10.24894/bf.2014.07020

Imperial, M. F., Morales, Y. B., & VERA Files. (2017, September 17). PWDs Left behind in Marikina's Disaster Preparedness Efforts. *ABS-CBN News.* https://news.abs-cbn.com/focus/09/28/17/pwds-left-behind-in-marikinas-disaster-preparedness-efforts

International Federation of Red Cross. (n.d.). *What Is a Disaster? | IFRC.* IFRC. https://www.ifrc.org/what-disaster

International Institute of Rural Reconstruction & Give2Asia. (2018). *Facilitating Inclusion in Disaster Preparedness: A Practical Guide for CBOs.* https://www.preventionweb.net/publication/facilitating-inclusion-disaster-preparedness-practical-guide-cbos

Ireni-Saban, L. (2012). Challenging Disaster Administration. *Administration & Society, 45*(6), 651–673. https://doi.org/10.1177/0095399712438375

Jerolleman, A. (2019). *Disaster Recovery Through the Lens of Justice* (1st ed., 2019 ed.). Palgrave Pivot.

Jha, S., Martinez, A., Quising, P., Ardaniel, Z., & Wang, L. (2018, March). *Natural Disasters, Public Spending, and Creative Destruction: A Case Study of the Philippines* (No. 817). Asia Development Bank Institute. https://www.adb.org/publications/natural-disasters-public-spending-and-creative-destruction-philippines

Kammerbauer, M., & Wamsler, C. (2017). Social Inequality and Marginalization in Post-disaster Recovery: Challenging the Consensus? *International Journal of Disaster Risk Reduction, 24,* 411–418. https://doi.org/10.1016/j.ijdrr.2017.06.019

Kulcsar, A. (2013, May). *Older People Disproportionately Affected by Typhoon Haiyan.* HelpAge International. Retrieved January 21, 2022, from https://www.helpage.org/newsroom/latest-news/older-people-disproportionately-affected-by-typhoon-haiyan/

Lee, A. C. K. (2016). Barriers to evidence-based disaster management in Nepal: A qualitative study. *Public Health, 133,* 99–106. https://doi.org/10.1016/j.puhe.2016.01.007

Luardo, P. E. N. (2017, October 16). *PWDs Emphasize Need to Involve in Disaster Risk Reduction Programs.* INQUIRER.Net. Retrieved January 22, 2022, from https://cebudailynews.inquirer.net/150751/pwds-emphasize-need-involve-disaster-risk-reduction-programs

Lukasiewicz, A., & Dovers, S. (2018, September). *The Emerging Imperative of Disaster Justice* (No. 405). Bushfire and Natural Hazards CRC. https://www.bnhcrc.com.au/sites/default/files/managed/downloads/405anna_lukasiewicz.pdf

Luna, F. (2020, December 6). *Advocates Laud 'Inclusive' Provisions in 2021 Budget, But Still a Long Way to Go for PWDs.* Phil Star. Retrieved from https://www.philstar.com/headlines/2020/12/06/2061896/advocates-laud-inclusive-provisions-2021-budget-still-long-way-go-pwds.

Maltais, D. (2019). Elderly People with Disabilities and Natural Disasters: Vulnerability of Seniors and Post Trauma. *Journal of Gerontology & Geriatric Medicine, 5*(4), 1–7. https://doi.org/10.24966/ggm-8662/100041

Manlapaz, A., & Center for Disaster Preparedness. (2019, September). *Making the Invisible Visible! The Significance of an Integrated Data Management System for Persons with Disabilities at National Level.* Philippine Statistics Authority. Retrieved from: https://psa.gov.ph/sites/default/files/8.3.3% 20Making%20 the%20Invisible%20Visible%21%20The%20Significance%20of%20an%20Integrated%20Data%20Management%20System%20for%20Persons%20with%20Disabilities%20.pdf

MDC. (n.d.). *When Disaster Strikes – Promising Practices.* From https://www.mdcinc.org/when-disaster-strikes/#:~:text=When%20Disaster%20Strikes%20%2D%20Promising%20Practices,help%20make%20these%20practices%20successful.

National Council on Disability Affairs. (2017). *Operational Framework of Disability Inclusive Development.* http://www.ncda.gov.ph/wp-content/uploads//2017/01/DID_Operational-Framework-2.pdf

National Disaster Risk Reduction and Management Council. (2020). *National Disaster Risk Reduction and Management Plan 2020–2030.* Office of Civil Defense - Policy Development and Planning Service. https://ndrrmc.gov.ph/attachments/article/4147/NDRRMP-Pre-Publication-Copy-v2.pdf

Nick, G. A., Savoia, E., Elqura, L., Crowther, M. S., Cohen, B., Leary, M., Wright, T., Auerbach, J., & Koh, H. K. (2009). Emergency Preparedness for Vulnerable Populations: People with Special Health-care Needs. *Public Health Reports (Washington, DC: 1974), 124*(2), 338–343. https://doi.org/10.1177/003335490912400225

Philippine Statistics Authority. (2005, March). *Senior Citizen Comprised Six Percent of the Population.* Retrieved January 2022, from https://psa.gov.ph/content/senior-citizen-comprised-six-percent-population

Republic Act 7277: Magna Carta for Disabled Persons. (1992, March 24). Official Gazette. https://www.officialgazette. gov.ph/ 1992/03/24/republic-act-no-7277/#:~:text=AN %20ACT%20PROVIDING%20FOR%20THE,SOCIETY%20AND%20FOR%20OTHER%20PURPOSES.&text=SECTION%20 1.,Magna%20Carta%20for%20Disabled%20Persons%E2%80%9D.

Republic Act 10121: Philippine Disaster Risk Reduction and Management Act of 2010. (2010, May 27). Official Gazette. https://www.officialgazette.gov.ph/2010/05/27/republic-act-no-10121/#:~:text=AN %20ACT%20 STRENGTHENING%20THE%20PHILIPPINE,THEREFOR%20AND%20FOR%20OTHER%20 PURPOSES.

Republic Act 10524 – An Act Expanding the Positions Reserved for Persons with Disability, Amending for the Purpose Republic Act No. 7277, As Amended, Otherwise Known as the Magna Carta for Persons with Disability. National Council on Disability Affairs. (2013, April 13). Official Gazette. https://www.ncda. gov.ph/disability-laws/republic-acts/republic-act-no-10524-an-act-expanding-the-positions-reserved-for-persons-with-disability-amending-for-the-purpose-republic-act-no-7277-as-amended-otherwise-known-as-the-magna-carta-for-persons/

Reyes, C., Arboneda, A., & Asis, R. (2019, September). *Silver Linings for the Elderly in the Philippines: Policies and Programs for Senior Citizens.* From https://pidswebs.pids.gov.ph/CDN/PUBLICATIONS/pidsdps1909.pdf

Seeking Social Justice in Disaster. (2021). UCI School of Social Ecology. Retrieved January 29, 2022, from https://socialecology.uci.edu/news/seeking-social-justice-disaster.

Serafica, R. (2015, March 10). *Where Are Persons with Disabilities during Disasters?* RAPPLER. from https://www.rappler.com/moveph/86256-persons-with-disability-disasters-cebu/

Shi, L., & Stevens, G. D. (2021). *Vulnerable Populations in the United States, 3rd Edition (Public Health/Vulnerable Populations)* (3rd ed.). Jossey-Bass.

Shrader-Frechette K. (2012). Nuclear Catastrophe, Disaster-related Environmental Injustice, and Fukushima, Japan: Prima-facie Evidence for a Japanese "Katrina". *Environmental Justice, 5*(3), 133–139.

Stephenson, J., Crane, S. F., Levy, C., & Maslin, M. (2013). Population, Development, and Climate Change: Links and Effects on Human Health. *Lancet (London, England), 382*(9905), 1665–1673. https://doi.org/10.1016/S0140-6736(13)61460-9

Strother, J. (2018, July 13). *For Filipinos with Disabilities: Climate Change and Natural Disasters Are a Dangerous Mix.* The World. From: https://theworld.org/stories/2018-07-13/disabled-community-coastal-philippine-city-feels-forgotten

The New Humanitarian. (2013, November 18). *Typhoon Leaves Elderly More Vulnerable.* https://www.thenewhumanitarian.org/news/2013/11/18/typhoon-leaves-elderly-more-vulnerable

Ton, K., & Adamson, C. (2020). Disaster Justice for People with Disabilities. *Disaster Prevention and Management: An International Journal, 30*(2), 125–136. https://doi.org/10.1108/dpm-08-2020-0248

United Nations. (2015). *Sendai Framework for Disaster Risk Reduction 2015–2030.* https://www.undrr.org/publication/sendai-framework-disaster-risk-reduction-2015-2030

United Nations Office for Disaster Risk Reduction. (2019). *Disaster Risk Reduction in the Philippines Status Report 2019*. United Nations Office for Disaster Risk Reduction (UNDRR), Regional Office for Asia and the Pacific. https://www.unisdr.org/files/68265_682308philippinesdrmstatusreport.pdf

United Nations Office for Disaster Risk Reduction. (2021, July 18). Faces of Resilience – Philippines. [Video]. YouTube. https://www.youtube.com/watch?v=OJeA3SMVySc

United Nations Office for Disaster Risk Reduction - Regional Office for Asia and Pacific. (2013). Haiyan Experiences Confirm Disability Survey Findings. From https://www.undrr.org/news/haiyan-experiences-confirm-disability-survey-findings

Verchick, R. R. M. (2012). Disaster Justice: The Geography of Human Capability. *Duke Environmental Law & Policy Forum, 23*(1), 23–71. https://scholarship.law.duke.edu/delpf/vol23/iss1/2/

What Is Social Justice? (2016). The San Diego Foundation. Retrieved 29 January 2022, from https://www.sdfoundation.org/news-events/sdf-news/what-is-social-justice/

10 Gender Dimension of Disasters in Africa

Building a Gender-Inclusive Culture of Preparedness

Goodness Ogeyi Odey, Ouma Atieno Sarah,
Samar Mohammed Alhaj, and Don Eliseo Lucero-Prisno III

Introduction

Disasters do not discriminate; they affect everyone. However, demographics and existing socioeconomic conditions differentiate how individuals and demographic groups survive and cope during and in the aftermath of disasters. The most vulnerable groups in communities often suffer the most. Gender is one of the key demographic factors that contributes to vulnerability (Halton, 2018). Each time a disaster occurs, it is undeniable that women and girls are more vulnerable, for many reasons. This being underlined by the fact that gender relations greatly influence how women and girls survive, go through, or cope with disasters. When disasters strike, gender inequalities are reinforced, perpetuated, and increased, especially in less developed countries in sub-Saharan Africa (Halton, 2018; Sellers, 2016). In fact, a gender vulnerability approach to disasters (Neumayer and Plümper, 2007) suggests that inequalities in exposure and sensitivity to risk as well as inequalities in access to resources, capabilities, and opportunities systematically disadvantage this group, rendering them more vulnerable to the impact of natural disasters.

Disasters have a cumulative effect on women's vulnerability by impacting on life expectancy. Social capital development is diminished over time particularly those affecting health, family composition, education, and accumulated assets. Economic capital development (such as employment, labor force re-entry, assets, wages, consumption) is also diminished across time. There is diminished political capital and agency (leadership roles, gender-based violence, women as agents of change) (Erman et al., 2021). Other disaster outcomes in which women are disproportionately affected include sexual and gender-based violence—a manifestation of systematic inequality between men and women, which is exacerbated in times of emergency (ARC, 2019; Erman et al., 2021; Yavinsky, 2012).

While discussing gender vulnerability in disasters, it is important to note that it is not a gendered tug of war, but rather a recognition of who needs the most help, in order to catch up with the rest of the post-disaster society. Other important points of emphasis are that disasters encompass a wide range of hazards and that women are a highly diverse group. Further, gender is not solely about women; it is about the relations between males and females and how these relations eventually affect vulnerability in disaster contexts (Erman et al., 2021; Goh, 2012). Understanding how gender relations shape the lives of men and women is critical for disaster risk reduction (DRR). This is due to the differences in men and women's roles, responsibilities, and access to resources, which influence how each will be affected by various hazards, as well as how they will cope with and recover from disaster. Due to unequal power relations between men and women, the latter face a variety of gender-specific vulnerabilities despite their resilience and capacity for survival in the face of disasters (Ciampi, et al., 2011).

DOI: 10.4324/9781003140245-10

In recognition of this vulnerability, gender intersectionality and DRR have been greatly discussed and researched worldwide, focusing on single or multiple disaster events or studying local, country, or international disasters. Previous studies present multi-level approaches, policies, and actions to reduce disaster risk to address the most vulnerable members of communities, including women and girls (ARC, 2019; Center for Research and Epidemiology of Disasters [CRED] Crunch, 2019; Denton, 2002; Dodson, 2007). There is a general consensus among policymakers, scholars, public and private agencies, and relevant stakeholders that understanding the gender implications of natural disasters and climate change is critical to effective disaster risk management that enables communities and countries to be disaster-resilient (ARC, 2019; CRED Crunch, 2019; García-vargas et al., 2008). However, even with this fairly recent interest and growing body of research on the topic of disaster and its gendered impact (Goh, 2012; Sellers, 2016; Schwerhoff and Konte, 2020), there is still a paucity of research and empirical information on sub-Saharan Africa. While most of the findings and scenarios of disaster vulnerability from around the world may apply to African women, it is important that African-centered studies fill a large gap in the literature.

According to Johnson (2011), literature about climate change and gender has so far been written mainly to advocate for a gender perspective within international politics, and that it has been marred by a lack of data and evidence. This signals that caution is necessary when examining evidence for gender-differentiated impacts of disaster to ensure that claims are supported by sound findings and data, and are not merely based on assumptions, projections, or speculations. With the paucity of data on the gendered effects of disaster in Africa, more research is needed. The bulk of the available information on gender and disaster in Africa comes from self-published literature by international organizations, nongovernmental organizations, and private foundations, as well as aid and disaster relief organizations. A smaller but slowly growing body of academic literature is looking into this area, especially in development and environment-related journals, with publications from around two decades or so (Annecke, 2002; Carvajal et al., 2007; García-Vargas et al., 2008; Denton, 2002; Hemmati and Rohr, 2009). While some publications provide a broad overview for navigating gender issues in the context of climate change, most of these are case studies specific to a certain area due to the highly contextual nature of the subject.

Recent literature reviews have mostly focused on gender and climate change-related disasters. Many explicitly cover links between natural disasters and gender (Goh, 2012; Sellers, 2016); others implicitly identify causes of women's vulnerability to climate change, including the increasing prevalence of natural disasters (Schwerhoff and Konte, 2020). Although a significant number of reviews are on climate change and gender, in-depth reviews of the literature on gender in the context of natural disasters are limited. This chapter hopes to deepen the gender equality and policy dialogue. It hopes to add to similar gender-focused work in thematic areas, i.e., DRR. This chapter reviews evidence and data on how men and women of all ages are impacted by and cope with disasters in Africa. Moreover, the chapter identifies the most important knowledge gaps in the channels through which African gender dynamics affect outcomes on the impact of disasters and resilience. In highlighting the scarcity of continent-specific data and current poignant issues, we hope that the review contributes to existing knowledge and practice in the field. It has a broad scope, covering almost all types of natural disasters, focusing on direct and indirect impacts and resilience, including both preparedness and coping capacity, and reviewing literature from developed and developing countries. We hope it calls attention to the need for deeper research into the gender vulnerabilities in disasters in Africa, in line with SDG 5 that advocates for gender equality, and SDG 11 that deals with cities and communities as we collectively and inclusively strive to achieve sustainable development.

Nature of Disasters in Africa

Every year, natural disasters occur on the African continent, and with a fast-growing population and the surging effect of climate change, the impact of disasters on Africa is anticipated to increase over the next few decades (CRED Crunch, 2019). The frequency and severity of natural disasters in the continent varies based on topography, season, and region. According to a 20-year review of disasters in Africa (CRED Crunch, 2019), since 2000, South Africa, Mozambique, and Kenya have experienced 54, 55, and 60 incidents of disaster, respectively, due to storms, droughts, and floods. Nigeria, Ethiopia, and the Democratic Republic of the Congo, three of the most populous countries south of the Sahara, have had 49, 43, and 41 disaster incidents, respectively, and are also among the top ten. Somalia ranks first, for the continent's highest death toll due to the 2010 drought, while Algeria is second in place with the highest number of deaths from a single earthquake (CRED Crunch, 2019).

Most recently, Africa has seen an increase in disaster incidents, mortality numbers, and population impacts. The World Population Prospects (United Nations, 2019) anticipates this problem to persist as Africa's share of the global population increases from around 13% in 2000 to 26% by 2050. Africa's population is expected to grow from 1.3 billion, at present, to 2.5 billion by 2050, roughly doubling the prospective group of people disasters will have an impact on (CRED Crunch, 2019). This high population growth increases the possibility of urbanization in places vulnerable to natural disasters and resource scarcity. Moreover, the Intergovernmental Panel on Climate Change (Hoegh-Guldberg et al., 2018) has declared that in previous decades due to climate change, sub-Saharan Africa has faced more regular and severe climate issues, a course that is likely to progress and worsen as the effects of climate change build up. Extreme heat, droughts, and heavy rains are projected to worsen across the region (Hoegh-Guldberg et al., 2018). All these projections augur poorly for sub-Saharan women, as they form at least half of the population, own less than a third of the property, and are demonstrably more vulnerable to disaster impact than their male counterparts.

Additionally, natural hazards, such as droughts, windstorms, floods, earthquakes, and landslides, damage or destroy a large number of people and economic assets (Ibarrarán et al., 2009). Africa's disasters are invariably the consequence of a mix of natural and human forces. When such conflict and drought combine, famine is a likely result. Soil erosion and vegetation depletion intensify the impact of flood or drought. Poverty and marginalization concentrate social vulnerability (Dodson, 2007). The International Strategy for Disaster Reduction (UNISDR, 2009) defines a disaster as a serious disruption of a community's or society's functioning at any scale as a result of hazardous events interacting with conditions of exposure, vulnerability, and capacity, leading to one or more of the following losses and impacts: human, material, economic, and environmental. Natural hazards become disasters when there is some form of vulnerability (Ibarrarán et al., 2009), with Africa experiencing 23 of the 100 most deadly natural disasters of the 20th century (Emergency Events Database [EM-DAT], 2004 as cited in Dodson, 2007).

Vulnerability of Women to Disaster in Africa

Vulnerability is a state defined by physical, social, economic, and environmental elements or processes that raise an individual's or a community's sensitivity to the effects of risks (UNISDR, 2009). It refers to the characteristics of a person or a group of people, as well as their circumstances that determine their ability to predict, cope with, resist, and recover from the effects of a natural disaster (Singh et al., 2014). Vulnerability determines the likelihood and magnitude of damage from the impact of a given hazard (United Nations Development Program [UNDP], 2004). It represents the physical, economic, political, or social susceptibility or predisposition of a community to damage in the case of a destabilizing phenomenon of natural or human origin (Cardona, 2003; Singh et al., 2014). The vulnerability of women increases dramatically during disaster situations (Caruson et al., 2014); they are likely to suffer more during such events, with women living alone even more at a disadvantage during the period of recovery from disaster (Wisner & Luce, 1993). A plethora of cyclones that have been wreaking havoc on the Southern African region since the 2000s mainly affected women (Chatiza, 2019; Matlakala et al., 2021). The post-evaluation of the effects of Cyclone Idai, which destroyed Mozambique, Zimbabwe, and Malawi in March 2019, revealed that women were more severely affected than men (Matlakala et al., 2021). Women are typically more vulnerable than men during disasters because of their socially created duties and responsibilities (Dankelman, 2008). Two aspects of vulnerabilities women experience as highlighted by Ibarrarán et al. (2009) are biophysical/environmental and social vulnerabilities.

At all levels of the disaster process, preparedness, mitigation, and recovery, gender discrimination occurs and African women have reduced access to essential resources (Dankelman, 2008; Islam, 2012). During disasters, women are often left behind in emergencies due to their lack of knowledge, mobility, and resources. Women refrain from going to shelters during a disaster due to loss of privacy, physical and mental abuse, and torture as their vulnerability further increases when a male head of the household dies (Islam, 2012). They are burdened even more by water, sanitation, and health issues when there is a collapse of livelihood, adding to the double strain of productive and reproductive work (Dankelman, 2008). These roles include food collection, household energy supply, caregiving tasks to children, the sick, and the elderly, and guarding the home and assets. During droughts, it becomes the responsibility of women to provide water for the household; they trek long distances in search of drinking water, and many girls drop out of school to assist the household with such tasks (Dankelman, 2008).

Women are vulnerable to reproductive and sexual health problems. Disasters cause women to experience miscarriages, premature delivery, and delivery-related complications (Islam, 2012). Girls in Malawi are married off early in times of drought mostly to older men with multiple sexual partners. They are forced to have sex in exchange for gifts or money and this increases the spread of HIV/AIDS in the country (Dankelman, 2008). A similar case was well reported in Uganda in which there was a surge in child marriage, domestic violence, and rape during drought (Opondo et al., 2016; Matlakala et al., 2021).

Cyclones, floods, and droughts typically affect the agricultural sector. Female farmers in South Africa reported that women are forced to stay at home because the disasters limit their progress and production, for example when crops are washed away during a flood (Matlakala et al., 2021). Livestock and poultry are also impacted. Women are unable to enter the market to sell items, such as milk, eggs, vegetables, or other products, due to damaged infrastructure and communication systems. They are forced to trade for lesser rates supplied by male purchasers. As a result, there is a net loss of income, making disaster recovery even more difficult for households (Islam, 2012).

The vulnerabilities of women to disasters in Africa are caused by a lack of integration of women into the disaster preparedness planning process, restriction to household tasks due to gender norms, a low social standing (Matlakala et al., 2021). Gendered inequalities in bargaining power in the community, labor market, and legal institutions also contribute to the vulnerability of women during disasters (Chant, 2007; Flatø et al., 2017). Women have less representation at all levels of decision-making (Wisner & Luce, 1993). The vulnerability of African women to gender-based violence during disasters is caused by a loss of the source of income. Men take advantage of women's social status during and after disasters, subjecting them to all sorts of discriminative treatments (Matlakala et al., 2021). In the aftermath of a disaster, surviving women living in poverty find it harder to recover because they had been typically living in a state of crisis before the advent of a disaster. Poor women are more likely to experience significant challenges to their livelihood security with deeper levels of poverty; they are often without the financial means to support themselves following a disaster.

Generally, women face obstacles to receiving relief services, and this is usually aggravated by religion and caste bias (Enarson et al., 2018). Women survivors also face harsh and sometimes violent socioeconomic conditions in the aftermath of a disaster, including increased exposure to domestic and sexual violence, inadequate compensation for losses, long-term economic hardship, long-term displacement, limited health care, and a lack of voice in recovery and rebuilding efforts (Caruson et al., 2014). The mental health status of women is also compromised after a disaster, especially on the death or disappearance of their husbands or children. This causes depression and post-traumatic stress due to feelings of solitude and isolation (Pan American Health Organization, [PAHO], 2004). Mental health care is unlikely to be received by low-income women (Caruson et al., 2014).

Men and women have different duties, roles, and capacities, so disasters affect them differently. Women, for example, have less access to factors of production, such as land and capital. Again, the nature of their work predisposes them to hazards, such as gathering firewood, air pollution from cooking with dirty energy, and general unemployment; these challenges impede their resilience in the aftermath of disasters. While Kenya has made progress toward gender mainstreaming, several gender inequality cracks remain (Maobe, 2021).

Disaster Risk and Gender in Africa

This section underlines the gender aspect of disaster risk and risk reduction, gender intersectionality perspectives, and ways of gender mainstreaming in disasters in Africa. According to the World Risk Report 2021, Oceania has the highest disaster risk, mainly due to its high exposure to extreme natural events. Africa is second, followed by the Americas, Asia, and Europe in descending order of disaster risk. Africa is also the continent with the highest overall societal vulnerability. Twelve of the 15 most vulnerable countries in the world are African, with the most vulnerable country in the world being the Central African Republic, followed by Chad, and the Democratic Republic of the Congo. With these levels of vulnerability to risk among the general population in Africa, it would be important to look closer at more vulnerable populations on the continent: in this case, women and girls.

One way to study the different group vulnerabilities to climate change is to take gender as an analytical category. As aforesaid, the common trend of the gender perspective is that women are more affected by adverse climate change than men (Matlakala et al., 2021; Neumayer & Plümper, 2007; Yavinsky, 2012). In fact, international policies and guidelines like the Paris Climate Agreement include specific provisions as seen in the Preamble, Article 7, paragraph 5 and Article 11, paragraph 2 to ensure women receive support to cope with the hazards of climate change (UNFCC, 2015).

Some of the different gendered impacts of the disaster are discussed below.

Increased Mortality Rates

Gender-focused quantitative analysis of mortality rates or summary mortality measures such as life expectancy can help determine whether the anecdotal evidence collected post disasters reflects a general trend. As pointed out by Neumayer and Plümper (2007), much of the existing literature on disaster mortality rates in Africa, either do not estimate gender-specific mortality rates and patterns at all, or are confined to single events such that no general conclusions can be drawn. In light of this, the only specific statistics for the African continent, with much of the data being anecdotal or only covering single events. And while the general/worldwide trends may apply to African women and or disasters, it is important to note that without actual figures, this may only speculate and not fully apply to this demographic.

According to the UNDP (2010), disasters reduce African women's life expectancy more so than men. Women, boys, and girls are 14 times more likely than men to die during a disaster (ARC, 2019). This might conflict with face value figures. For example, men account for 70% of flood-related deaths in Europe and the United States. This is for various reasons, including an overrepresentation of men in rescue professions. In less developed countries, similar to those on the African continent, more women tend to die from disasters. This is because gender gaps in access to information on disaster preparedness, access to public shelters, and limits to mobility contribute more to gendered mortality outcomes, putting women at a disadvantage (Neumayer & Plümper, 2007).

More women dying in disasters is reported in the findings of Neumayer and Plümper (2007), spanning across 141 countries in 20 years, including African countries, such as Mozambique, Zimbabwe, South Africa, and Malawi as found in older studies (Ager et al., 1995). More recent research (Chatiza, 2019; Matlakala et al., 2021) discovered that natural disasters and their aftermath on average kill more women than men or kill women at an earlier age than men, narrowing the gender gap in life expectancy. The more fatal the disaster, the stronger this effect on the gender gap in life expectancy. That is, major calamities lead to more severe impacts on female life expectancy (relative to that of males) than do smaller disasters. Women's vulnerability to disaster has been worsened due to their low socioeconomic status. While no one cause was clear, besides the aforesaid, similar patterns have shown that men were more likely to evacuate faster (physical strength), while women lost precious evacuation time trying to look after dependants, were inhibited from moving/evacuating by pregnancy, clothing, and religio-cultural practices that required them to either be accompanied by a male relative or have their permission to move (Neumayer & Plümper, 2007; Yavinsky, 2012). To elaborate further, in cultural communities that require modest clothing, women and girls may find it harder to run away from danger (i.e., an approaching tsunami or a collapsed building) because of the barriers their clothing may create. Additionally, modest dress and/ or cultural norms may mean females engage in different cultural and recreational activities. This could mean girls may not be taught how to swim or to climb trees. This creates barriers that make it difficult to take care of themselves when trying to survive flooding.

In contrast, some literature argues that disasters do not portend disadvantages to women's life and health. Rivers (1982) asserts that in principle, women are physiologically at an advantage in famines and droughts because, unless they are pregnant or lactating, they can better cope with food shortages due to their lower nutritional requirements and higher body fat (Rivers, 1982). Toole et al. (1997), in their review of the literature, state that on the whole, there is no reason to suspect that diseases related to natural disasters will systematically disadvantage women. This would partly explain why overall mortality rates for females are often lower in many famines, particularly the very severe ones of the 19th and early 20th centuries, than for men (Macintyre, 2002). Contributing to the trend, in some African famines like the Ethiopian famines during the 1970s and 1984–1985, more female than male famine victims died at a very young age or in infancy, which was attributed to a discriminatory access to food resources in times of famine with a bias against female babies and children (Kidane, 1989, 1990; Greenough, 1982). Another explanation is the association between post-disaster female childhood mortality and maternal mortality and their detriment to the social infrastructures causing reduced access to food, hygiene, health services, and clean water (Toole et al., 1997). When this basic health care infrastructure is severely damaged or health expenditures are reduced to reallocate public funds for immediate disaster response purposes, obstetrical care is usually reduced, leading to maternal and infant mortality. This, as could be informedly guessed, would be crippling for a continent like Africa that already faces high infant and maternal mortality rates (Neumayer & Plümper, 2007).

Displacement

Worldwide, U.N. figures indicate that 80% of people displaced by climate change are women (Halton, 2018). According to the Internal Displacement Monitoring Centre's report on Women in Displacement (IDMC, 2020), the African continent is home to 1/3 of the world's refugee population. The highest proportion of these are refugee children and females, at 51% and 59% respectively. Kenya, Uganda, and Ethiopia are among the top ten countries worldwide for refugee and displaced persons populations, and even then, they house a greater proportion of girls than boys.

While boys and girls are affected by crisis and conflict, the face of displacement in Africa is undoubtedly and disproportionately that of women and girls (IDMC, 2020). As for internally displaced persons, estimates by the Centre show that at least 21 million women and girls were uprooted within their countries by disasters, conflict, and violence by the end of 2018. This formed more than half of the 41 million IDPs in the world at the time. Two-thirds of these internally displaced women and girls were in Africa and the Middle East. Further, five of the nine countries worldwide with over one million internally displaced women and girls were African countries. They included the Democratic Republic of the Congo, Somalia, Nigeria, Ethiopia, and Sudan. Keeping up with those figures, the Centre estimates that, in many cases, the proportion of women and girls in displaced populations is higher than that of men and boys, and also higher than in the national population. In Burkina Faso, for instance, where violence led to a ten-fold increase in displacements in 2019, 65% of adult IDPs are women. This is likely because many men are forcibly recruited to fight by armed groups, so were unable to flee with the women (IDMC, 2020).

In recognition of the pertinence of this issue, the 32nd African Union Summit in February marked 2019 as "The 'Year of the Refuges, Returnees and Internally Displaced Persons" and sought to find "durable solutions to forced displacement" (GPE, 2019). Together with its partners, the AU tabled discussions on the gender dimensions of forced displacement, especially of its impact on girls. Further initiatives toward this end include Gender Is My Agenda (GIMAC) launched before the 33rd AU Summit. The 33rd GIMAC, under the theme "Towards Gender-Responsive Durable Solutions to Forced Displacement" provided a unique Pan-African platform for civil society to leverage its influence and their partners' on the AU gender equality agenda across six areas (governance, peace and security, human rights, health, education, and economic empowerment) (GPE, 2019). As an accountability platform, GIMAC also monitored the implementation of the AU's Solemn Declaration on Gender Equality in Africa. The AU's 3rd High Level Dialogue on Gender, Education, and Protection of Schools in Humanitarian Settings also addressed the vulnerability of displaced girls and boys to ensure their continued schooling in humanitarian and emergency situations (GPE, 2019). With all the aforeseen political and regional commitments to address the gender needs of displaced populations, it is important that the scale shifts from intention and strategy to actual action and accountability.

Work and Labor

Globally, women are more likely to experience poverty, and to have less socioeconomic power than men. This makes it difficult to recover from disasters that affect infrastructure, jobs, and housing (Halton, 2018). This shows that women are more adversely affected economically, by disasters. This could therefore explain why women having a greater socioeconomic power has a protective effect in the face of climate change and associated disasters, both mortality-wise and adaptability and survival post event. However, African women own less than 1/3 of land and property on the continent and that has created a bleak scenario. They own significantly less land than men, averaging 15% in sub-Saharan Africa, ranging from less than 8.8% in DRC, and just over 30% in Botswana and Malawi. As a result, when a man dies, women and family are often left without land, leaving them highly vulnerable to falling into poverty when disaster strikes (Neumayer and Plümper, 2007; Yavinsky, 2012; World Risk Report, 2021).

Results from Neumayer and Plümper's (2007) analysis reveals that the deleterious impact of disasters on women particularly on the gender gap in life expectancy reduced with women's access to socioeconomic opportunities. Gender disproportionalities in labor post-disaster in Africa can also influence resilience to future disasters, creating a negative feedback loop. For example, in the context of frequent flood exposure, prevailing social norms may drive women to stay close to their homes so they can salvage belongings when the flood comes, while men pick up employment outside the community. Therefore, the nearby labor opportunities available to women may not offer the income and stability they need to respond efficiently to flood exposure, which in turn affects their capacity to cope with future shocks (World Risk Report, 2021).

Changes in Socioeconomic Status

Climate change-related disasters have a significant impact on securing basic needs like food, water, and fuel—domestic responsibilities mostly done by women and girls. Extremes of climate often force women and girls to walk farther, work harder, and spend more of their time collecting water and fuel, and caring for plants and livestock, often for much lower yields. According to Oxfam, women have a harder time accessing and providing water and WASH amenities for their families after hydro meteorological disasters (OXFAM, 2018). Girls may have to drop out of school to help their mothers with these tasks, continuing the cycle of poverty and inequity (Yavinsky, 2012).

Reports as recent as 2021 (World Risk Report, 2021) show that boys and girls are affected differently by disasters. For health outcomes, boys are disadvantaged when affected *in utero* or during early life due to biological factors. However, the preferred treatment of boys means that girls are worse off when their families face disaster-related scarcity. Girls are more likely to be taken out of school if their families cannot afford tuition or the domestic burden increases after a disaster. They are also more likely to be married off so that their dowry ensures family socioeconomic security. On the other hand, if labor needs increase—for example, in agriculture—boys are more likely to be taken out of school (World Risk Report, 2021). Economically, disasters have different effects for men and women, with women largely disadvantaged.

In African countries, agriculture is the most important economic sector for female employment, and women farmers tend to be more vulnerable to disasters than male farmers. The domestic burden also tends to increase after a disaster, and women usually bear the brunt of this, at the cost of missing out on other income-generating activities. In some cultures, women are forbidden from owning property, being in charge of finances or having bank accounts. With this cultural practices and limited access to bank accounts, their assets are less protected than men's. For example, women end up holding a larger share of their assets in tangible form, and are therefore at greater risk of losing their assets than men, which would worsen economic inequality (Yavinsky, 2012; World Risk Report, 2021).

During recovery, women and girls may have to work harder to carry out the functions of daily living for their families. This can include lining up for relief supplies, having to travel farther to access water or cooking under challenging conditions. These activities often happen during the day, limiting the access women and girls have to education or employment. After a disaster, women will likely be responsible for caring for the sick and injured while still maintaining their daily chores; and if the main breadwinner is killed during the disaster, women often need to seek outside employment, especially in an international context, girls are pulled from school to take care of the household (World Risk Report, 2021).

Increased Incidence of Sexual and Gender-Based Violence

Increased incidence of violence against women, including sexual assault and rape, have also been documented in the wake of disasters. According to the UNFPA, disasters create conditions that intensify and drastically heighten pre-existing SGBV risk factors and incidences due to reduced coping capacities, pressure, and strain (Yavinsky, 2012). What happens is that disaster-affected people often spend long periods in collective or evacuation centers, where living conditions are routinely cramped, with little private space for couples and families. For example, women living in relief centers were reportedly being violently forced into sex by their husbands despite their reluctance due to concerns about over-crowding and lack of privacy (Yavinsky, 2012).

Girls got taken out of school to generate cash through sex work, and during periods of drought, women and children who were forced to walk farther to water wells reported instances of rape and abuse. Some SGBV centers record increases in new domestic violence cases reported after hydro meteorological disasters. They also see an increased incidence of child trafficking and prostitution, entry into commercial sex work, and increasing child brides in the region (ARC, 2019). Following a disaster, it is more likely that women will be victims of domestic and sexual violence; many even avoid using shelters for fear of being sexually assaulted.

Discrimination and Reduced Emergency Preparedness to Support Women Affected by Disasters

In societies with existing patterns of gender discrimination, like the mostly patriarchal African societies, males are likely to be given preferential treatment in rescue and humanitarian efforts (Neumayer and Plümper, 2007). When natural disaster strikes, these pre-existing discriminatory practices become exacerbated ending in discrimination and reduced access to resources by women and girls, intensifying the detriment to their health and wellbeing. African women are marginalized in their access to relief resources and services like rescue services, relief food, and sanitation packages in climatic disasters. Despite the relief efforts intended for the entire population of a disaster-affected area, the existing patriarchal structure of resource distribution within the society and the unequal power structure are considered a reflection of gender inequality in the context of disasters (Neumayer and Plümper, 2007). One example is during famine where men accessed and were allocated assistance to families, distributing resources with a distinct sex bias against females and an age bias against children. Concomitantly, female children were more adversely affected by the famine. Even in the absence of natural disasters, the report found that

> there is a good deal of evidence from all over the world that food is often distributed very unequally within the family—with a distinct sex bias (against the female) and also an age bias (against the children). When natural disaster strikes, these pre-existing discriminatory practices become exacerbated and their detrimental health impact on women and girls is intensified
>
> (Neumayer & Plümper, 2007)

Again, such findings would not be foreign to the African context; in fact, they would fit it since most sub-Saharan communities are patriarchal, with men as the head of the family. That means that the decision-making structure heavily depends on and is influenced by men, even as regards post-disaster relief. This is supported by a study of Mozambican refugees in Malawi in the late 1990s wherein policies on relief were biased in favor of refugee men (Neumayer & Plümper, 2007).

The PAHO (2002) suggests that this anecdotal evidence from a few natural disasters might be representative of a more general trend, further suggesting unequal power structures as the underlying cause:

> The majority of relief efforts are intended for the entire population of a disaster affected area; however, when they rely on existing structures of resource distribution that reflects the patriarchal structure of society, women are marginalized in their access to relief resources.

Disaster researchers agree, noting that in most countries, relief efforts are almost exclusively managed and controlled by men, systematically excluding women, their needs, competencies, and experiences from contributing to these efforts (Bradshaw, 2004; Enarson, 2000). The net effect of this patriarchal system is that women have reduced access to essential services that affect their health and wellbeing, like food, water, health, and sanitation products. Women would also have restricted access to post-disaster relief funds and resources. This means that women have reduced chances of surviving and coping from disasters. This could easily be remedied, as found by Neumayer and Plümper (2007). In principle, recovery assistance could be preferentially aimed at those most vulnerable groups to protect them from the negative effects of increased discrimination. Yet, as mentioned above, instead of being granted a preferential role, African women are still often marginalized in their access to relief resources.

Underrepresentation in Disaster Risk Management Planning and Policy

The average representation of women in national and global climate negotiating bodies is below 30% (Halton, 2018). Gender inequality at the community and international level hampers women's capacity and potential to be actors of climate action. The inequalities in access to information and control over resources and the decision-making processes define and limit what women can do in the context of climate change and disaster risk management and policy (Halton, 2018). Nevertheless, according to the UNIDSR 2009 report, disasters could also create opportunities for women as change agents. Disasters can provide opportunities to redress gender disparities. Gender-sensitive programming can lead men and women to challenge long-standing gender biases, thereby providing an opportunity to transform discriminatory and harmful practices inherent in society. However, such opportunities will be lost if women are left out of planning for disaster response or risk reduction measures (UNISDR, 2009). Unfortunately, as recognized by the African Risk Capacity Group Gender Strategy and Action Plan (ARC, 2019), and as trends across the globe show, disaster management and response are traditionally viewed as 'men's business' – planned by men, for men. As a result, African women's different and specific needs during a disaster are often not understood or addressed. Thus, while women's vulnerability to disasters is often highlighted, their role in fostering a culture of resilience and their active contribution to building disaster resilience has often been overlooked and has not been adequately recognized.

Women are largely marginalized in the development of DRM policy- and decision-making processes and their voices go unheard (UNISDR, 2009). In developing countries of African continent, women are often given no education or independence and they lack employment opportunities. As a result, they are under-represented in society. Globally, the proportion of seats held by women in national parliaments was only 24% as of 2019. The UN Climate Change Conference COP24 in 2018 had only 38% representation of women, indicating only 1% increase from the previous year

(CDP, 2021). These numbers demonstrate the lack of participation of women in key policy and decision-making, limiting their ability to advocate for climate solutions. Two-fifths of countries worldwide limit women's property rights; in 19 countries, women still do not have equal ownership rights to immovable property (CDP, 2021). Disregarding half of the world's population and their needs will not bring sustainable, inclusive, or holistic climate-mitigation actions.

Conclusions/Recommendations

Amid these vulnerabilities discussed thus far, women have shown resilience in disaster situations. They have created coping strategies as individuals and found ways to adapt to these situations as a community. Coping mechanisms could be indigenous or modern with most communities using indigenous methods based on socioeconomic status (Mavhura et al., 2013). Because of the major role of women as primary care providers for both the young and the elderly, women play a key part in a community's ability to mitigate, prepare for, and recover from disasters all over the world (Caruson et al., 2014). A study by Dayour et al., (2014) reported that to adapt to flooding in Ghana that destroys farmlands close to riverbanks, farmers worked on highlands, avoiding the valleys. To face droughts, women adapted by planting drought-resistant seeds to increase a household's food security or by resorting to livestock rearing; to face rainstorms, they planted trees around houses that serve as windbreaks (Dayour et al., 2014). Other strategies include raising the kitchen and storeroom platforms during flooding, reducing food consumption and dependence on inexpensive foods, collecting wild fruits, searching for alternative sources of income, selling financial assets, and obtaining loans from moneylenders as well as from financial institutions (Mavhura et al., 2013).

Gender relations are part of the human experiences that arise from disasters each time a disaster occurs. Therefore, the inclusion and advancement of gender mainstreaming or responsiveness into DRR is a pertinent need, especially when the world faces numerous disasters, including emerging ones, such as COVID-19. While it is encouraging that most African countries and regional and economic blocks have plans and guidelines on gender and disaster risk management, it is important that we shift the weight from the intent and plan to action. We need to create and implement interventions that fit the African situation and evolve disaster responses in ways that capitalize on solving inequality. These efforts call for training, a community leadership network, and a rethink of policies for research and practice to address the local people's sufferings in the face of disasters and lost livelihoods. There is a need for gender mainstreaming in incorporating local technical resources, such as knowledge, insights, skills, personnel, desires, and needs, in identifying problems and proffering solutions to disaster preparedness, mitigation, and management. The goal is to reduce urgent and long-term vulnerability, both in terms of natural disaster risk and social vulnerability. Additionally, in disaster research and mitigation approaches, priority should be given to generating Africa-specific empirical data. There should also be institutional development in disaster research, and infrastructural systems strengthening, encouraging, and supporting women's political representation and disaster risk management leadership are also vital to have a continent where no one is left behind even in the face of present or future catastrophes.

References

African Risk Capacity [ARC]. (2019). *Gender strategy and action plan*. https://arc.int/sites/default/files/2021-09/ARC_Gender-Strategy_2019.pdf

Ager, A., Ager, W., & Long, L. (1995). The differential experience of Mozambican refugee women and men. *The Journal of Refugee Studies*, 8(3), 265–287. doi: 10.1093/jrs/8.3.265. PMID: 12291584.·

Annecke, W. J. (2002). Climate change, energy-related activities and the likely social impacts on women in Africa. *International Journal of Global Environmental Issues*, 2, 207–222.

Bradshaw, S. (2004). *Socioeconomic impacts of natural disasters: a gender analysis.* Serie Manuales 33. United Nations Economic Commission for Latin America and the Caribbean.

Cardona, O. D. (2003). *The need for rethinking the concepts of vulnerability and risk from a holistic perspective: a necessary review and criticism for effective risk management.* Bankoff.

Carjaval Escobar, Yesid, Quintero-Angel, Mauricio, & García-Vargas, M. (2007). *The women's role in the adaptation to climate variability and climate change: its contribution to the risk management.* AGU Spring Meeting Abstracts. https://www.researchgate.net/publication/252560515_The_Women's_Role_in_the_Adaptation_to_Climate_Variability_and_Climate_Change_Its_Contribution_to_the_Risk_Management

Caruson, K., Alhassan, O., Ayivor, J., & Ersing, R. (2014). Disaster and development in Ghana: improving disaster resiliency at the local level. In N. Kapucu & K. Liou (Eds.), *Disaster and development: environmental hazard* (pp. 213–287). Springer, Cham. https://doi.org/10.1007/978-3-319-04468-2_16

CDP-Centre for Disaster Philanthropy (2021). *Women and girls in disasters.* https://disasterphilanthropy.org/resources/women-and-girls-in-disasters/

Center for Research and Epidemiology of Disasters [CRED] Crunch. (2019). *Disasters in Africa: 20 year review (2000–2019*)*, issue No. 56. https://www.google.com/url?q=https://cred.be/sites/default/files/CredCrunch56.pdf&sa=D&source=docs&ust=1641497135754204&usg=AOvVaw3FiQEEXoaYUyxAwpPXhgtc

Chant, S. H. (2007). *Gender, generation and poverty: exploring the feminisation of poverty in Africa, Asia and Latin America.* Edward Elgar Publishing. ISBN: 978 1 84376 992 7. http://www.e-elgar.co.uk/

Chatiza, K. (2019). *Cyclone Idai in Zimbabwe: An analysis of policy implications for post-disaster institutional development to strengthen disaster risk management.* OXFAM. https://doi.org/10.21201/2019.5273

Ciampi, Maria Caterina, Gell, Fiona, Lasap, Lou, & Turvill, Edward (2011). *Gender and disaster risk reduction: a training pack.* https://docs.google.com/document/d/1h0CuciCqjBDyHgKXNYZiwOjVtZZmcQ9lYf5o5AIqxdQ/edit

Clack, Zoanne, Keim, Mark, Macintyre, Anthony, & Yeskey, Kevin (2002). Emergency health and risk management in sub-Saharan Africa: a lesson from the embassy bombings in Tanzania and Kenya. *Prehospital and Disaster Medicine*, 17, 59–66. 10.1017/S1049023X00000194. https://www.researchgate.net/publication/10974220_Emergency_Health_and_Risk_Management_in_Sub-Saharan_Africa_A_Lesson_from_the_Embassy_Bombings_in_Tanzania_and_Kenya

Dankelman, I. E. M. (2008). *Gender, climate change and human security lessons from Bangladesh, Ghana and Senegal.* Gender and Disaster Network, Newcastle upon Tyne. https://hdl.handle.net/2066/72456

Dayour, F., Yendaw, E. and Jasaw, G.S. (2014). "Local residents' perception and adaptation/coping strategies to climate-induced disasters in Bankpama, Wa West District, Ghana", International Journal of Development and Sustainability, Vol. 3 No. 12, pp. 2186–2205.

Denton, Fatima. (2002). Climate change vulnerability, impacts, and adaptation: why does gender matter? *Gender & Development,* 10, 10–20. https://doi.org/10.1080/13552070215903

Dodson, B. (2007). Natural disasters in Africa. In J. Lidstone, L. M. Dechano, & J. P. Stoltman (Eds.), *International perspectives on natural disasters: occurrence, mitigation, and consequences. Advances in natural and technological hazards research* (vol. 21, pp. 231–245) Springer, Dordrecht. https://doi.org/10.1007/978-1-4020-2851-9_12

Enarson, E. (2000). *Gender and natural disasters: working paper no. 1 in focus programme on crisis response and reconstruction.* International LabourOrganisation, Recovery and Reconstruction Department.

Enarson, E., Fothergill, A., & Peek, L. (2018). Gender and disaster: foundations and new directions for research and practice. In H. Rodríguez, W. Donner, & J. Trainor (Eds.), *Handbook of disaster research* (pp. 205–223). Springer, Cham. https://doi.org/10.1007/978-3-319-63254-4_11

Erman, Alvina, De VriesRobbe, Sophie Anne, Thies, Stephan Fabian, Kabir, Kayenat, & Maruo, Mirai (2021). *Gender dimensions of disaster risk and resilience: existing evidence.* © *World Bank.* https://openknowledge.worldbank.org/handle/10986/35202 License: CC BY 3.0 IGO. https://openknowledge.worldbank.org/handle/10986/35202

Flatø, M., Muttarak, R., & Pelser, A. (2017). Women, weather, and woes: the triangular dynamics of female-headed households, economic vulnerability, and climate variability in South Africa. *World Development*, 90, 41–62. https://doi.org/10.1016/j.worlddev.2016.08.015

García-Vargas, M., Escobar, Yesid, & Quintero-Angel, Mauricio (2008). *Women's role in adapting to climate change and variability.* AdvGeosci. 14. 10.5194/adgeo-14-277–2008. https://www.researchgate.net/publication/29631622_Women's_role_in_adapting_to_climate_change_and_variability

Goh Amelia, H. X. (2012). *A literature review of the gender-differentiated impacts of climate change on women's and men's assets and well-being in developing countries.* https://www.worldagroforestry.org/sites/default/files/4.pdf

GPE (2019). *Forced displacement in Africa has a female face: Africa's bold steps to address the gender dimension of forced displacement and its impact on the education of girls.* Global Partnership for Education Secretariat.

Greenough, P. R. (1982). *Prosperity and misery in modern Bengal – the famine of 1943–1944.* Oxford University Press, Oxford.

Halton, M. (2018). *Climate change 'impacts women more than men'.* BBC News. https://www.bbc.com/news/science-environment-43294221

Hemmati, Minu, & Rohr, Ulrike (2009). Engendering the climate-change negotiations: experiences, challenges, and steps forward. *Gender & Development*, 17, 19–32. 10.1080/13552070802696870. https://www.researchgate.net/publication/240536735_Engendering_the_climate-change_negotiations_Experiences_challenges_and_steps_forward

Hoegh-Guldberg, O., Jacob, D., Taylor, M., Bindi, M., Brown, S., Camilloni, I., Diedhiou, A., Djalante, R., Ebi, K. L., Engelbrecht, F., Guiot, J., Hijioka, Y., Mehrotra, S., Payne, A., Seneviratne, S. I., Thomas, A., Warren, R., & Zhou, G. (2018). *Impacts of 1.5C global warming on natural and human systems.* IPCC. https://www.ipcc.ch/site/assets/uploads/sites/2/2019/06/SR15_Chapter3_Low_Res.pdf

Ibarrarán, M. E., Ruth, M., Ahmad, S., & London, M. (2009). Climate change and natural disasters: macroeconomic performance and distributional impacts. *Environment, Development and Sustainability*, 11(3), 549–569. https://doi.org/10.1007/s10668-007-9129-9

Internal Displacement Monitoring Centre [IDMC]. (2020). *Thematic series- hidden in plain sight, women and girls in internal displacement.* 202003-twice-invisible-internally-displaced-women.pdf (internal-displacement.org)

Islam, M. R. (2012). Vulnerability and coping strategies of women in disaster: a study on coastal areas of Bangladesh. *Arts Faculty Journal*, 4, 147–169. https://doi.org/10.3329/afj.v4i0.12938

Johnson, Cassidy (2011). *Creating an enabling environment for reducing disaster risk: recent experience of regulatory frameworks for land, planning and building in low and middle-income countries.* https://www.preventionweb.net/english/hyogo/gar/2011/en/bgdocs/Johnson_2011.pdf

Kidane, A. (1989). Demographic consequences of the 1984–1985 Ethiopian famine. *Demography*, 26(3), 515–522.

Kidane, A. (1990). Mortality estimates of the 1984–85 Ethiopian famine. *Scandinavian Journal of Social Medicine*, 18(4), 281–286.

Matlakala, F. K., Nyahunda, L., & Makhubele, J. C. (2021). Population's vulnerability to natural disasters in Runnymede Village at Tzaneen Local Municipality, South Africa. *Humanities and Social Sciences Reviews*, 9(4), 160–166. https://doi.org/10.18510/hssr.2021.9423

Maobe, Atela (2021). *Gender intersectionality and disaster risk reduction- Context Analysis: Tomorrow's cities urban risk in transition.* https://docs.google.com/document/d/1-MTkTngKgKXgWmE0AW5ybfYfIhlSkL3U7u5wHmkKb3c/edit

Mavhura, E., and Mucherera, B. (2020). Flood survivors' perspectives on vulnerability reduction to floods in Mbire district, Zimbabwe. *Jàmbá J. Disaster Risk Stud.* 12, 1–12. doi: 10.4102/jamba.v12i1.663

Neumayer, E., & Plümper, T. (2007). The gendered nature of natural disasters: the impact of catastrophic events on the gender gap in life expectancy, 1981–2002. *Annals of the Association of American Geographers*, 97(3), 551–566. https://doi.org/10.1111/j.1467-8306.2007.00563.x

Opondo, M., Abdi, U., & Nangiro, P. (2016). Assessing gender in resilience programming: Uganda. *BRACED Resilience Intel*, 2(2), 1–16. https://assets.publishing.service.gov.uk/media/57a08964e5274a27b2000069/Assessing_gender_in_resilience_programming-Uganda_10215.pdf

OXFAM. (2018). *The weight of water on women: the long wake of hurricane María in Puerto Rico: identi-fying and analysing the gendered impacts of Hurricane María on WASH practices in rural communities of Puerto Rico.* https://www.oxfamamerica.org/explore/research-publications/research-backgrounder-wash-gender-report-puerto-rico/

Pan-American Health Organization [PAHO]. (2002). *Gender and natural disasters.* Pan-American Health Organization, Washington DC.

Pan American Health Organization, [PAHO]. (2004). *Management of dead bodies in disaster situations.* https://iris.paho.org/handle/10665.2/6252

Rivers, J. (1982), Women and children last: an essay on sex discrimination in disasters. *Disasters*, 6, 256–267. https://doi.org/10.1111/j.1467-7717.1982.tb00548.x

Schwerhoff, Gregor, & Konte, Maty (2020). *Gender and climate change: towards comprehensive policy options.* 10.1007/978-3-030-14935-2_4. https://www.researchgate.net/publication/334125576_Gender_and_Climate_Change_Towards_Comprehensive_Policy_Options

Sellers (2016) *Gender and age inequality of disaster risk.* https://reliefweb.int/sites/reliefweb.int/files/re-sources/Gender%20and%20age%20inequality%20of%20disaster%20risk.pdf

Singh, S. R., Eghdami, M. R., & Singh, S. (2014). The concept of social vulnerability: a review from disasters perspectives. *International Journal of Interdisciplinary and Multidisciplinary Studies*, 1(6), 71–82. http://www.ijims.com/

Toole, Michael J., & Noji, Eric K. (1997). The historical development of public health responses to disasters. *Disasters*, 21(4), 366–376. https://www.burnet.edu.au/system/publication/file/750/Noji_and_Toole_1997.pdf

United Nations. (2019). *World population prospects.* https://population.un.org/wpp/

United Nations Development Programme [UNDP] (2004). *Reducing disaster risk: a challenge for development-a global report.* Bureau for Crisis and Recovery. https://www.undp.org/sites/g/files/zsk-gke326/files/publications/Reducing%20Disaster%20risk%20a%20Challenge%20for%20development.pdf

United Nations Development Programme [UNDP]. (2010). *Gender and disasters.* https://www.undp.org/content/dam/undp/library/crisis%20prevention/disaster/7Disaster%20Risk%20 20Reduction%20-%20Gen-der.pdf

United Nations Framework Convention on Climate Change [UNFCC]. (2015). *Adoption of the Paris agree-ment conf. of the parties on its twenty-first session §.* United Nations, Paris. https://unfccc.int/sites/default/files/english_paris_agreement.pdf

Wisner, B., & Luce, H. R. (1993). Disaster vulnerability: scale, power and daily life. *Geo Journal*, 30(2), 127–140. https://doi.org/10.1007/BF00808129

World Risk Report. (2021). Bündnis Entwicklung Hilft & Ruhr University Bochum – Institute for International Law of Peace and Armed Conflict (IFHV). https://reliefweb.int/sites/reliefweb.int/files/resources/2021-world-risk-report.pdf

Yavinsky, R. (2012). *Women more vulnerable than men to climate change: Racheal Yavinsky.* Populations Reference Bureau (PRB). https://www.prb.org/resources/women-more-vulnerable-than-men-to-climate-change/

11 Pre-Existing Sociodemographic and Health Characteristics and Trends in Confirmed COVID-19 Cases in Louisiana

Hui Liew and Leslie Green

Background

The Lower Mississippi Delta (LMD) comprises Arkansas, Louisiana, Mississippi, and Tennessee. Decades after the Civil Rights Movement, a number of critical issues and obstacles to overcoming inequality remain inadequately addressed in this region. This region remained one of the persistently poor and unhealthy regions in the United States. Persistent problems included low income and education, high poverty rates, stagnant economies, inequality, rural isolation, and poor health (Green et al., 2015). The high rates of poverty, unemployment, and burden of disease, as well as the limited success in removing the barriers to health improvements in the LMD might be attributable to the multifaceted forces that impact health, the longstanding historical and cultural factors, and the lack of coordination among stakeholders (Liew, 2016).

HIV infection remained a major public health challenge in Louisiana. In 2018, Louisiana ranked 4th in the nation for HIV case rates and 11th for the estimated number of HIV diagnoses (Louisiana Department of Health, 2019). The number of persons living with HIV infection (PLHIV) increased from 15,733 in 2009 to 21,744 in 2018 (Louisiana Department of Health, 2019). Among the largest metropolitan areas in the nation, New Orleans and Baton Rouge ranked 6th and 4th for HIV case rates (24.6 and 27.5 per 100,000, respectively) (Louisiana Department of Health, 2019). Racial and ethnic minorities bore the overwhelming burden of HIV infection. In 2019, African American men and women represented about 63.1% and 81.2% of those with PLHIV infection, followed by Whites (about 29.7% for men and 14.5% for women), and Hispanics (about 5.6% for men and 3.2% for women) (Louisiana Department of Health, 2019). In 2018, those aged 24 and under constituted about 23.5% of the new HIV diagnoses (Louisiana Department of Health, 2019).

The 2019 novel coronavirus (2019-nCov or COVID-19) was first detected in Louisiana on March 9, 2020 (Office of the Governor, 2020). Two days later, Governor John Be Edwards declared a public health emergency when 13 residents from Orleans, Jefferson, Iberia, St. Tammany, Caddo, and Lafourche parishes tested positive (Louisiana Department of Health, 2020a). He also expedited emergency preparedness and other preventive measures among residents in the state. On March 12, 2012, the Louisiana 211 statewide network was established to answer queries concerning this pneumonia of unknown source (Louisiana Department of Health, 2020b) and visits to healthcare facilities were restricted to those deemed essential (Louisiana Department of Health, 2020c). A day later, the Governor prohibited gatherings of more than 250 people and closed all K-12 public schools statewide (Louisiana Department of Health, 2020d). A statewide stay-at-home order was issued on March 26, 2020 (Louisiana Department of Health, 2020e). To date, Louisiana remains one of the hardest hit states by COVID-19 in the United States (USA Facts, 2021). The number of confirmed cases in Louisiana continued to increase remarkably in most parishes

DOI: 10.4324/9781003140245-11

(Louisiana Department of Health, 2021), raising great concern among local and state leaders for the health and well-being of residents.

Deaths associated with COVID-19 disproportionately affected Blacks, which constituted about 32% of the state's total population (Deslatte, 2020). The chronic disease and health behavioral profiles in Louisiana could imply a high prevalence of risk factors for COVID-19. For instance, in 2019, 35.90% and 35% of the population in Louisiana was either overweight or obese and 12.60% of population had diabetes (Center for Disease Control and Prevention, 2017). During the same year, 25.90% and 12.40% of male and female population in Louisiana self-identified as binge drinkers (Center for Disease Control and Prevention, 2017).

Review of Relevant Literature

In Louisiana, the body of literature focused independently on either COVID-19 or HIV/AIDS. Published works on COVID-19 focused on projecting the number of infections, hospitalizations, and deaths in the New Orleans Metropolitan Statistical Area (Straif-Bourgeois & Robinson, 2020), comparing the Black–White hospitalization and mortality rates (Price-Haywood et al., 2020), estimating the impact of school closures on the healthcare workforce (Bayham & Fenichel, 2020), and detecting the clusters of COVID-19 (Desjardins et al., 2020). Published works on HIV/AIDS have focused on nonadherence to high active antiretroviral therapy (Mohammed et al., 2004), examining the determinants of HIV disclosures (Mohammed & Kissinger, 2006), examining the interrelationships among race, incarceration, and risky sexual behaviors (Arp III, 2009), assessing the effectiveness of partner counseling and referral services (Shrestha et al., 2009), hospital length of stay among infected individuals (Santella et al., 2010), examining the interrelationships between discrimination and HIV-related risk behaviors (Kaplan et al., 2016), preferences for home-based testing (Robinson et al., 2017), exploring the accessibility of HIV medical care (Brewer et al., 2018, 2019a), and durable viral suppression among criminal justice-involved Black men (Brewer et al., 2019b).

The few case studies that focused on the coinfections of the COVID-19 and HIV epidemics found mixed findings. All these studies were based on small samples of COVID-19/HIV coinfected patients. When compared to their non-coinfected counterparts, a study conducted in Bronx, New York (Suwanwongse & Shabarek, 2020) found relatively high mortality rates among HIV/COVID-19 co-infected patients. Likewise, a study conducted in Madrid, Spain found higher rates of confirmed cases among people living with HIV (PLWH) than the general population, while the reverse was true for suspected cases (Vizcarra et al., 2020). Still, a study conducted in Barcelona, Spain found no difference in the mortality and severity (Blanco et al., 2020) and hospitalization rates (Shalev et al., 2020) of COVID-19 among patients with HIV than their non-infected counterparts. In contrast, another study conducted in Spain found lower risks for hospitalization among HIV/COVID-19 co-infected patients than patients with COVID-19 if they received TDF/FTC regiment (del Amo et al., 2020).

To date, only one study in the United States, France, Mexico, and Columbia focused on the sociodemographic and health determinants of COVID-19 confirmed cases (i.e. Rozenfeld et al., 2020) and deaths (Prado-Galbarro et al., 2020; Rodriguez-Villamizar et al., 2020; Smati et al., 2021; Tai et al., 2021; Tartof et al., 2020). None of these studies focused on a southern state like Louisiana. Additionally, no empirical research known to date has provided a spatial-temporal cluster analyses to assess trends in the number of COVID-19 confirmed cases and HIV prevalence rates. To fill these research gaps, this study sought to:

1 Examine how the longitudinal changes in the number of COVID-19 confirmed cases and HIV prevalence rates differ across parishes in Louisiana by assigning each to distinctive spatial-temporal clusters.

2 Look at the role of HIV prevalence rate, behavioral health patterns, and pre-existing sociodemographic conditions in determining the parish's resilience and susceptibility to COVID-19.

Data and Methodology

Measures

Data on the number of confirmed COVID-19 cases from March 11, 2020 to August 15, 2021 for each parish was obtained from USA Facts (2021). Even though annual data on HIV prevalence rates and other data pertaining to the pre-existing sociodemographic and health behavioral conditions originated from different sources, they were compiled by the County Health Rankings website maintained by the University of Wisconsin Population Health Institute (County Health Rankings, 2021). Annual data on HIV prevalence rates from 2007 to 2017 originated from the National Center for HIV/AIDS, Viral Hepatitis, STD, and TB Prevention. This variable was the dependent variable used in the ordinary least squares (OLS) models described below.

Information pertaining to the 2018 estimates of the population and the percentages of population that was non-Hispanic Black or African American and population living in a rural area were obtained from the Census Bureau's Population Estimates Program (PEP). The population of a given parish referred to the number of people who were the residents in that parish. The percentage of the population living in a rural area was obtained from the 2010 estimates of the Census's PEP program. The Black–White segregation indices were obtained from 2014 to 2018 estimates of The American Community Survey (ACS). Information pertaining to the percentages of adults of ages 25–44 with some post-secondary education were obtained from 2014 to 2018 ACS estimates.

Excessive drinking referred to the percentage of adult population who reported binge or heavy drinking in the past 30 days in a given parish. Data on alcohol use were obtained from the 2017 Behavioral Risk Factor Surveillance System. Data on adult obesity and diabetes prevalence were obtained from the 2016 United States Diabetes Surveillance System. The former was measured as the percentage of the adult population (age 20 and older) that reports a body mass index greater than or equal to 30 kg/m^2. The latter was measured as the percentage of adults of ages 20 and above with diagnosed diabetes.

Analytic Strategies

All analyses were conducted using the R Statistical Programming Software. Spatial-temporal cluster analysis proceeded in three steps. The *diss* function under the *TSclust* library was first used to calculate the dissimilarity measures/distances among the COVID-19 and HIV trends of these parishes using the dynamic time warping (DTW) metric. DTW was an appropriate metric for the purposes of this study because it sought to compare two time series by identifying the best alignment that minimizes the dissimilarities or distances between them in a given distance matrix. Because of that, DTW provided more robust measures of dissimilarities/distances than the Euclidean method as it facilitated a way to compare two time series over similar time frames even if their trends did not "sync up" perfectly.

After that, the Elbow Method was used to determine the optimal number of clusters. Results from the Elbow Method revealed that there was an "elbow" at two clusters even though the total within-clusters sum of squares changed slowly and remained less changing after five clusters for both COVID-19 and HIV trends. Finally, hierarchical agglomerative clustering was performed using the *hclust* function under the *cluster* library to classify and assign the different parishes into their distinctive spatial-temporal clusters based on their longitudinal changes in the confirmed

COVID-19 cases from March 11, 2020 to August 15, 2021. Hierarchical agglomerative clustering initially performed using $K = 2$ resulted in uneven clusters with one cluster having a couple of unusual samples from the rest (provided upon request). Thus, to obtain meaningful clusters, the *cutree* function was used to separate observations into five groups for these trends.

Because of the insignificant Moran I's statistic, OLS regression was used to examine the effects of the 2017 HIV prevalence rate, the pre-existing sociodemographic characteristics and health behaviors on the number of confirmed COVID-19 cases on August 15, 2021. Since the principal concern of this analysis was to examine the potential impacts of HIV prevalence rates on the number of confirmed COVID-19 cases, the analysis began by including the 2017 HIV prevalence rate in the first (baseline) model. The second model is built on the first model to add the percentage of non-Hispanic Black population and the extent of Black–White segregation. The third model is built on the first model to add the percentages of adults who were excessive drinkers, obese, and diagnosed with diabetes. The fourth model is built on the first model to add the estimated population and the percentage of adults with post-secondary education.

Results

Spatial-Temporal Cluster Analyses for COVID-19 Trends

Spatial-temporal cluster analysis yielded five distinct clusters based on the trends in COVID-19. Cluster assignment of each parish is provided in Table 11.1. Slightly over half of the parishes (i.e. 34) were assigned to the cluster characterized by *mild-to-moderate* case growth (figure provided upon request). Most of these parishes registered no more than 10 confirmed cases before April 2020 but experienced a mild-to-moderate increase with cases ranging from slightly over 400 (i.e. Tensas) to slightly over 4,000 in some parishes (i.e. Beauregard, Evangeline, and Vernon) in mid-August 2021.

Nearly a fourth of the parishes (i.e. 14) were assigned to the *slightly severe* case growth cluster. As shown in Figure 11.1, these parishes registered no more than 10 confirmed cases during the first few weeks of March 2020 but experienced a noticeable increase by mid-August of the following year with cases growing to slightly over 8,000 in Acadia and 10,000 in Iberia.

As shown in Figure 11.2, Ascension, Bossier, Lafourche, Livingston, Rapides, St. Landry, Tangipahoa, and Terrebonne were assigned to the *moderately severe* case growth cluster, with no more than five cases before March 20, 2020, to slightly about 20,000 cases in Ascension, Livingston, and Tangipahoa by mid-August of the following year.

Caddo, Calcasieu, Lafayette, Orleans, Ouachita, and St. Tammany were assigned to the *severe* case growth cluster, with no more than 10 cases (except for Orleans) before March 20, 2020 to between 24,000 and 40,000 cases by mid-August of the following year (see Figure 11.3).

East Baton Rouge and Jefferson were assigned to the *drastic* case growth cluster, with no more than 100 cases before March 20, 2020 to slightly over 53,000 cases in East Baton Rouge and nearly 60,000 cases in Jefferson by mid-August of the following year (see Figure 11.4).

Spatial-Temporal Cluster Analyses for HIV Trends

Most parishes were assigned to the first cluster, which was characterized as having *mild* increases in HIV prevalence rates (figure provided upon request). The HIV prevalence rates for these parishes were no more than 200 in 2007 (except for Caldwell and Richland) but increased to no more than 300 for most parishes in 2017.

Except for La Salle, the other 12 parishes assigned to the second cluster were characterized as having *somewhat moderate but slow increases* in HIV prevalence rates over time. HIV prevalence

Table 11.1 Cluster Assignment of Parishes

Parish	COVID-19 Cluster	HIV Cluster
Acadia	Slightly severe	Mild
Allen	Mild to moderate	High and drastic increase
Ascension	Moderately severe	Mild
Assumption	Mild to moderate	Mild
Avoyelles	Slightly severe	Moderate
Beauregard	Mild to moderate	Mild
Bienville	Mild to moderate	Somewhat moderate
Bossier	Moderately severe	Mild
Caddo	Severe	Moderate
Calcasieu	Severe	Somewhat moderate
Caldwell	Mild to moderate	Mild
Cameron	Mild to moderate	Mild
Catahoula	Mild to moderate	Somewhat moderate
Claiborne	Mild to moderate	Moderate
Concordia	Mild to moderate	Somewhat moderate
De Soto	Mild to moderate	Mild
East Baton Rouge	Drastic	High and drastic increase
East Carroll	Mild to moderate	Moderate
East Feliciana	Mild to moderate	High and drastic increase
Evangeline	Mild to moderate	Mild
Franklin	Mild to moderate	Mild
Grant	Mild to moderate	Mild
Iberia	Slightly severe	Mild
Iberville	Slightly severe	High and drastic increase
Jackson	Mild to moderate	Mild
Jefferson	Drastic	Moderate
Jefferson Davis	Mild to moderate	Mild
Lafayette	Severe	Somewhat moderate
Lafourche	Moderately severe	Mild
La Salle	Mild to moderate	Somewhat moderate
Lincoln	Slightly severe	Mild
Livingston	Moderately severe	Mild
Madison	Mild to moderate	Moderate
Morehouse	Mild to moderate	Somewhat moderate
Natchitoches	Slightly severe	Somewhat moderate
Ouachita	Severe	Moderate
Orleans	Severe	Relatively high but declining
Plaquemines	Mild to moderate	Mild
Pointe Coupee	Mild to moderate	Somewhat moderate
Rapides	Moderately severe	Moderate
Red River	Mild to moderate	Mild
Richland	Mild to moderate	Mild
Sabine	Mild to moderate	Mild
St. Bernard	Slightly severe	Moderate
St. Charles	Slightly severe	Mild
St. Helena	Mild to moderate	Mild
St. James	Mild to moderate	Somewhat moderate
St. John the Baptist	Slightly severe	Somewhat moderate
St. Landry	Moderately severe	Somewhat moderate
St. Martin	Slightly severe	Mild
St. Mary	Slightly severe	Mild
St. Tammany	Severe	Mild

(Continued)

Table 11.1 (Continued)

Parish	COVID-19 Cluster	HIV Cluster
Tangipahoa	Moderately severe	Somewhat moderate
Tensas	Mild to moderate	Mild
Terrebonne	Moderately severe	Mild
Union	Mild to moderate	Mild
Vermilion	Slightly severe	Mild
Vernon	Mild to moderate	Mild
Washington	Slightly severe	Moderate
Webster	Slightly severe	Mild
West Baton Rouge	Mild to moderate	Moderate
West Carroll	Mild to moderate	Mild
West Feliciana	Mild to moderate	High and drastic increase
Winn	Mild to moderate	Moderate

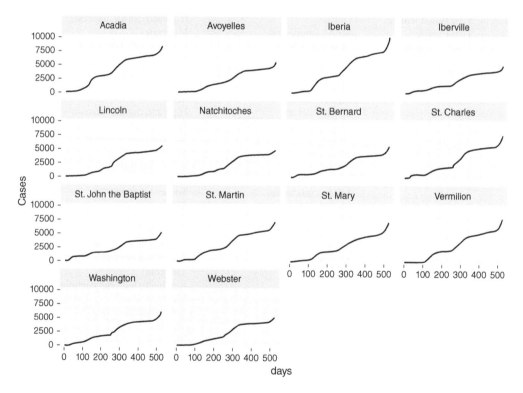

Figure 11.1 Parishes with *slightly severe* COVID-19 case growths.

rates for these parishes remained somewhat unchanged during the period of observation. As shown in Figure 11.5, the HIV prevalence rates for these parishes were no more than 300 in 2007 (except for Calcasieu) but increased to no more than 500 in 2017. In La Salle, HIV prevalence rates nearly tripled from 2007 to 2008, nearly doubled from 2008 to 2009, remained unchanged from 2009 to 2011, increased somewhat from 2011 to 2013, declined somewhat from 2013 to 2016, and slightly increased from 2016 to 2017.

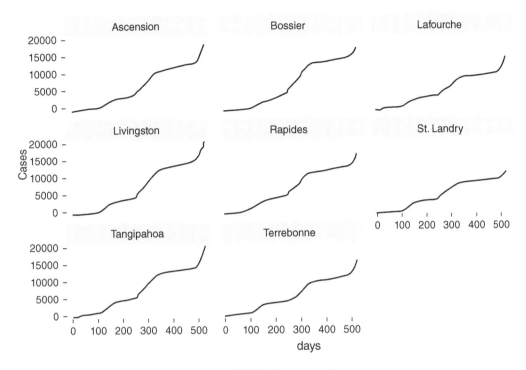

Figure 11.2 Parishes with *moderately severe* COVID-19 case growths.

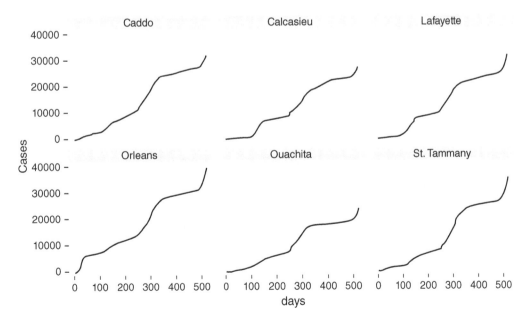

Figure 11.3 Parishes with *severe* COVID-19 case growths.

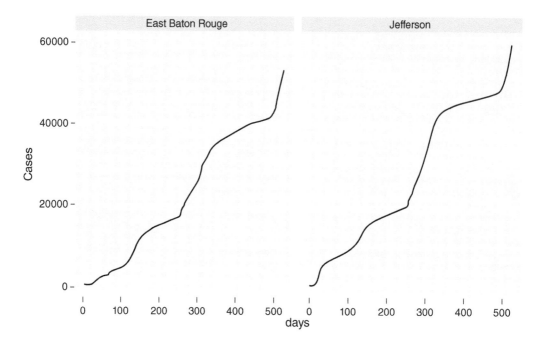

Figure 11.4 Parishes with *drastic* COVID-19 case growths.

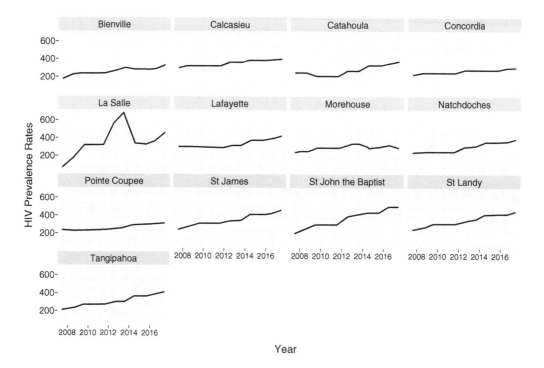

Figure 11.5 Parishes with *somewhat moderate* HIV prevalence rates.

As shown in Figure 11.6, two-thirds of the parishes assigned to the third cluster were character-ized as having *moderate but slow* (i.e. Avoyelles, Jefferson, Ouachita, Rapides, St. Bernard, and Washington) or *drastic* (i.e. Caddo and Claiborne) *increases* in HIV prevalence rates. Another three were characterized as having *moderate but drastic declines* in HIV prevalence rates (i.e. East Carroll, Madison, and Winn) while the rates remained *moderate but relatively unchanged* in West Baton Rouge. As shown in the top panel of Figure 11.1, the HIV prevalence rates for these parishes were no more than 400 in 2007 (except for East Carroll, Madison, and West Baton Rouge) but increased to no more than 600 in 2017.

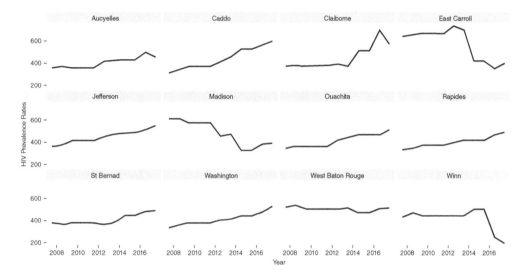

Figure 11.6 Parishes with *moderate* HIV prevalence rates.

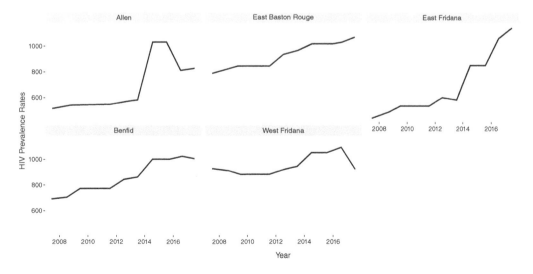

Figure 11.7 Parishes with *high and drastic increase* in HIV prevalence rates.

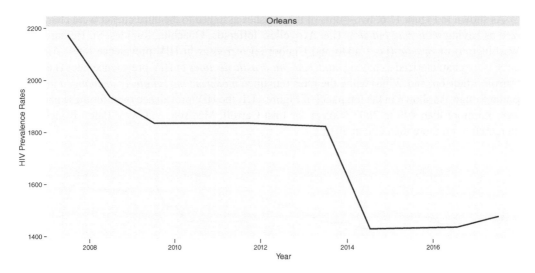

Figure 11.8 Parishes with *relatively high but declining* HIV prevalence rates.

As shown in Figure 11.7, half of the parishes (i.e. 6) assigned to the fourth cluster were characterized as having a *high and drastic increase* in HIV prevalence rates except for West Feliciana. The HIV prevalence rates in these parishes nearly or more than doubled during the period of observation. In West Feliciana, the HIV prevalence rates remained relatively unchanged from 2007 to 2013, slightly increased thereafter until 2016, and somewhat declined from 2 to 16 in 2017.

Orleans was assigned to the fifth cluster, characterized by *relatively high but declining* HIV prevalence rates over time. As shown in Figure 11.8, HIV prevalence rates decreased from slightly over 2,100 in 2007 to nearly 1,500 in 2017.

Descriptive Statistics

Descriptions for each of these variables are provided in Table 11.2. As shown in the same table, on average, HIV prevalence rates were relatively high in the parishes characterized by *severe* and *drastic*, and to a lesser extent, *moderately severe* case growths. In general, the percentages of non-Hispanic Black population were relatively low in the parishes characterized by *moderately severe* case growth. The extent of Black–White segregation was relatively high in parishes characterized by *severe* and *drastic* case growths.

The percentages of adults who were excessive drinkers were slightly higher in parishes characterized by *severe* and *drastic* case growths while the reverse was true for the percentages of adults who were obese. The percentages of adults with diabetes were slightly higher in parishes characterized by *mild-to-moderate* case growths. On average, the estimated population was relatively high in parishes characterized by *drastic* and *severe* case growths, and to a lesser extent, in parishes characterized by *moderately severe* case growths. On average, the percentages of adults with some post-secondary education were slightly higher in the parishes characterized by *severe* and *drastic* case growth, and to a lesser extent, in parishes characterized by *moderately severe* case growths.

Table 11.2 Descriptive Statistics (Standard Deviations in Parentheses)

Variables	Mild to Moderate (n = 35)	Slightly Severe (n = 13)	Moderately Severe (n = 8)	Severe (n = 6)	Drastic (n = 2)
# HIV prevalence rates (2017)	3,014.57 (2,335.46)	6,601.15 (1,540.56)	18,619.75 (5,999.17)	26,824.67 (13,379.07)	56,558.00 (4,552.35)
% of non-Hispanic Black population (2018)	32.77% (15.43%)	31.81% (11.59%)	25.09% (10.19%)	32.58% (19.47%)	36.65% (13.93%)
Extent of Black–White segregation (2014–2018)	42.91 (14.20)	40.46 (9.34)	40.88 (8.97)	59.33 (9.24)	54.50 (3.54)
% of adults with excessive drinking (2017)	18.06% (2.13%)	18.77% (1.54%)	20.00% (2.07%)	19.67% (2.16%)	21.00% (1.41%)
% of adults who were obese (2016)	37.63% (4.99%)	39.31% (3.45%)	35.88% (4.22%)	34.33% (4.49%)	32.50% (0.71%)
% of adults with diabetes (2016)	15.86% (4.19%)	13.38% (3.55%)	11.88% (1.96%)	13.00% (2.77%)	13.00% (1.41%)
Population (2018)	22,377 (5,327)	49,608 (12,152)	136,541 (27,951)	210,757 (79,202)	437,504 (4,883)
% of adults ages 25–44 with some post-secondary education (2014–2018)	42.37% (8.70%)	47.69% (8.81%)	55.50% (10.07%)	58.50% (10.29%)	63.00% (5.66%)

OLS Regression

Results from Model 1 of Table 11.3 suggested that the logged number of confirmed COVID-19 cases increased with the HIV prevalence rates. The addition of the percentage of non-Hispanic Black population and the extent of Black–White segregation in Model 2 did not affect the significance of the HIV prevalence rates variable but did change its magnitude. A comparison of the coefficients for HIV prevalence rates between the first two models suggested that exclusion of the percentage of non-Hispanic Black population and the extent of Black–White segregation in Model 2 exerted a suppressing effect on the association between HIV prevalence rates and the logged number of confirmed COVID-19 cases. Results from Model 2 also revealed that the logged number of confirmed COVID-19 cases increased with the extent of Black–White segregation while the reverse was true for the percentage of non-Hispanic Black population.

The addition of the percentages of adults who were excessive drinkers, obese, and diagnosed with diabetes in Model 3 did not affect the significance but slightly changed the magnitude of the HIV prevalence rates. A comparison of the first and third models suggested that the percentages of adults who were excessive drinkers, obese, and diagnosed with diabetes in Model 3 exerted a slight mediating effect on the association between HIV prevalence rates and the logged number of confirmed COVID-19 cases. Results from Model 3 also revealed that the logged number of confirmed COVID-19 cases increased with the percentage of adults who were excessive drinkers while the reverse was true for the percentage of adults with diabetes.

The effect of HIV prevalence rates on the logged number of confirmed COVID-19 cases became insignificant with the addition of the estimated population and the percentage of adults with

Table 11.3 Results from OLS Regression

Variables	Model 1	Model 2	Model 3	Model 4
Intercept	8.056*	7.604*	4.901*	−2.026*
HIV Rate (2017)	0.001*	0.002*	0.001*	0.0001
% of non-Hispanic Black population (2018)		−0.030*		−0.002
Extent of Black–White segregation (2014–2018)		0.026*		0.001
% of adults with excessive drinking (2017)			0.189*	−0.015
% of adults who were obese (2016)			0.028	0.008
% of adults with diabetes (2016)			−0.089*	−0.005
Population (log)				1.022*
% of adults ages 25–44 with some post-secondary education (2014–2018)				−0.004
Adj. R^2	0.088	0.268	0.353	0.983

* $p<=.05$

post-secondary education in Model 4. Results from Model 4 also revealed that the logged number of confirmed COVID-19 cases increased with logged population of a given parish. A comparison of the first and fourth models revealed that the effects of the percentage of non-Hispanic Black population and the extent of Black–White segregation on the logged number of confirmed COVID-19 cases were mediated by the percentages of adults who were excessive drinkers, diagnosed with diabetes, and adults with post-secondary education and the logged estimated population. Similarly, the effects of the percentages of adults who were excessive drinkers and diagnosed with diabetes on the logged number of confirmed COVID-19 cases were mediated by the percentages of non-Hispanic Black population and adults with post-secondary education, the extent of Black–White segregation, and the logged estimated population.

Discussion

Results from the OLS regression revealed that the logged number of confirmed COVID-19 cases increased with the estimated population of a given parish. Results from the spatial-temporal cluster analysis also revealed that the estimated population tended to be relatively high in parishes with severe and drastic increases in the number of confirmed COVID-19 cases. In 2018, the estimated population in these parishes were as follows: Caddo 242,922; Calcasieu 203,112; East Baton Rouge 440,956; Jefferson 434,051; Lafayette 242,782; Ouachita 154,475; Orleans 391,006; and St. Tammany 258,111 (County Health Rankings, 2020). East Baton Rouge also experienced a high and drastic increase in HIV prevalence rates. HIV prevalence rates in Orleans were still relatively high even though it showed a declining trend over time. The metropolitan areas like New Orleans-Metairie-Kenner, Baton Rouge, and Shreveport-Bossier City were also located in these parishes. The relatively high population densities increased the susceptibility to coronavirus and HIV infections for those living in these parishes.

The extent of Black–White to White segregation were somewhat higher in parishes assigned to the *severe* (i.e. Caddo [60] and Ouachita [68]) and *drastic* (i.e. East Baton Rouge [57] case growth clusters). The percentages of adults who were obese were somewhat higher in parishes assigned to the *severe* COVID-19 case growth cluster (i.e. Caddo and Ouachita [both 40%]). The percentages of adults with excessive drinking problems were somewhat higher in Jefferson and West Feliciana (both 20%, the former characterized by *drastic* COVID-19 case growth clusters and the latter characterized by *moderately severe* COVID-19 case growth clusters). The percentages of adults with diabetes were also somewhat higher in parishes assigned to the *slightly* (i.e. East Feliciana [17%]) and *moderately severe* (i.e. Bienville [24%], Claiborne [21%], Grant [21%], West Carroll [25%], and Winn [22%]) and *slightly severe* (i.e. Evangeline [20%] and Washington [23%]) COVID-19 case growth clusters.

Results from OLS regression models revealed that HIV prevalence rates were associated with the logged number of confirmed COVID-19 cases even after taking the percentages of non-Hispanic Black population, adults who were excessive drinkers, adults who were obese, adults diagnosed with diabetes, and adults with post-secondary education, the extent of Black–White segregation, and the estimated population of a given parish into account.

Results from OLS regression revealed that the logged number of confirmed COVID-19 cases decreased with the percentages of non-Hispanic Black population and adults who were diagnosed with diabetes. Because of that, identifying the obstacles faced by these individuals in testing and treatment seeking would be crucial to mitigate the negative consequences of COVID-19. These efforts should also focus on parishes with somewhat higher percentages of non-Hispanic Black population: Caddo (49.4%), East Baton Rouge (46.5%), East Feliciana (42.5%), Iberville (48.3%), Orleans (59.1%), and West Feliciana (44.3%) parishes (County Health Rankings, 2020). As of August 19, 2021, the number of Blacks reported to have died of this pneumonia of unknown origin was relatively high in some of these parishes (476 in Caddo, 560 in East Baton Rouge, 375 in Jefferson, and 701 in Orleans) (Louisiana Department of Health, 2021).

Results from OLS regression also revealed that the logged number of confirmed COVID-19 cases increased with the extent of Black–White segregation and the percentages of adults who were excessive drinkers. This finding corroborated with an earlier study that found that residential segregation increased the risks of low birth weight (Grady, 2006). This finding was also related to an earlier study that found that nursing home segregation decreased the odds of getting vaccinated which in turn increased Black resident's susceptibility to seasonal flu (Whoriskey et al., 2020). Thus, residential segregation might have increased a person's risk of getting infected by this pneumonia of unknown source. Because alcohol consumption was associated with numerous physical (Da et al., 2020), neurological (Meredith et al., 2020), and psychiatric (Castillo-Carniglia et al., 2019) comorbidities, it was plausible that increased alcohol consumption during the pandemic could increase one's vulnerability to COVID-19.

Some of the parishes assigned to the *slightly* and *moderately severe* COVID-19 case growths had relatively low percentages of adults with post-secondary education (i.e. Tensas [26%], East Carroll [30%], East Feliciana [35%], Jackson [35%], Madison [34%], and St. Mary [34%]). Bivariate regression analysis also revealed that the logged number of confirmed COVID-19 cases increased with the percentage of adults with post-secondary education (provided upon request). This finding was related to a study conducted in Nepal that found women with formal education are more likely to be aware of human papillomavirus (HPV) and its vaccine (Johnson et al., 2014). This finding was also in line with results from a recent study conducted in Speu Province, Cambodia, by Touch and Oh (2018) who found that women with at least a secondary education were more likely to undergo a Pap test and to receive the HPV vaccination. It was logical to assume that educated individuals might be more informed about the risks associated with COVID-19 and were therefore more inclined to get tested. It seemed equally likely that accessibility and affordability to COVID-19 testing increased with the level of education.

Conclusion

This study was timely and warranted because the 2019-nCov and HIV/AIDS remain the most taxing epidemic diseases in Louisiana to date. This pioneering study used spatial-temporal cluster analyses to explore how the pre-existing sociodemographic conditions and health behavioral patterns affect the parish's resilience and susceptibility to the 2019-nCov and to examine how trends in the number of confirmed coronavirus cases differ across the 64 parishes in Louisiana. This clustering technique could be used to delineate parishes with similar trends in 2019-nCov and HIV/AIDS into distinct clusters. Because of that, results from this study could guide health policymakers and practitioners as they tailor policies and delivery according to the behavioral health patterns and pre-existing sociodemographic conditions in each spatial-temporal cluster.

Results from spatial-temporal cluster analyses and OLS regression suggested that COVID-19 and HIV prevention and testing should be integrated. Attempts to improve the accessibility and affordability of harm reduction supplies, expanding venue-based testing for STI and HIV, increasing remote provision of HIV pre-exposure prophylaxis, and viral suppression among HIV-positive individuals (Shoptaw et al., 2020) should remain essential for 2019-nCov prevention and treatment in Louisiana. Information pertaining to HIV and COVID-19 should be made accessible through various avenues (e.g. public service commercials, television health announcements, billboards, workshop, and so on) and conveyed using terminologies appropriate to these populations. Attempts to recruit health workers and contracted staff to work in various mobile syringe services programs should also be continued (Eisinger et al., 2019). Priority should be given to parishes that face double jeopardy in COVID-19 and the number of PLHIV such as East Baton Rouge, Jefferson, and Orleans. These parishes were characterized by drastic COVID-19 case growth with 4,152, 2,129, and 5,309 PLHIV respectively in 2019 (Louisiana Department of Health, 2019). The number of PLHIV was also somewhat higher in other parishes assigned to the *severe* case growth cluster (i.e. 1,305 in Caddo, 884 in Lafayette, 684 in Ouachita, 723 in Calcasieu, and 554 in St. Tammany) (Louisiana Department of Health, 2019).

A recent study demonstrated that diabetes might hasten the progression of COVID-19 due to higher susceptibility to uncontrolled inflammatory responses (Guo et al., 2020). Because of that, expanding the coverage for testing and screening should concentrate on individuals living in parishes with *slightly* and *moderately* severe case growths. Attempt to improve preventive measures against the coronavirus should also focus on parishes with a large population, high levels of Black–White segregation, and high percentages of non-Hispanic Black population, adults who were excessive drinkers, adults among whom were fewer educated individuals. These might also be the parishes characterized by a high unmet need for commercial and state testing and vaccination. Therefore, governments at the state and local levels should seek to drive screening, testing, and vaccination efforts in a more inclusive and sustainable manner. Policy measures and mitigation efforts to expand coverage for testing, screening, and vaccination should focus on redesigning existing program delivery approaches to focus on the structural barriers that existed in these highly populated, highly segregated, and majority Black parishes. The successful implementation of these endeavors should not only be well-planned with clearly defined objectives, but they should also be tailored to the specific cultural contexts of these parishes. Because of that, it is important to garner support from health practitioners, policymakers, the local and state medical associations, and community groups to ensure successful implementation of these disease-preventive mechanisms. Efforts to promote resilience in the COVID-19 pandemic in Louisiana should also focus on increasing people's awareness about the detrimental effects of excessive drinking on the functioning of lung and respiration system, which can in turn increase the health complications associated with COVID-19. Because of that, attempts to reduce and avert the health complications associated with excessive drinking should be continued and priorities should be given to parishes with high percentages of adults who were excessive drinkers.

References

Arp III, W. (2009). Race, incarceration and HIV/AIDS in Louisiana: risky sexual behavior demands mandatory testing. *Race, Gender & Class, 16*(1/2), 228–237.

Bayham, J., & Fenichel, E. P. (2020). Impact of school closures for COVID-19 on the US health-care workforce and net mortality: a modelling study. *Lancet Public Health, 5*(5), e171–e178.

Blanco, J. L., Ambrosioni, J., Garcia, F., Martínez, E., Soriano, A., Mallolas, J., & Miro, J. M. (2020). COVID-19 in patients with HIV: clinical case series. *The Lancet HIV, 7*(5), e314–e316. doi: 10.1016/S2352-3018(20)30111-9

Brewer, R. A., Chrestman, S., Mukherjee, S., Mason, K. E., Dyer, T. V., Gamache, P., Moore, M., & Gruber, D. (2018). Exploring the correlates of linkage to HIV medical care among persons living with HIV infection (PLWH) in the deep south: results and lessons learned from the Louisiana positive charge initiative. *AIDS and Behavior, 22*(8), 2615–2626.

Brewer, R., Issema, R., Moore, M., Chrestman, S., Mukherjee, S., Odlum, M., & Schneider, J. A. (2019a). Correlates of durable viral suppression (DVS) among criminal justice-involved (CJI) black men living with HIV in Louisiana. *AIDS and Behavior, 23*(11), 2980–2991.

Brewer, R., Daunis, C., Ebaady, S., Wilton, L., Chrestman, S., Mukherjee, S., Moore, M., Corrigan, R., & Schneider, J. (2019b). Implementation of a socio-structural demonstration project to improve HIV outcomes among young black men in the deep south. *Journal of Racial and Ethnic Health Disparities, 6*(4), 775–789.

Castillo-Carniglia, A., Keyes, K. M., Hasin, D. S., & Cerdá, M. (2019). Psychiatric comorbidities in alcohol use disorder. *The Lancet Psychiatry, 6*(12), 1068–1080.

Center for Disease Control and Prevention. (2017, September 13). BRFSS Prevalence & Trends Data. *National Center for Chronic Disease Prevention and Health Promotion, Division of Population Health.* https://www.cdc.gov/brfss/brfssprevalence/

County Health Rankings. (2021). *Nebraska.* https://www.countyhealthrankings.org/app/nebraska/2020/overview

Da, B. L., Im, G. Y., & Schiano, T. D. (2020). Coronavirus disease 2019 hangover: a rising tide of alcohol use disorder and alcohol-associated liver disease. *Hepatology, 72*(3), 1102–1108.

del Amo, J., Polo, R., Moreno, S., Díaz, A., Martínez, E., Arribas, J. R., Jarrín, I., & Hernán, M. A. (2020). Incidence and severity of COVID-19 in HIV-positive persons receiving antiretroviral therapy: a cohort study. *Annals of Internal Medicine, 173*(7), 536–541.

Desjardins, M. R., Hohl, A., & Delmelle, E. M. (2020). Rapid surveillance of COVID-19 in the United States using a prospective space-time scan statistic: detecting and evaluating emerging clusters. *Applied Geography, 118*, 102202. doi: 10.1016/j.apgeog.2020.102202

Deslatte, M. (2020, April 7). Louisiana Data: Virus Hits Blacks, People with Hypertension. *U.S. News & World Report.* https://www.usnews.com/news/best-states/louisiana/articles/2020-04-07/louisiana-data-virus-hits-blacks-people-with-hypertension

Eisinger, R. W., Dieffenbach, C. W., & Fauci, A. S. (2019). HIV viral load and transmissibility of HIV infection: undetectable equals untransmittable. *JAMA, 321*(5), 451–452.

Green, J., Greever-Rice, T., & Glass Jr., G. D. (2015). Sociodemographic snapshots of the Mississippi delta. In J. Collins (Ed.), *Defining the delta: multidisciplinary perspectives on the lower Mississippi River Delta* (pp. 107–119). Fayetteville, AR: University of Arkansas Press.

Guo, W., Li, M., Dong, Y., Zhou, H., Zhang, Z., Tian, C., Qin, Renjie, Wang, Haijun, Shen, Yin, Du, Keye, Zhao, Lei, Fang, Heng, Luo, Shanshan, & Hu, D. (2020). Diabetes is a risk factor for the progression and prognosis of COVID-19. *Diabetes/metabolism Research and Reviews, 36*(7), e3319. doi: 10.1002/dmrr.3319

Grady, S. C. (2006). Racial disparities in low birthweight and the contribution of residential segregation: a multilevel analysis. *Social Science Medicine, 63*(12), 3013–3029.

Johnson, D. C., Bhatta, M. P., Gurung, S., Aryal, S., Lhaki, P., & Shrestha, S. (2014). Knowledge and awareness of human papillomavirus (HPV), cervical cancer and HPV vaccine among women in two distinct
Nepali communities. *Asian Pacific Journal of Cancer Prevention, 15*(19), 8287–8293.

Kaplan, K. C., Hormes, J. M., Wallace, M., Rountree, M., & Theall, K. P. (2016). Racial discrimination and
HIV-related risk behaviors in southeast Louisiana. *American Journal of Health Behavior, 40*(1), 132–143.
doi: 10.5993/AJHB.40.1.15.

Liew, H. (2016). Challenges to sustainable development in Mississippi. *Community Development, 47*(5),
620–637.

Louisiana Department of Health. (2019, September 30). Louisiana HIV, AIDS, and Early Syphilis Surveillance Quarterly Report September 30, 2019. http://www.ldh.la.gov/assets/oph/HIVSTD/HIV_Syphilis_
Quarterly_Reports/2019Reports/ThirdQuarter2019HIVSyphilisReport.pdf

Louisiana Department of Health. (2020a, March 24). Gov. Edwards Declares Public Health Emergency in
Response to COVID-19. https://ldh.la.gov/index.cfm/newsroom/category/6?pn=37

Louisiana Department of Health. (2020b, March 12). Questions about COVID-19 Now Being Answered by
Louisiana 211 Statewide Network. http://ldh.la.gov/index.cfm/newsroom/detail/5471

Louisiana Department of Health. (2020c, March 12). State Health Department Orders Healthcare Facilities to
Restrict Visitors. http://ldh.la.gov/index.cfm/newsroom/detail/5475

Louisiana Department of Health. (2020d, March 13). Gov. Edwards Signs Proclamation Aimed to Slow the
Spread of COVID-19 in Louisiana. https://gov.louisiana.gov/index.cfm/newsroom/detail/2403

Louisiana Department of Health. (2020e, March 22). Gov. Edwards Issues Statewide Stay at Home Order to
Further Fight the Spread of COVID-19 in Louisiana. https://gov.louisiana.gov/order/

Louisiana Department of Health. (2021, September 30). Coronavirus (COVID-19). http://ldh.la.gov/
coronavirus/

Meredith, L. R., Lim, A. C., & Ray, L. A. (2020). Neurocognitive performance in alcohol use disorder using
the NIH toolbox: role of severity and sex differences. *Drug and Alcohol Dependence, 216*(1), 108269.

Mohammed, H., Kieltyka, L., Richardson-Alston, G., Magnus, M., Fawal, H., Vermund, S. H., Rice, J., &
Kissinger, P. (2004). Adherence to HAART among HIV-infected persons in rural Louisiana. *Aids Patient
Care and STDs, 18*(5), 289–296.

Mohammed, H., & Kissinger, P. (2006). Disclosure of HIV serostatus to sex partners in rural Louisiana. *AIDS
Care, 18*(suppl), 62–69.

Office of the Governor. (2020, March 9). Gov. Edwards Confirms Louisiana's First Presumptive Positive Case
of COVID-19. http://gohsep.la.gov/portals/0/News/Covid-Release03092020.pdf

Prado-Galbarro, F. J., Sanchez-Piedra, C., Gamiño-Arroyo, A. E., & Cruz-Cruz, C. (2020). Determinants of
survival after severe acute respiratory syndrome coronavirus 2 infection in Mexican outpatients and hospi-
talised patients. *Public Health, 189*, 66–72.

Price-Haywood, E. G., Burton, J., Fort, D., & Seoane, L. (2020). Hospitalization and mortality among black
patients and white patients with Covid-19. *New England Journal of Medicine, 382*(26), 2534–2543.

Robinson, W. T., Zarwell, M., & Gruber, D. (2017). Preferences for home-based HIV testing among hetero-
sexuals at increased risk for HIV/AIDS: New Orleans, Louisiana, 2013. *JAIDS Journal of Acquired Immune Deficiency Syndromes, 75*, S352–S356.

Rodriguez-Villamizar, L. A., Belalcazar-Ceron, L. C., Fernández-Niño, J. A., Marin-Pineda, D. M., Rojas-
Sánchez, O. A., Acuna-Merchan, L. A., Ramirez-Garcia, N., Mangones-Matos, S. C., Vargas-Gonzalez, J.
M., Herrera-Torres, J., Agudelo-Castaneda, D. M., Jiminez, J. G. P., Rojas-Roa, N. Y., & Herrera-Galindo,
V. M. (2020). Air pollution, sociodemographic and health conditions effects on COVID-19 mortality in
Colombia: an ecological study. *Science of The Total Environment, 756*, 144020.

Rozenfeld, Y., Beam, J., Maier, H., Haggerson, W., Boudreau, K., Carlson, J., & Medows, R. (2020). A model
of disparities: risk factors associated with COVID-19 infection. *International Journal for Equity in Health,
19*(1), 1–10.

Santella, A., Shi, L., & Campbell, C. (2010). Factors associated with hospital length of stay among HIV-
infected adults in Louisiana. *Journal of Louisiana State Medical Society, 162*, 325–326.

Shalev, N., Scherer, M., LaSota, E. D., Antoniou, P., Yin, M. T., Zucker, J., & Sobieszczyk, M. E. (2020).
Clinical characteristics and outcomes in people living with HIV hospitalized for COVID-19. *Clinal Infectious Diseases, 71*(16), 2294–2297.

Shoptaw, S., Goodman-Meza, D., & Landovitz, R. J. (2020). Collective call to action for HIV/AIDS community-based collaborative science in the era of COVID-19. *AIDS and Behavior, 24*(7), 2013–2016. doi: 10.1007/s10461-020-02860-y

Shrestha, R. K., Begley, E. B., Hutchinson, A. B., Sansom, S. L., Song, B., Voorhees, K., Busby, A., Carrel, J., & Burgess, S. (2009). Costs and effectiveness of partner counseling and referral services with rapid testing for HIV in Colorado and Louisiana, United States. *Sexually Transmitted Diseases, 36*(10), 637–641.

Smati, S., Tramunt, B., Wargny, M., Caussy, C., Gaborit, B., Vatier, C., Verges, B., Ancelle, D., Amadou, C., Bachir, L. A., Bourron, O., Coffin-Boutreux, C., Barraud, S., Dorange, A., Fremy, B., Gautier, J., Germain, N., Larger, E., Laugier-Robiolle, S., … & CORONADO investigators. (2021). Relationship between obesity and severe COVID-19 outcomes in patients with type 2 diabetes: Results from the CORONADO study. *Diabetes, Obesity and Metabolism, 23*(2), 391–403. doi: 10.1111/dom.14228

Straif-Bourgeois, S., & Robinson, W. (2020). About Coronavirus disease 2019 (COVID-19). *Journal of Health Care Finance, 46*(4), 5–10.

Suwanwongse, K., & Shabarek, N. (2020). Clinical features and outcome of HIV/SARS-CoV-2 co-infected patients in the Bronx, New York City. *Journal of Medical Virology, 92*(11), 2387–2389. doi: 10.1002/jmv.26077

Tai, D. B. G., Shah, A., Doubeni, C. A., Sia, I. G., & Wieland, M. L. (2021). The disproportionate impact of COVID-19 on racial and ethnic minorities in the United States. *Clinical Infectious Diseases, 72*(4), 703–706.

Tartof, S. Y., Qian, L., Hong, V., Wei, R., Nadjafi, R. F., Fischer, H., Li, Z., Shaw, S. F., Caparosa, S. L., Nau, C. L., Saxena, T., Rieg, G. K., Ackerson, B. K., Sharp, A. L., Skarbinski, J., Naik, T. K., & Murali, S. B. (2020). Obesity and mortality among patients diagnosed with COVID-19: results from an integrated health care organization. *Annals of Internal Medicine, 173*(10), 773–781.

Touch, S., & Oh, J. (2018). Knowledge, attitudes, and practices toward cervical cancer prevention among women in Kampong Speu Province, Cambodia. *BMC Cancer, 18*(1), 294. doi: 10.1186/s12885-018-4198-8

USA Facts. (2021, August 17). *Coronavirus Locations: COVID-19 Map by County and State*. https://usafacts.org/visualizations/coronavirus-covid-19-spread-map/

Vizcarra, P., Pérez-Elías, M. J., Quereda, C., Moreno, A., Vivancos, M. J., Dronda, F.,... & Vivancos, M. J. (2020). Description of COVID-19 in HIV-infected individuals: a single-centre, prospective cohort. *The lancet HIV, 7*(8), e554–e564. doi: 10.1016/S2352-3018(20)30164-8

Whoriskey, P., Sacchetti, M., & Webster, R. A. (2020, March 21). Coronavirus Cases Surge at Nursing Homes as Workers Battle 'almost Perfect Killing Machine. *The Washington Post*. https://www.washingtonpost.com/business/2020/03/21/nursing-home-coronavirus-deaths/

12 Social Inequality, COVID-19, and the Delta Wave

Intersections of Race, Gender, and Education

Omar Bird

Introduction

At the time of this writing, and for most of the pandemic, the United States has led the world in COVID-19 reported cases and deaths. As of June 2022, there have been over 1 million reported deaths and over 86 million reported cases (CDC, 2022). Within this number, racial and gender differences show significant variation in who contracts COVID-19 and who ultimately dies from the disease. For instance, a report published in February 2022 by the Kaiser Family Foundation shows the risk of COVID-19 infection, hospitalization, and death for Black, Hispanic, American Indian/Alaskan Native, and Asians compared with Whites in the United States. Unsurprisingly, results indicate that Hispanic, Black, and American Indian/Alaskan Native people are twice as likely to be hospitalized and die from COVID-19 compared with Whites *(COVID-19 Cases and Deaths, Vaccinations, and Treatments by Race/Ethnicity as of Fall 2022 KFF, 2022)*. Among categories of gender, though men might be more susceptible to the disease, women report more pandemic-related difficulties, such as mental health concerns and food and economic insecurities (Zhang, Walkover, & Wu, 2021). Regarding disease prognosis, both biological and behavioral factors help explain some differences between men and women. Estrogen, for example, promotes adaptive immune responses that result in greater vaccine efficacy and quicker clearance of disease pathogens within the body. Conversely, testosterone has more suppressive effects on the immune system leading to greater susceptibility to disease (Maleki Dana et al., 2020). From a behavioral standpoint, more men are likely to believe that mask wearing is infringing on personal freedom and less likely to wear a mask during shopping, which could also help explain some gendered differences on disease contraction (Haischer et al., 2020). Though racial and gender differences exist in the pandemic, more research is needed on the interplay between COVID-19-related factors, social status, and socioeconomic status.

In the United States, there is no question that the pandemic has widened pre-existing health and socioeconomic gaps among individual and social groups. In the quest to understand this elusive disease, less knowledge centers around how categories of race, gender, and socioeconomic status *intersect* with one another and social structures to show the nuance of pandemic-related social inequality across *and within* such categories. Research has shown that there is more variation in health status within groups than between them. Perhaps some of those patterns are observed through social circumstances linked to the pandemic (e.g., loss of employment and recent food insufficiency). The data presented here are intended to show the patterns and distribution of the social determinants of health through an analysis on the effect of the Delta variant during the summer of 2021. The Delta variant was first detected in India in 2020. By the summer of 2021, Delta became the dominant variant in the United States and by November of 2021, the Delta variant was detected in over 170 countries. Examining specific points in time during the pandemic provides researchers the opportunity to retroactively examine social circumstances and pandemic-related outcomes with greater accuracy and detail.

DOI: 10.4324/9781003140245-12

This chapter employs the concept of *intersectionality* to theorize and empirically analyze COVID-19 data from the U.S. Census House Pulse Survey (HPS). Tenets of intersectionality will ground empirical evidence to improve social scientific analysis and policy recommendations aimed at investigating disparities in health and building more resilient communities for the future. For purposes of this study, the COVID-19 pandemic is framed as an "eco-pandemic injustice" that provides an analysis of disaster capitalism and social despair and its connection to intersectional theory. Viewing the effects of COVID-19 as an "eco-pandemic injustice" means extending our understanding beyond isolated environmental or health risks and identify the links between environmental injustices and social inequities that also include "a lack of access to basic human needs, social recognition, and political and participatory rights" (Powers et al., 2021, p. 223).

As an analytical tool, intersectionality offers researchers the ability to see how various institutions and structures of power within society (e.g., capitalism, globalization, nationalism, racism, xenophobia, sexism, and patriarchy) shape the health and well-being of individuals and communities. Using an intersectional analysis with survey data means that though data presented may reveal patterns and distributions of social inequality at the individual level, the implication of such evidence has direct linkages to macro processes of society and social policy.

Background

In nearly every report regarding the connection between social inequality and COVID-19, data show that non-White communities bear the brunt of infection, hospitalization, and death. Such reports also include a smattering of research that illustrate the pre-existing social inequities of racialized and gendered groups in the United States prior to the pandemic (Holst, Fessler and Niehoff, 2020). For instance, according to a report from the Common Wealth Fund, evidence shows that Hispanics and Blacks fair worse in comparison with Whites across a list of social indicators that include, but are not limited to, the following: median household income from 2003 to 2019, poverty distribution in accordance with the United States Federal Poverty Line, household wealth at every level of educational attainment, and rate of uninsured individuals among the elderly and children (Baumgartner et al., 2021).To enact a more comprehensive and effective social policy aimed at addressing social disparities through the pandemic, incorporating an intersectional approach is needed in health research to examine how COVID-19 has been equally a health *and* social disaster (Maestripieri, 2021). Hospitalization and/or death is not the result for every person who contracts the virus. Maestripieri (2021) outlines three distinct ways in which the pandemic has become a social catastrophe that has direct effects on our collective social experiences and individual survival outside of direct bodily harm.

According to Maestripieri (2021), one way that a pandemic is a social catastrophe is by exposing existing vulnerabilities such as economic instability and food insecurity pre-pandemic. Second, pandemics can be understood as a social catastrophe by reinforcing current inequalities that stem from the social conditions pre-pandemic. The process of "reinforcing" or "reproducing" current inequalities means that, compared with financially stable individuals and communities, those people and places that experience significant economic hardship are more likely to experience financial insecurity throughout a crisis. Lastly, Maestripieri (2021) argues that social disasters also amplify social differences in the future due to inadequate policy. Understanding pandemics as a health *and* social dilemma widens the net on who becomes impacted by global crises, especially those who do not contract COVID-19. Paying close attention to national pandemic responses, social policy, and individual social behavior is critical to capturing a comprehensive understanding of social pandemic effects. For example, in the United States, hundreds of thousands of people were thrusted into unemployed because of national lockdowns and disruptions in global, national, and local economic flows. Additionally, "stay at home" mandates meant that many local stores, corporations, and restaurants closed, and thus directly harming the employees who lost work, regardless of infection. To this end, combining the social and biological impacts of a pandemic is a more inclusive and holistic approach that can influence local, state, national, and global responses to pandemics.

Unsurprisingly, the U.S. response to the pandemic has reinforced current inequities and thus explains why disparities in social conditions continue to persist. According to Monte and Perez-Lopez's (2021), a national study of Black and White households, researchers found that the compounded effect of job loss, food insufficiency, and financial insecurity were most felt among Black households, after pre-existing socioeconomic factors, such as income, age, gender, and educational attainment were considered. Globally, Mude and colleagues (2021) conducted a meta-analysis of studies that reported the prevalence, hospitalizations, and deaths from COVID-19 by racial groups between January 1, 2020 and April 15, 2021, and they found overwhelming support that racial minorities in western countries experience disproportionate socioeconomic and social disadvantages compared with Whites. They conclude by arguing that their study "underscores the need to address inequities in these communities to improve overall health outcomes" (Mude et al., 2021, p. 1).

To capture the extent to which social factors combine to exacerbate the effects of the pandemic, a deeper analysis of the social impact is needed. What follows is a brief description of two prominent medical sociological theories that have been used to investigate linkages between social determinants of health and social status (e.g., race, gender, and education) and research that argues for an intersectional approach to improve sociological theory and pandemic-related research.

The Social Stress Process Model and Fundamental Cause Theory: Gaps in Health Disparities Research

Over the past 50 years, medical sociology and stress and health research have made strides in understanding the connections between social determinants of health and social status markers, especially regarding race and racism (Mossakowski, 2008; Williams, 1997, 2018). Several dominant theories emerged such as the *Social Stress Process Model* and *Fundamental Cause Theory* of health. The Social Stress Process Model is used to understand the impact of dealing with acute and chronic stressors on the health of individuals and communities (Pearlin et al. 1981). The Social Stress Process Model posits that the more stressors one experiences in life, the more likely individuals are to report poor mental and physical health (Pearlin et al., 1981; Williams, 2018). Due to the prevalence of severe social inequality, those who have a disadvantaged or marginalized status in society (e.g., non-White compared with White, women compared with men, low status compared with high status), are more likely to experience a higher level of stressors and therefore be more vulnerable to them. As a result, the resources available to individuals to address the stress of long bouts of poverty, for example, become less effective, the lower you are in SES (Mossakowski, 2008).

Research on COVID-19 and social status overwhelmingly confirms the social inequality foundation of the stress process. However, to improve upon these associations, research needs to consider the multiple social statuses that people occupy and the given social context in which disparities arise. We do not yet know the nuances in pandemic-related outcomes for specific groups or contexts such as Black American women with high educational attainment compared with Black

American women who have low educational attainment. We do not yet know if the social inequality foundation of the Stress Process Model follows a similar distribution among White men with limited education compared with Black men with limited education.

Another dominant medical sociological theory is the *Fundamental Cause Theory*. Bruce Link and Jo Phelan (2004) identified one's socioeconomic status as a fundamental cause of disease and later argue for processes of racism as a distinct feature of the Fundamental Cause Theory that helps explain racial differences in health disparities when SES is controlled. In short, racism as a fundamental cause of disease borrows Feagin's (2000) concept of systemic racism in the United States. In this case, systemic racism is situated in the economic advantages of Whites during slavery and how these economic and social advantages over time have been engrained within institutions and reproduces racial stereotypes, emotions, ideas, and institutional practices (Feagin, 2000). These processes of systemic racism have also been instrumental in fueling interpersonal conflict, hate crimes, and acts of violence against non-Whites.

According to racism as a fundamental cause of disease, social factors that have benefited Whites over time, are three-fold: (1) structural factors such as the representation of Whites in local, state, and national levels of government; (2) personal resources of money, power, and social and occupational prestige that have historically benefited Whites; and (3) social psychological resources such as the expectation that Whites will dominate and Whites are generally the "superior race". Racism is a fundamental cause of disease because "the broad range and flexibility of the resources that racism provides Whites facilitate the reproduction of SES inequalities by race" (Phelan and Link, 2015, p. 315). One stark limitation of this theoretical perspective is an analysis that encompasses the role of other social status markers in connection to one's reported racial status. Moreover, Phelan and Link (2015) do not account for the variation of health status among White individuals in the United States. As it is a stereotype to assume that Black people are disadvantaged and therefore must have poor health, it is equally hyperbolic to say that White people, because of their social advantages, inherently or automatically have good health. The effect of whiteness as a function of systemic racism must be seriously interrogated (Malat, Mayorga-Gallo and Williams, 2018). Without a comprehensive analysis of COVID-19 data by social status, we have a limited understanding of the social consequences of COVID-19.

Together, these two theories represent a significant portion of racial health disparities research. The existing gap in quantitative analysis emphasizes an approach that seeks to underscore the mechanisms that link social status to health and the continuation of "cataloguing and quantifying" such factors, especially among people of color (Williams, 2018). Though there is a consensus that exposure to acute or chronic stressors linked to the living and working conditions of people of color and disadvantaged Whites can significantly impact one's mental health (Malat et al., 2018; Mossakowski, 2008, 2013; Pearlin et al., 2005; Williams, 2018), COVID-19 has shown us that the multiple ways in which people are affected by disease and its politics are too vast and complex to be relegated to one theory or approach. At present,

> we do not currently have a clear sense of either the determinants of the levels of mental health status for the major racial-ethnic groups in the United States or the patterning of the various indicators of mental health status for all of these minority populations
>
> (Williams, 2018, p. 467)

To address these gaps in the literature, an intersectional analysis is integral to disentangling the connections between and within Black and White racial groups, health, and other pandemic-related outcomes of COVID-19.

Intersectionality and COVID-19

The intersectional approach has been very influential in feminist scholarship and the Critical Race Theory. Intersectionality posits that social categories like "race", "class", and "gender", or, systems of oppression, are "mutually constituted and work together to produce inequality" (Viruell-Fuentes et al., 2012, p. 2100). For example, in theorizing about one's immigrant and racial status and the socio-cultural implications of assimilating into American society, intersectional theory calls on scholars to attend to the "unequal power relations that underlie social categories, such as race, class, and gender, and to move beyond treating them merely as demographic variables" (Viruell-Fuentes et al., 2012, p. 2103). Intersectionality was made popular within sociology by two Black feminist scholars, Patricia Hill Collins and Kimberlé Crenshaw and is integral to theories such as the Critical Race Theory. However, incorporating intersectional approaches to health disparities and health inequality is rather limited but has seen a more prominent role over the last 15 years (Brown, 2018; Ferrer et al., 2017, Hargrove et al., 2020; Kelly, 2009; Rosenthal and Lobel, 2011; Viruell-Fuentes et al., 2012). By using the concept of "race" as the focus of this analysis, the inclusion of an intersectional analysis will provide new insights that can foster new questions about the social consequences of human and environmental crises. Hence, intersectionality can help researchers better analyze empirical data and provide a framework for several theories and policy initiatives to build a collective and anti-racist approach to issues of environmental health (Powers et al., 2021).

From a theoretical perspective, the intersectionality approach does not treat social status categories as additive in explaining inequality (Brown, 2018; Hargrove et al., 2020). An additive approach holds that there is a "double negative" or compounded set of disadvantages. The additive approach assumes that all Black women, for example, should have worse health outcomes based on their disadvantaged status within the gender hierarchy and within the racial hierarchy. This additive approach to health disparities does not account for other types of intersections that produce a dynamic relationship between advantaged and disadvantaged identities. For instance, Black men may experience advantages within gendered social experiences while also experiencing disadvantages in racialized circumstances.

With the passage of nearly three years since COVID-19 reached the shores of the United States and even after vaccine distribution, millions of people throughout the country are still experiencing deleterious effects from this global crisis. From the beginning of the pandemic in the United States in March 2020, millions of Americans filed for unemployment and those who were poor, less educated, women, and people of color experienced the most negatives effects (Kochhar, 2020). Intersectionality requires a deeper understanding of how social categories of differences are linked to social structures that together produce inequality through environmental crises. According to the Critical Environmental Justice Theory (Pellow, 2017), one major component is recognizing the multiple forms in which oppression and inequality are presented, thus the importance of utilizing the analytical tool of intersectionality which can aid in bringing us closer to a more equitable future.

Data and Measures

The following analysis will be conducted using data from the national HPS administered by the U.S. Census Bureau. The HPS measures household experiences in the United States during the coronavirus pandemic. HPS data seeks to track the social and economic effects of the crises across three distinct "phases". The current analysis uses Phase 3.2, which was collected between July 21, 2021 and October 11, 2021. This time period represents the emergence of the Delta variant in the United States. The HPS dataset is part of the U.S. Census Bureau's "Experimental Data Series" because it produces survey results in two-week intervals allowing for a short turnaround to aid in pandemic recovery policy. The HPS dataset is a unique dataset in that it allows researchers to separately and/or collectively analyze social conditions throughout the pandemic as new variants emerge under rapid social change. Pandemic-related outcomes will be stratified by measures of race, gender, and educational attainment. These data will be used to describe the prevalence and patterns of social conditions experienced during the pandemic over the course of the Delta summer surge of 2021.

Key Measures

Levels of symptoms of anxiety and depression are measured using a two-item modified version of the Generalized Anxiety Disorder (GAD-2) (alpha = 0.90) and a two-item Patient Health Questionnaire (PHQ-2) (alpha = 0.92). A summed scale was constructed to measure *anxiety* where respondents were asked to what extent did they experience anxiousness and feeling worried over the last two weeks. Symptoms of depression, also known as psychological distress, were measured with a summed scaled where respondents were asked to what extent they had "little interest in things" or "feeling depressed". Scales were coded so that higher values reflected higher levels of anxiety and depression. Other measures of mental health measures include prescription drug use and use of mental health services. Socioeconomics and financial hardship were measured by household income, educational attainment, employment, difficulty paying bills, and housing stability and food insufficiency.

Results

Table 12.1 shows the prevalence of pandemic-related outcomes of the Delta summer surge among the overall sample and the full sample of Black and White Americans. Results show that, overall, most respondents surveyed during the Delta surge graduated from college with an associates (AA) or bachelor's (BA) degree and a little over 60% of respondents had a household income of 99K or less in 2020 (29.73% with 49K or less and 31.71% between 50K and 99K) and about 67% reported having health insurance at the time. The remaining seven measures reflect pandemic-related outcomes such as a scaled symptoms of anxiety and depression score over the previous two weeks; prescription drug use and mental health services over the last four weeks; loss of employment over the last four weeks; caught up on rent and mortgage payments; and food insufficiency over the previous week.

Black Americans are more likely to be at a disadvantage on measures of socioeconomics and at an advantage on both mental health measures. Black people are more likely to have a high school degree or less; less likely to have an AA or BA degree (22.3% compared with 29.32%); and less likely to have a graduate or professional degree (21.99% compared with 25.76%). Regarding household income pre-pandemic, Blacks are more impoverished and less likely to be in the middle–upper (100K–149K) and upper-income (>150K) brackets. For income, Black and White Americans share comparable representation in the 50K to 90K income bracket (Black = 29.87% compared with White = 31.88%). What is most striking is the nearly 20% difference between Blacks and Whites at the lowest income tier. Within the Black population, 46.6% had a household income of less than 49K compared with 28.26% of White Americans. Relatedly, difficulty with paying expenses shows a similar trend. Within the Black population, 38.29% reported having no difficulty in paying expenses over the last 7 days compared with 62.08% of Whites, nearly a 23% difference. On the other end of the spectrum regarding difficulty with expenses, 6.75% of Whites

Table 12.1 Prevalence of Social Conditions among the Full Sample and Sub-sample of Black and White Americans during the Summer 2021 Delta Surge

Age Group	Full Sample		Full Black Sample		Full White Sample	
	%	n	%	n	%	n
Emerging Adults (18–24)	2.85	9,837	2.89	902	2.84	8,935
Young Adults (25–44)	28.31	97,813	32.5	10,148	27.89	87,665
Middle-Aged Adults (45–64)	39.19	135,419	43.94	13,722	38.72	121,697
Older Adults (65–88)	29.65	102,437	20.67	6,456	30.54	95,981
Total				31,228		314,278
Educational Attainment						
HS Grad/GED or Lower	13.51	46,661	17.98	5,616	13.06	41,045
Some College	21.65	74,794	25.97	8,110	21.22	66,684
Associates AA/AS	10.74	37,106	11.76	3,671	10.64	33,435
Bachelor BA	28.69	99,117	22.3	6,963	29.32	92,154
Graduate/Professional Degree	25.42	87,828	21.99	6,868	25.76	80,960
Household Income (2020)						
Less Than US$49,000	29.73	81,547	46.6	10,243	28.26	71,304
US$50,000–US$99,000	31.71	86,984	29.87	6,565	31.88	80,419
US$100,000–US$149,000	18.64	51,128	12.61	2,771	19.17	48,357
US$150,000 or Higher	19.91	54,610	10.92	2,400	20.69	52,210
Economic Hardship (Last 7 Days) Difficulty w/ Expenses						
Not at All	60.03	191,612	38.29	10,559	62.08	181,053
A Little Difficult	20.28	64,733	24.78	6,833	19.85	57,900
Somewhat Difficult	12.07	38,529	20.12	5,548	11.31	32,981
Very Difficult	7.62	24,329	16.8	4,633	6.75	19,696
Loss Employment (Last 4 Weeks) Anyone in household						
Yes	11.43	38,369	19.71	5,919	10.62	32,450
No	88.57	297,290	80.29	24,118	89.38	273,172
Housing Security						
Caught Up on Rent Payments						
Yes	89.32	54,761	78.22	7,247	91.29	47,514
No	10.68	6,551	21.78	2,018	8.71	4,533
Caught Up on Mortgage Payments						
Yes	95.23	133,024	87.86	8,435	95.77	124,589
No	4.77	6,667	12.14	1,165	4.23	5,502
Mental Health (Last 2 Weeks)						
Symptoms of Anxiety	3.25/8	342,608	3.13/8	30,920	3.26/8	311,688
Symptoms of Depression	2.94/8	342,332	2.87/8	30,911	2.95/8	311,421
Prescription Drug Use (Last 4 Weeks) for Emotions, Concentration Behavior, or Mental Health						
Yes	24.84	75,453	16.88	4,277	25.57	71,176
No	75.16	228,275	83.12	21,054	74.43	207,221
Mental Health Counseling (Last 4 Weeks)						
Yes	11.23	34,121	10.94	2,775	11.26	31,346
No	88.77	269,740	89.06	22,586	88.74	247,154
Health Insurance Status						
Yes	66.62	193,797	65.67	16,098	66.71	177,699
No	33.38	97,094	34.33	8,415	33.29	88,679

(Continued)

Table 12.1 (Continued)

	Full Sample		Full Black Sample		Full White Sample	
Food Insufficiency (Last 7 Days)						
Describe the Type of Food in Household						
Enough of the Food (I/We) Wanted to Eat	79.61	248,699	63	16,751	81.15	231,948
Enough, but Not Always the Kinds of Food (I/We) Wanted to Eat	15.38	48,049	24.86	6,609	14.5	41,440
Sometimes Not Enough to Eat	3.93	12,272	9.64	2,562	3.4	9,710
Often Not Enough to Eat	1.08	3,381	2.51	667	0.95	2,714

reported having a "very difficult" time paying expenses compared with 16.8% of Blacks, which is more than double. Black people also were much more likely than Whites to report either themselves or someone else in their household losing employment over the previous month, 19.71% compared with 10.62%, respectively. Lastly, at every level of food insufficiency, Black people were worse off compared with Whites. Among Blacks, 63% reported having "enough of the food (I/we) wanted to eat", compared with 81.15% of Whites. At the highest indicator of lacking nutrition, 2.51% of Black households reported "often not enough to eat" compared with 0.95% of Whites. These results show striking differences of social conditions by categories of race.

Despite all these social disadvantages, Black people, on average, reported better mental health outcomes for psychological distress (Blacks mean score = 2.87 out of 8 compared with Whites mean score = 2.95 out of 8) and symptoms of anxiety (Blacks mean score = 3.13 out of 8 compared with Whites mean score = 3.26 out of 8). Supplementary analysis (not shown) of independent t-test sampling confirms a statistically significant difference between Blacks and Whites ($p <$ 0.001). White Americans (25.57%) were much more likely than Black Americans (16.88%) to use prescription drugs to manage "emotions, concentration, behavior, or mental health" over the previous 4 weeks, notwithstanding reporting similar results for having health insurance and using mental health counseling during the sampling period.

Rather than examining differences *between* or *across* independent racial categories, Table 12.2 shows the same distribution of social indicators but broken down by race *and* gender. In this way, comparisons can be made between Black men/Black women and White women/White men. The first set of results described here will be between Black women and Black men followed by a description of White women compared with White men. Regarding intersectionality, this level of analysis will show a more nuanced pattern of the social determinants of health and social outcomes. According to Table 12.2, Black women and men have a similar distribution of educational outcomes at every level of educational attainment; however, differences emerge when comparing income. Black men have significantly better income than Black women. More than half of Black women, 51.26%, made less than 50k, compared with 36.53% of Black men. Black women were more likely to report having a "very difficult" time (18.3%) paying expenses over the last 7 days compared with Black men (13.59%). Regarding mental health, despite having similar access to healthcare (e.g., currently having health insurance), 18.98% of Black women compared with 12.36% of Black men reported using prescription drugs over the last month and have a higher prevalence of mental health issues.

Similar to the Black sample, White women and men share an even distribution across educational attainment; however, White women are more likely to be impoverished compared with

Table 12.2 Prevalence of Social Conditions among the Full Sample and Sub-sample of Black and White Americans during the Summer 2021 Delta Surge

Age Group	Black Men %	n	Black Women %	n	White Women %	n	White Men %	n
Emerging Adults (18–24)	2.78	592	3.13	310	2.67	4,994	3.09	3,941
Young Adults (25–44)	34.82	7,422	27.5	2,726	29.31	54,726	25.82	32,939
Middle-Aged Adults (45–64)	43.11	9,188	45.74	4,534	39.92	74,529	36.97	47,168
Older Adults (65–88)	19.3	4,113	23.64	2,343	28.09	52,451	34.12	43,530
Total		21,315		9,913		186,700		127,578
Educational Attainment								
HS Grad/GED or Lower	17.65	3,762	18.7	1,854	13.52	25,242	12.39	15,803
Some College	26.25	5,595	25.37	2,515	21.37	39,907	20.99	26,777
Associates AA/AS	17.65	3,762	18.7	1,854	11.75	21,934	9.01	11,501
Bachelor BA	21.34	4,549	24.35	2,414	28.41	53,050	30.65	39,104
Graduate/Professional Degree	22.39	4,773	21.13	2,095	24.94	46,567	26.96	34,393
Household Income (2020)								
Less Than US$49,000	51.26	7,705	36.53	2,538	31.38	46,682	23.78	24,622
US$50,000–US$99,000	29.21	4,391	31.29	2,174	32.62	48,515	30.81	31,904
US$100,000–US$149,000	10.8	1,624	16.51	1,147	18.09	26,902	20.72	21,455
US$150,000 or Higher	8.73	1,312	15.66	1,088	17.91	26,643	24.69	25,567
Economic Hardship (Last 7 Days) Difficulty w/ Expenses								
Not at All	34.75	6,536	45.91	4,023	58.88	101,761	66.74	79,292
A Little Difficult	25.48	4,793	23.28	2,040	21.07	36,410	18.09	21,490
Somewhat Difficult	21.47	4,039	17.22	1,509	12.47	21,548	9.62	11,433
Very Difficult	18.3	3,442	13.59	1,191	7.58	13,106	5.55	6,590
Loss Employment (Last 4 Weeks) Anyone in Household								
Yes	20.12	4,122	18.82	1,797	10.71	19,424	10.49	13,026
No	79.88	16,367	81.18	7,751	89.29	161,991	89.51	111,181
Housing Security Caught Up on Rent Payments								
Yes	77.64	5,241	79.76	2,006	90.5	29,272	92.58	18,242
No	22.36	1,509	20.24	509	9.5	3,072	7.42	1,461
Caught Up on Mortgage Payments								
Yes	12.87	812	10.73	353	95.45	74,290	96.24	50,299
No	87.13	5,498	89.27	2937	4.55	3,539	3.76	1,963
Mental Health (Last 2 Weeks)								
Symptoms of Anxiety	3.27/8	21,115	2.81/8	9,805	3.46/8	185,221	2.97/8	126,467
Symptoms of Depression	2.96/8	21,106	2.68/8	9,805	3.04/8	185,067	2.81/8	126,354

(*Continued*)

Table 12.2 (Continued)

	Black Men		Black Women		White Women		White Men	
Prescription Drug Use (Last 4 Weeks) for Emotions, Concentration, Behavior, or Mental Health								
Yes	18.98	3,285	12.36	992	31.34	51,681	17.18	19,495
No	81.02	14,021	87.64	7,033	68.66	113,243	82.82	93,978
Mental Health Counseling (Last 4 Weeks)								
Yes	12.12	2,100	8.4	675	13.46	22,218	8.04	9,128
No	87.88	15,229	91.6	7,357	86.54	142,804	91.96	104,350
Health Insurance Status								
Yes	64.85	10,890	67.45	5,208	66.56	105,507	66.93	72,192
No	35.15	5,902	32.55	2,513	33.44	53,017	33.07	35,662
Food Insufficiency (Last 7 Days) Describe the Type of Food in Household								
Enough of the Food (I/We) Wanted to Eat	60.43	10,969	68.54	5,782	79.18	134,088	84.02	97,860
Enough, but Not Always the Kinds of Food (I/We) Wanted to Eat	26.49	4,809	21.34	1,800	16.05	27,186	12.24	14,254
Sometimes Not Enough to Eat	10.43	1,894	7.92	668	3.77	6,385	2.85	3,325
Often Not Enough to Eat	2.65	481	2.2	186	1	1,686	0.88	1,028

White men, 31.38% compared with 23.78%, respectively. White women are also less likely to be in the upper-income tier compared with White men, 17.91% compared with 24.69%, respectively. Through the intersection of race and gender, Tables 12.1 and 12.2 show that women do not make as much money as men; however, even at the lowest income tier, more Black women occupy a much larger share of their population who are poor (51% compared with 31%). Unlike the Black population, White men and women have a similar distribution of economic hardship over the past 7 days; however, Black women are at the lower end compared with White men and White women reporting less hardship. White women and White men additionally report similar percentages regarding loss of employment over the previous month and being caught up on mortgage and rent payments.

Pertaining to health and nutrition, despite having similar rates of health insurance, White women and White men differ in prescription drug use over the past month. With the highest percentage of 31.34%, White women reported needing to use prescription drugs to manage their mental health over the past month compared with White men at 17.18%. In reference to food over the past week, 79.18% of White women reported having "enough of the food (I/we) wanted to eat" compared with 84.02% of White men, which is a significant improvement compared with Black women and Black men at 60.43% and 68.54%, respectively. In sum, Table 12.2 demonstrates how patterns of social conditions change when considering the multiple social statuses that people occupy, but the gap between gender categories are starker within the Black community compared with the White community.

Discussion

In our collective local, regional, national, and global memories, there is no precedent on how nations and individuals would respond to a coronavirus pandemic. This study was designed to inform researchers and policymakers on the patterns and distribution of social conditions and pandemic-related outcomes during the surge of the summer Delta wave. A contribution of this study is to bring awareness to the complexity of categories of difference and how individual experiences differ depending on the intersections of race, gender, and educational attainment. That is, minorities, women, and those with limited education experience the brunt of the social consequences of this global crisis. These findings show that pre-pandemic inequalities were exacerbated during Delta's surge. One key theme in the data presented here is that despite Black Americans reporting worse socioeconomic status than Whites, Black people reported better overall mental health. This evidence is in line with research that challenges the social inequality foundation of the stress process model (Farmer and Ferraro 2005; Louie and Wheaton, 2019), which argues that a disadvantaged or marginalized social status leads to poor health due to higher levels of stress exposure and stress vulnerability. The intersectional approach also demonstrates the legitimacy in examining within-group variation in health and pandemic-related outcomes by revealing disparities between White men and women and Black men and women. The level of vulnerability and exposure to acute and chronic stressors will vary by the intersecting categories of race, gender, and education. Supplementary analysis of regression data show that when all social factors included in the study are controlled, Blacks compared to Whites, women compared to men, and low-educated Blacks and Whites compared to highly educated Blacks and Whites, have a higher prevalence of symptoms of anxiety, psychological distress, and loss of employment. Future research should consider further regression analysis of COVID-19 data to make better predictions about the social consequences of COVID-19. Statistical models using interactions effects between social status can better operationalize intersectional research designs.

Despite the contributions, no study is conducted without its limitations. First and foremost, this study is not longitudinal therefore causal inferences or temporal ordering of social conditions could not be considered. Another limitation is that this study did not include measures of citizenship status or other social status markers such as disability status. Future research would benefit from an analysis of pandemic effects on migrants and/or those with limited mobility. Though outside of the scope of this chapter, future research should also consider occupational prestige and occupational status. The sharp increase in teleworking underscores pre-existing labor marker inequalities as many white-collar jobs were essentially protected throughout the peaks and valleys of the pandemic whereas blue-collar and other "essential jobs" remained precarious and routinely faced with high levels of virus exposure. We must not forget that hundreds of thousands of individuals benefited from policy shifts during the pandemic. In this way, intersectional research designs can examine the impact of pandemics and other environmental issues between individuals and communities by helping to influence policy responses that alleviate the unequal distribution of stress, deleterious social circumstances, and social advantages throughout a crisis (Maestripieri, 2021).

Policy and Recommendations

As COVID-19 exposes deep structural inequalities, the present moment provides opportunities to address them. During a pandemic, at the individual level, this means the federal government and state legislatures must work together to extend eviction moratoriums and provide better-paid family leave protections among those who do not have the privilege of remote work. If the logic of neoliberal politics is to emphasize "personal responsibility", it would benefit the government to construct policy that gives individuals and families the ability to make the *best* possible opportunity to make appropriate decisions. Welfare recipients should see expansions of food establishments that accept SNAP benefits. Rather than pulling money away from public assistance, more federal dollars need to strengthen food programs, especially in times of crises. At the structural level, large corporations *and* small businesses and entrepreneurs should get routine subsidies so business owners can withstand the storm of rising case rates, understaffing, and disruptions in import and export flows. Policies that create safety nets can buffer the external effects of institutions during a crisis so that those effects do not trickle down to the microlevel. As a result, such policies would increase individual agency to navigate the ebb and flow of rapid social change.

Relatedly, macro-level policies should also understand context-specific issues. For example, in the United States, there are geographic and political ideologies that are correlated with vaccination status. Awareness campaigns that are specifically designed to demystify vaccines should be top priority to help limit the spread of a deadly respiratory illness. As time goes on, the immediate health impact of COVID-19 will dissipate resulting in an endemic disease that, at the very least, will cause disruptions in daily life that are easier to manage. Understanding where vulnerable populations and communities are located, along with their specific socioeconomic and health-related concerns, will drastically improve the lives of those who live there.

Powers and colleagues (2021) note "despite openings for greater social and environmental justice with the next presidential administration, the pandemic may still result in greater neoliberal entrenchment and the exacerbation of inequality" (p. 226). Beyond the social sciences, evidence from this chapter can be used to guide state- and local-level policies to safeguard against less inclusive neoliberal social policy. *Before* the next local, state, national, or global crises ensue, there must be institutional linkages that enable local health professionals, grassroots organizations, and local politicians to exchange information on the needs and issues within communities. Understanding, for example, how low-income Black men and women from southern states experience the transition from education systems to the labor market compared with low-income White men and women in the Midwest, which would significantly improve initiatives, such as SNAP education programs, career workshops, vocational schooling opportunities, and the like. Evidence from this chapter can also be elevated to influence national policy during a crisis by way of revealing the social consequences that thousands of people negatively experience in such a short period of time. Without a strong national safety net in place, preventable inequalities will remain or worsen without fundamental change at the policy level. As a result, future research on social disasters and community-building must be aware of the contentious relationships among local, state, and national politics and their connection to social policy.

References

Brown, T. H. (2018). Racial stratification, immigration, and health inequality: A life course-intersectional approach. *Social Forces*, *96*(4), 1507–1540. https://doi.org/10.1093/sf/soy013

Baumgartner, J. C., Aboulafia, G. N., Getachew, Y., Radley, D. C., Collins, S. R., & Zephyrin, L. (2021). (rep.). *Inequities in Health and Health Care in Black and Latinx/Hispanic Communities: 23 Charts* (pp. 1–31). The Commonwealth Fund.

COVID-19 Cases and Deaths, Vaccinations, and Treatments by Race/Ethnicity as of Fall 2022 | KFF. (2022, November 17). KFF. https://www.kff.org/racial-equity-and-health-policy/issue-brief/covid-19-cases-and-deaths-vaccinations-and-treatments-by-race-ethnicity-as-of-fall-2022/

Farmer, M. M., & Ferraro, K. F. (2005). Are racial disparities in health conditional on socioeconomic status? *Social Science & Medicine*, *60*(1), 191–204. https://doi.org/10.1016/j.socscimed.2004.04.026

Ferrer, I., Grenier, A., Brotman, S., & Koehn, S. (2017). Understanding the experiences of racialized older people through an intersectional life course perspective. *Journal of Aging Studies*, *41*, 10–17. https://doi.org/10.1016/j.jaging.2017.02.001

Haischer, M. H., Beilfuss, R., Hart, M. R., Opielinski, L., Wrucke, D., Zirgaitis, G., Uhrich, T. D., & Hunter, S. K. (2020). Who is wearing a mask? gender-, age-, and location-related differences during the COVID-19 pandemic. *PLoS One, 15*(10). https://doi.org/10.1371/journal.pone.0240785

Hargrove, T. W., Halpern, C. T., Gaydosh, L., Hussey, J. M., Whitsel, E. A., Dole, N., Hummer, R. A., & Harris, K. M. (2020). Race/ethnicity, gender, and trajectories of depressive symptoms across early- and mid-life among the add health cohort. *Journal of Racial and Ethnic Health Disparities, 7*(4), 619–629. https://doi.org/10.1007/s40615-019-00692-8

Holst, H., Fessler, A., & Niehoff, S. (2020). Covid-19, social class and work experience in Germany: inequalities in work-related health and economic risks. *European Societies, 23*(suppl 1), S495–S512. https://doi.org/10.1080/14616696.2020.1828979

Kelly, U. A. (2009). Integrating intersectionality and biomedicine in health disparities research. *Advances in Nursing Science, 32*(2), E42–E56. https://doi.org/10.1097/ans.0b013e3181a3b3fc

Kochhar, R. (2020, August 26). *Unemployment rose higher in three months of COVID-19 than it did in two years of the great recession.* Pew Research Center. https://www.pewresearch.org/fact-tank/2020/06/11/unemployment-rose-higher-in-three-months-of-covid-19-than-it-did-in-two-years-of-the-great-recession/

Louie, P., & Wheaton, B. (2019). The black-white Paradox revisited: Understanding the role of counterbalancing mechanisms during adolescence. *Journal of Health and Social Behavior, 60*(2), 169–187. https://doi.org/10.1177/0022146519845069

Maestripieri, L. (2021). The Covid-19 pandemics: Why intersectionality matters. *Frontiers in Sociology, 6.* https://doi.org/10.3389/fsoc.2021.642662

Malat, J., Mayorga-Gallo, S., & Williams, D. R. (2018). The effects of whiteness on the health of whites in the USA. *Social Science & Medicine, 199*, 148–156. https://doi.org/10.1016/j.socscimed.2017.06.034

Maleki Dana, P., Sadoughi, F., Hallajzadeh, J., Asemi, Z., Mansournia, M. A., Yousefi, B., & Momen-Heravi, M. (2020). An insight into the sex differences in COVID-19 patients: What are the possible causes? *Prehospital and Disaster Medicine, 35*(4), 438–441. https://doi.org/10.1017/s1049023x20000837

Monte, L. M., & Perez-Lopez, D. J. (2021). (rep.). *How the Pandemic Affected Black and White Households.* United States Census. Retrieved from https://www.census.gov/library/stories/2021/07/how-pandemic-affected-black-and-white-households.html.

Mossakowski, K. N. (2008). Dissecting the influence of race, ethnicity, and socioeconomic status on mental health in young adulthood. *Research on Aging, 30*(6), 649–671. https://doi.org/10.1177/0164027508322693

Mossakowski, K. N. (2013). Disadvantaged family background and depression among young adults in the United States: The roles of chronic stress and self-esteem. *Stress and Health, 31*(1), 52–62. https://doi.org/10.1002/smi.2526

Mude, W., Oguoma, V. M., Nyanhanda, T., Mwanri, L., & Njue, C. (2021). Racial disparities in COVID-19 pandemic cases, hospitalisations, and deaths: A systematic review and meta-analysis. *Journal of Global Health, 11.* https://doi.org/10.7189/jogh.11.05015

Pearlin, L. I., Menaghan, E. G., Lieberman, M. A., & Mullan, J. T. (1981). The stress process. *Journal of Health and Social Behavior, 22*(4), 337. https://doi.org/10.2307/2136676

Pearlin, L. I., Schieman, S., Fazio, E. M., & Meersman, S. C. (2005). Stress, health, and the life course: Some conceptual perspectives. *Journal of Health and Social Behavior, 46*(2), 205–219. https://doi.org/10.1177/002214650504600206

Phelan, J. C., Link, B. G., Diez-Roux, A., Kawachi, I., & Levin, B. (2004). "Fundamental causes" of social inequalities in mortality: A test of the theory. *Journal of Health and Social Behavior, 45*(3), 265–285. https://doi.org/10.1177/002214650404500303

Pellow, D. N. (2017). *What Is Critical Environmental Justice?* (1st ed.). Polity.

Powers, M., Brown, P., Poudrier, G., Ohayon, J. L., Cordner, A., Alder, C., & Atlas, M. G. (2021). Covid-19 as eco-pandemic injustice: Opportunities for collective and antiracist approaches to environmental health. *Journal of Health and Social Behavior, 62*(2), 222–229. https://doi.org/10.1177/00221465211005704

Rosenthal, L., & Lobel, M. (2011). Explaining racial disparities in adverse birth outcomes: Unique sources of stress for Black American women. *Social Science & Medicine, 72*(6), 977–983. https://doi.org/10.1016/j.socscimed.2011.01.013

Viruell-Fuentes EA, Miranda PY, Abdulrahim S. (2012). More than culture: structural racism, intersectionality theory, and immigrant health. *Social Science & Medicine*, *75*(12), 2099–2106. https://doi.org/10.1016/j.socscimed.2011.12.037. Epub 2012 Feb 9. PMID: 22386617.

Williams, D. R. (1997). Race and health: Basic questions, emerging directions. *Annals of Epidemiology*, *7*(5), 322–333. https://doi.org/10.1016/s1047-2797(97)00051-3

Williams, D. R. (2018). Stress and the mental health of populations of color: Advancing our understanding of race-related stressors. *Journal of Health and Social Behavior*, *59*(4), 466–485. https://doi.org/10.1177/0022146518814251

Zhang, W., Walkover, M., & Wu, Y. Y. (2021). The challenge of covid-19 for adult men and women in the United States: Disparities of psychological distress by gender and age. *Public Health*, *198*, 218–222. https://doi.org/10.1016/j.puhe.2021.07.017

13 Convergence of COVID-19 Pandemic Disaster, Mental Health, and Substance Use Disorder

Paul Archibald, Anthony T. Estreet, and Len Price, Jr.

The relationship between substance use and disasters have been examined extensively over the past 15 years with research demonstrating a link between disaster-exposure and post-event substance use (Parslow & Jorm, 2006; Cerdá, Vlahov, Tracy, & Galea, 2008; Flory, Hankin, Kloos, Cheely, & Turecki, 2009; Cerdá, Tracy, & Galea, 2011; Alexander & Ward, 2018; Alexander, Ward, Forde, Stockton, & Read, 2019; Wainwright et al., 2020; Capasso et al., 2021). The coronavirus disease 2019 (COVID-19) pandemic was declared a disaster for all states, tribes, territories, and the District of Columbia (The White House, 2020), which has implications for substance use prevention and treatment (Kopak & Brown, 2020). For instance, there have been research that demonstrated an increase in substance use and drug overdoses in the United States since the declaration of the COVID-19 pandemic as a disaster by former President Donald Trump on March 13, 2020 (Grossman, Benjamin-Neelon, & Sonnenschein, 2020; The White House, 2020; Wainwright et al., 2020; Capasso et al., 2021; Niles, Gudin, Radcliff, & Kaufman, 2021). A recent systematic review was conducted to determine the impact of the COVID-pandemic disaster on the prevalence, incidence, and severity of substance use (Schmidt et al., 2021). The researchers summarized 53 studies published by March 2021 and reported a consensus in study results that demonstrated an increase in frequency, quantity, and severity of substance use, with most related to changes in alcohol use. In a span of four months prior to COVID-19 being declared as a disaster to four months after, a population of individuals diagnosed with or deemed at risk for a substance use disorder (SUD), had a dramatic increase in urine drug test positivity for non-prescribed cocaine, fentanyl, heroin, and methamphetamine (Wainwright et al., 2020). A diagnosis of SUD requires a pattern of symptoms resulting from the use of alcohol, caffeine, cannabis, hallucinogens, inhalants, opioids, sedatives, hypnotics, or anxiolytics, stimulants, tobacco, and other known or unknown substances that an individual continues to take, despite experiencing problems as a result (American Psychological Association, 2013). Similar research conducted by Niles and colleagues (2021) reported that when comparing urine drug test specimens pre-COVID-19 and during COVID-19, urine drug test positivity increased by 35% and 44% for non-prescribed fentanyl and heroin, respectively. They also identified that when examining individuals impacted by polysubstance use issues that included fentanyl and another drug, the urine drug test positivity increased by 89%, 48%, 34%, and 39% for amphetamines, benzodiazepines, cocaine, and opiates, respectively (Niles et al., 2021). This revealed that there was an increase in combining fentanyl with other drugs during the COVID-19 pandemic disaster. In addition, the Overdose Mapping Application Program's (ODAP) report showed that fatal drug overdoses increased by 11.4% and nonfatal drug overdoses increased by 18.6% during 2020 (ODAP, 2020).

To gain a better understanding of the role that the COVID-19 pandemic disaster plays in substance use, this chapter gives a brief overview of the relationship between disasters and SUD with a focus on the COVID-19 pandemic disaster. We discuss how the COVID-19 pandemic disaster

DOI: 10.4324/9781003140245-13

has exacerbated challenges for individuals impacted by SUD. We use concepts from the life stress process, environmental affordances model, and self-medication hypothesis, to provide some explanations for the pathways to SUD during the COVID-19 pandemic disaster. We conclude with a call to action for substance use service delivery during this COVID-19 pandemic disaster.

Disaster and SUD

A disaster is a phenomenon caused by an environmental event that is a natural occurrence, manmade, technological, or armed conflict that results in multiple fatalities, injuries, stress, physical damage, potential trauma, and economic strains (McFarlane & Norris, 2006). To be considered a disaster, that phenomenon is expected to have an acute onset, be time-limited, and have a profound effect on the resources of the disaster-affected area requiring external disaster-relief (Perry, 2018). Just like there is an unequal distribution of wealth in the United States (Bhutta, Chang, Dettling, & Hsu, 2020), there is an unequal exposure to disasters that have an influence on the varied coping responses to the deleterious effects of a disaster (Yeeles, 2018). This unequal exposure and varied coping responses tend to be associated with the differential vulnerability to disaster among the exposed population (Brown, Kopak, & Marie-Hinkel, 2019). The most vulnerable members of the population include those impacted by SUD or those who have developed trauma symptoms or other psychopathology associated with exposure to a disaster (Norris, Friedman, Watson, Byrne, & Kaniasty, 2002; North et al., 1999; Moise & Ruiz, 2016). For example, after the Oklahoma City bombing in 1995, researchers found that greater than 15% of survivors reported using alcohol to cope with their experience (North et al., 1999).

Extensive disaster research has been conducted on the impact of the September 11, 2001 terrorist attacks (9/11 attacks) on SUD. Vlasov and colleagues (2002) found that, among New York City residents, there was a significant increase in self-reported tobacco, alcohol, and marijuana use after the 9/11 attacks. A more recent study evaluated alcohol- or drug-related hospitalizations among persons exposed to the 9/11 attacks and found that traumatic events and post-traumatic stress disorder (PTSD) were independently associated with substance use-related hospitalizations (Hirst, Miller-Archie, Welch, Li, & Brackbill, 2018). Admissions to the hospital required hospitalizations for an alcohol-related diagnosis (53.4%) and a drug-related diagnosis (46.6%) of the patients. Of those patients, exposure as a witness to three or more traumatic events related to 9/11 increased the risk of having a drug-related hospitalization. Having a diagnosis of PTSD was significantly associated with having alcohol- or drug-related hospitalizations.

After Hurricane Katrina in 2005, Moise and Ruiz (2016) examined the hospital admission in New Orleans between 2004 and 2008 to compare the hospitalization rate of individuals afflicted with SUDs. They found that substance use-related hospitalization rates rose from 7.13 per 1,000 population in 2004 to 9.65 (almost one-third) in 2008. Researchers also explored the effects of Hurricane Sandy in 2012 on individuals impacted by SUDs (Pouget, Sandoval, Nikolopoulos, & Friedman, 2015). They found that withdrawal symptoms were prevalent among 60% of the study population. Some of the study participants (27%) also disclosed that they engaged in needle-sharing with unfamiliar people. Approximately 70% of study participants who were on opioid maintenance reported that they could not obtain adequate doses.

These studies demonstrate that substance use is an important area of inquiry when examining the effects of disasters. There seems to be a direct link between the disaster-effects and substance use initiation and increase. Additionally, we can infer that disasters seem to happen at the intersection of physical, psychological, and social environments. When considering the physical crosswalk of disasters, physical damages to the built environment, including houses, buildings, and other structure, loss of power, and diseases are common occurrences. Disasters have also been found to be associated with symptoms of behavioral health problems, encompassing mental health and SUDs, both in the short term and long term. Some of those symptoms that are linked to depression, anxiety, PTSD, and SUD are symptoms, such as uncontrollable stress and anxiety, prolonged feelings of grief and sadness, emotional instability, shock, denial, or disbelief, confusion, difficulty concentrating, anger, irritability, mood swings, adjustment problems, and inability to control the use of legal or illegal substances, alcohol, or medications (Makwana, 2019). Included in this discussion is the social vulnerability of individuals impacted by SUDs (Brown et al., 2019). Social vulnerability in this context refers to the capacity of individuals impacted by SUD to cope with and recover from disaster-effects (Wisner, Blaikie, Cannon, & Davis, 2004). We will discuss this further in the next sections, with a focus on the COVID-19 pandemic disaster.

The COVID-19 Pandemic Disaster and SUD

The COVID-19 pandemic disaster has been extremely devastating to the SUD population (Wang, Kaelber, Xu, & Volkow, 2021). For instance, the risk of COVID-19 exposure was increased for patients with a SUD diagnosis within the past year compared with those with no SUD diagnosis; especially among those with an opioid use disorder and tobacco use disorder. Compared with patients without a SUD, patients with a SUD diagnosis had a higher prevalence of three of the top COVID-19 underlying chronic medical conditions: lung diseases, obesity, and diabetes. African American patients with SUD were at a greater risk for COVID-19, COVID-19 hospitalization, and COVID-19 death than White Americans with SUD, which increased when opioid use disorder was considered. In addition, overall, COVID-19 patients with a SUD diagnosis were more at risk for death and hospitalization than COVID-19 patients without SUD. This demonstrates that individuals impacted by SUD, and more specifically African Americans impacted by SUD, are vulnerable populations in regard to the COVID-19 pandemic disaster, which may be influenced by the traumatic stress exposures associated with the disaster (Grant et al., 2016; Berenz et al., 2017; Rogers et al., 2020; Archibald & Thorpe, 2021).

When examining the association between the COVID-19 pandemic disaster and trauma, COVID-19 has been found to be associated with symptoms of PTSD prevalence rates of 64–75.5% for vicarious traumatization; 46.5–57% for psychological responses; 13–15% for behavioral responses; and 15–19% for emotional responses. The symptoms associated with these responses included poor appetite, sleep problems, irritability, inattention, fatigue, numbing, fear, and despair (Rogers et al., 2020). COVID-19-related trauma and stressors have implications for people experiencing SUDs. For instance, research demonstrates a strong link between exposure to traumatic events and substance use problems, and this comorbidity is associated with poorer treatment outcomes (Grant et al., 2016; Berenz et al., 2017). Although a large proportion of people with histories of SUD will demonstrate resilience to the stress effects of COVID-19, there will be a proportion that is more susceptible to subsequent substance use. Those most at risk for increased substance use may be those whose post-traumatic stress exposures exceed their coping capacity (Brooks et al., 2020; Lai et al., 2020). Also, there have been studies that link acute and chronic stress to substance use initiation and relapse through the pathways of genetic predispositions. These genetic predispositions can make structural changes in the brain that predispose specific individuals to substance use and determine their ability to abstain (De Mar Capella & Adan, 2017; Levran et al., 2018).

The COVID-19 Pandemic Disaster's Impact on Individuals Impacted by SUDs

So, the question remains, how are individuals impacted by SUD being affected by the COVID-19 pandemic disaster? The lives of marginalized individuals, such as vulnerable individuals impacted by SUD, have been disrupted by the COVID-19 pandemic disaster. The COVID-19 pandemic disproportionately disrupted the daily lives of marginalized populations in the form of broken access to substance abuse prevention and treatment services (American Society of Addiction Medicine, 2020) (ASAM). Individuals impacted by SUD are a particularly vulnerable population because of their unique social and health care needs. The unique health care needs for individuals impacted by SUD stem from the likelihood of having comorbid medical or psychiatric conditions (e.g., suicidality) coupled with physical and cognitive disabilities and risk for mortality due to accidents or diseases (e.g., human immunodeficiency virus and human papillomavirus) as a result of continued substance use (Daley, 2013). Many individuals impacted by SUD, experience co-occurring social issues such as unemployment or underemployment, criminal justice exposure as a victim or as a perpetrator, poverty, and low socioeconomic status, limited or no transportation, homelessness, or housing instability, or do not have adequate access to basic needs such as food and medical insurance (Walker & Druss, 2017). The COVID-19 pandemic disaster illuminated financial barriers that prevented many individuals impacted by SUD from obtaining the necessary technology or equipment like smartphones, laptops, computers, or internet services that could enhance or help maintain their recovery process. Moreover, as many state and local governments were following public health requirements for stay-at-home, many individuals were prevented from accessing the necessary services to apply for essential benefits. This disruption forced individuals not to be able to complete the appropriate application or experience severe delays. For those that had an online application process, many were ill-prepared to process the increase of online applications that ultimately impacted the overall access to care and benefits such as Unemployment, Temporary Cash Assistance, Medical Assistance, and Food Stamps (Walker & Druss, 2017; McCarthy, Carter, Jansson, Benoit, & Finnagan, 2018).

Due to unique health care and social needs of individuals impacted by SUD, their lives have been affected in many ways that are centered on the pathway of the *stay-at-home* orders. Stay-at-home extends further than the requirements of social distancing as it is a directive that requires individuals to stay at home, leaving only for specifically authorized activities until the identified hazard or disaster has passed (Mervosh, Lu, & Swales, 2020). The first stay-at-home Executive Order was signed into law on March 19, 2020, by Governor Newsom in the State of California (Mervosh et al., 2020). By April 1, 2020, it was estimated that approximately 316 million people from 42 states, 3 counties, 10 cities, Washington, DC, and Puerto Rico had issued stay-at-home Executive Orders (Mervosh et al., 2020). We can estimate that approximately 96% of the population was affected by the Executive Orders, with 18.9 million individuals impacted by SUD engaged in stay-at-home (SAMHSA, 2019).

Although the stay-at-home orders impact the lives of all residents, it is challenging for individuals experiencing SUD. When examining the effects of the stay-at-home orders on individuals impacted by SUD, the legal or illegal access to the substance of choice for individuals experiencing SUD were restricted, which may have forced many into increased panic, anxieties, and possibly withdrawal (Brooks et al., 2020; Volkow, 2020). In addition, most individuals experiencing SUD require a daily structure and routine aimed at recovery enhancement (Polcin & Henderson, 2008); however, this was interrupted by the COVID-19 pandemic disaster. One of the highly structured areas for many individuals experiencing SUD is group counseling and support groups like Narcotics Anonymous or Alcoholics Anonymous. Due to the COVID-19 pandemic disaster, many of the treatment and support groups resorted to conducting remote and virtual individual and group sessions, even though many individuals may experience technological deficits, such as poor, weak, or no internet services and are not as digitally literate to engage appropriately. Although technology can help mitigate the impact of the COVID-19 pandemic disaster for individuals who are seeking SUD treatment services, it is expected that many individuals impacted by SUD will experience some level of *technostress*, which is an adverse emotional reaction, such as anxiety to using new technology (Brod, 1984; Ragu-Nathan, Tarafdar, Ragu-Nathan, & Tu, 2008). Because of the quick progression of COVID-19, there was not much time allotted to teach clients the skills required to engage some of the technology that was being used without adding increased stress and anxiety.

The COVID-19 Pandemic Disaster's Impact on Treatment for Individuals Impacted by SUDs

In addition to the challenges of restrictive access, daily routines, and structure, technology, and *technostress* associated with it, and socioeconomic challenges, individuals impacted by SUD were also faced with barriers to essential services that would grant them access to effective treatment. SUDs are chronic health co-occurring conditions that have been minimally discussed compared with medical conditions, such as hypertension and diabetes, when addressing the health impact of the COVID-19 pandemic disaster. However, many people experiencing SUDs typically have high-risk experiences that are often identified and addressed when people enter into treatment. These conditions, as discussed earlier, include co-occurring chronic health concerns, poverty, involvement with the criminal justice system, food insecurity, homelessness or housing instability, and lack of financial stability, including unemployment and underemployment (Walker & Druss, 2017; McCarthy et al., 2018). Consequently, as a result of the COVID-19 pandemic disaster, millions of people in SUD treatment and recovery will be impacted more acutely than the general public.

People in SUD treatment and recovery are likely to have an increased vulnerability to the stressors and impact of the various social distancing, safer at home, and stay-at-home requirements. In particular, due to increased isolation, people may experience an increase in substance use and the worsening of symptoms related to depression, anxiety, other psychiatric disorders, and trauma. Consistent with previous research, the increased uncertainty about the health implication of the COVID-19 pandemic disaster has resulted in increased stress responses globally (Brooks et al., 2020; Lai et al., 2020). Research has also demonstrated that increased stress leads to the onset and increase in symptoms for many mental health conditions. In people with depressive disorder, we have seen increases in mood dysregulation and sleep disturbances.

Moreover, individuals with anxiety disorders may find their symptoms are increasing during the COVID-19 pandemic disaster as a result of the public health response but also mixed messages from mainstream media (Brooks et al., 2020; Rogers et al., 2020). With the ongoing requirements for social distancing in place, people in SUD treatment and recovery may find it difficult to remain connected to their support network. For example, if they are not able to effectively navigate remote treatment options and peer support self-help, it could lead to increased isolation and possible triggers for relapse. Similarly, the impact of COVID-19 pandemic disaster on treatment providers has resulted in the sudden large-scale transitions from a typical face-to-face interaction to primarily remote. This has resulted in many practitioners feeling underprepared and ill-equipped to provide services using online technologies. As a result, the COVID-19 pandemic disaster has created a "perfect storm" for increased issues of retention and engagement for providers.

For individuals in SUD treatment, the biggest threat from the COVID-19 pandemic disaster is the treatment disruption caused by the coordinated pandemic suppression activities. This is especially true for those in opioid treatment programs (OTPs) that utilize medication-assisted therapy (MAT) (Samuels et al., 2020; Wakeman, Green, & Rich, 2020). Historically, programs that dispense methadone have been tightly regulated, often requiring daily administration of methadone, which is directly observed. To prevent treatment disruption, SAMHSA provided guidance for increasing take-home methadone, which supported the ongoing pandemic activities by decreasing the number of sessions needed for face-to-face contact (SAMHSA, 2020). Consequently, those in the initial assessment and early engagement phase of OTP still need to conduct initial face-to-face evaluations. These requirements were further complicated due to the reduced or limited services provided by public transportation services, which were also following public health guidelines and often operated at limited capacity and scheduled for "essential workers" only. As a result, many individuals experiencing financial hardships or poverty and relying on public transportation to access SUD treatment were forced to find other means of transportation at their expense.

Consequently, the added stress of transportation compounded with poverty and financial barriers further exacerbated the COVID-19 pandemic disaster's impact on individuals seeking treatment and increased the risk of relapse (Walker & Druss, 2017). Fortunately for individuals in OTPs who utilized buprenorphine/naloxone for MAT, treatment disruption was less of an issue regarding medication administration. This was mainly due to fewer barriers to access such as the medication distribution by pharmacies and the length of prescriptions could be up to 30 days. On the other hand, treatment disruption for people in SUD counseling was still a threat. This was primarily due to both client and provider experiencing challenges with adapting to the use of technology, such as Zoom, Google Meet, GoToMeeting, and other video-conferencing approaches.

Overall, individuals impacted by SUD and their treatment providers were unprepared for the changes required for remote or socially distant treatment provision caused by the COVID-19 pandemic. Still, due to the social distancing measures enforced by public health officials, mutual support groups are available online, but barriers to accessing these services remain for some groups (American Society of Addiction Medicine, 2020). Treatment groups that did provide services in-person were forced to develop protocols to comply with the social distancing and mask-wearing requirements; requiring at least 6-feet distance between individuals; and capping group size to accommodate the necessary distancing. At the same time, treatment providers were forced with the task of quickly developing protocols and informing clients regarding online support and treatment groups, netiquette for the online support groups, confidentiality, and protection for online meetings on platforms, such as Zoom, Cisco WebEx, or Microsoft Teams. These changes may serve as another layer of acute and chronic stress stimuli for individuals impacted by SUD, further disrupting their SUD recovery process.

In an attempt to assist with the level of unpreparedness, the ASAM, one of the leading developers of clinical guidelines and standards for SUD treatment, convened the ASAM Caring for Patients during the COVID-19 (CPDC) Task Force (American Society of Addiction Medicine, 2020). They identified 13 areas of treatment that have been affected by the COVID-19 pandemic and require consideration: *(1) access to buprenorphine; (2) access to care in opioid treatment facilities; (3) SUD treatment in hospital settings; (4) drug testing protocols; (5) SUD treatment in criminal justice systems; (6) infection mitigation in outpatient settings; (7) infection mitigation in residential treatment facilities; (8) consideration of COVID-19 in medication dosage formulation; (9) varied national and state regulations; (10) support group participation; (11) SUD treatment for persons experiencing homelessness; (12) telehealth access for SUD treatment; and (13) opioid use disorder treatment for pregnant women.* These treatment areas require ongoing resource assessment since this is a fluid crisis in which the COVID-19 pandemic disaster information changes daily. To address this, the ASAM CPDC Task Force provides continuously revised resources in real-time at https://www.asam.org/Quality-Science/covid-19-coronavirus.

Pathways to SUDs during the COVID-19 Pandemic Disaster

We have discussed how the COVID-19 pandemic disaster can be considered a stressful and of-tentimes traumatic event, causing individuals impacted by SUD to attempt to cope with being at a greater risk of COVID-19, hospitalization, and death than individuals without SUD by engaging in substance use. We reviewed how individuals impacted by SUD are also coping with the strain caused by their unique health care and social needs and the stressors associated with access to drugs and to substance use treatment. An integrative approach to explain the increase of SUD during the COVID-19 pandemic disaster is now provided.

Life Stress Process and Affordances Model

As indicated earlier, although the affective responses to these stressors may not cause an individual to engage in substance use, it seems to activate their life stress response (Lazarus & Folkman, 1984; Lazarus, 1991). In this context, the experiences of the COVID-19 pandemic disaster are the stress stimuli, which may be perceived as either not stressful (*no stress*) or as stressful depending on whether an individual impacted by SUD finds the event desirable or not. The individuals impacted by SUD then appraise whether they have the required resources available to cope with the COVID-19 pandemic disaster-stress-exposure.

The imbalance between the demands placed on the individual impacted by SUD and the available resources to adaptively cope will determine the subsequent type of COVID-19 pandemic disaster-stress-response. Individuals impacted by SUD may have insufficient resources to cope with the COVID-19 pandemic disaster-stress-exposures. However, individuals impacted by SUD who have sufficient resources may respond in a number of different ways. For example, if the lack of available resources is not perceived as a threat, then the individual impacted by SUD may generate adaptive solutions to remedy the effects of the stressor. Alternatively, if there are insufficient resources to remedy the effects of the stressor, the individual by SUD may focus on developing the necessary resources to cope, rather than identifying ways to reduce the deleterious effects of the COVID-19 pandemic disaster-stress-exposure.

Unfortunately, some individuals impacted by SUD may also use maladaptive coping methods to deal with the stress associated with the lack of resources, including substance use. The Environment Affordances Model hypothesizes that individuals utilize self-regulatory coping strategies that are affordable, accessible, and acceptable in their communities (Jackson, Knight, & Rafferty, 2010; Mezuk et al., 2013). This seems to influence the availability of coping strategies linked to poor health behaviors such as substance use that may provide momentary relief from COVID-19 pandemic disaster stressors while simultaneously increasing risk for chronic medical conditions. Environmental affordances are the possibilities and opportunities within an individual impacted by SUD environment to alleviate stress (Gibson, 1977). However, Mezuk and colleagues (2013) provide a sound argument for including both affordances (opportunities) and constraints (barriers) in the model. Therefore, included in the environment that is being formed by the COVID-19 pandemic disaster are sources of opportunities and barriers to relieve the stress. These opportunities and barriers are influenced by sociopolitical-cultural-historical factors such as stigma in the SUD realm, SUD discourse throughout U.S. history used to institute and determine cultural and political ideals, and religious beliefs; and sociodemographic factors such as race/ethnicity, gender, and age, and socioeconomic factors, such as education, employment, and income. It is the synergy and interplay of these factors that influence substance use as a coping strategy for individuals impacted by SUD.

Self-Medication Hypothesis

Even further, the self-medication hypothesis seems to provide some potential pathways for understanding the relationship between substance use and the COVID-19 pandemic disaster. An extensive literature review identified a large body of research that supported the self-medication hypothesis (Berenz et al., 2017) that proposes that individuals cope with their psychological distress by using substances (Khantzian, Mack, & Schatzberg, 1974; Khantzian, 2003). It is theorized that individuals who use substances prescribe to a belief system that supports the use of psychoactive drugs as a way to relieve psychological suffering (Khantzian, 1997). In addition, whether an individual chooses to use a stimulant, depressant, or hallucinogen depends on past experiences with the drug to effectively interrupt the affective responses to a traumatic stressor. For instance, Alexander and Ward (2018) reported that depressants, such as alcohol and cannabis, are most often used to achieve a sedating effect with the intention of alleviating the feelings associated with intense anxiety and fear. On the other hand, individuals attempting to avoid the stressor or are depressed may gravitate more to stimulants, such as nicotine or cocaine, to increase their energy level and improve mood and confidence (Khantzian, 1997; Khantzian, 2003). However, coping with the affective responses to the COVID-19 pandemic disaster is not the only catalyst in greater substance use because there is a portion of the SUD population who did not increase their substance use (Nordløkken, Pape, Wentzel-Larsen, & Heir, 2013; Alexander & Ward, 2018). The experiences of the COVID-19 pandemic disaster may activate the life stress process of an individual impacted by SUD, influencing the sympathetic nervous system, which prepares the body for a "flight or fight response" (von Rosenberg et al., 2017). The individual impacted by SUD, may then identify a set of coping strategies, including substance use, to influence the parasympathetic nervous system, which restores the body to a calm state and functions to regulate stress arousal to a state of homeostasis (von Rosenberg et al., 2017). Based on the information provided above, substance use can be considered a COVID-19 pandemic disaster self-medication strategy where individuals engage in substance use to alleviate the traumatic stress associated with the COVID-19 pandemic disaster-exposure (Alexander & Ward, 2018).

These theories indicate that the traumatic stress associated with the COVID-19 pandemic disaster may be predicting subsequent SUD rather than vice versa. Thus, initiating substance use and relapse can be the consequences of the COVID-19 pandemic disaster-coping strategies used to manage acute and chronic stress associated with the COVID-19 pandemic disaster (De Mar Capella & Adan, 2017).

Call to Action

Individuals suffering SUDs are at an increased risk of the negative consequences of the COVID-19 pandemic disaster. Although many public health social work agencies were able to rise to the occasion and develop innovative treatment services for individuals experiencing SUDs, the COVID-19 pandemic disaster exposed cracks in our current service delivery system to the point that access to services was interrupted in many ways (American Society of Addiction Medicine [ASAM], 2020). This vulnerability is related to SUD practitioners' ability to respond to viral disasters in the United States while simultaneously utilizing varied forms of technology to deliver competent services to individuals experiencing SUD (Brod, 1984; Ragu-Nathan et al., 2008). The COVID-19 pandemic disaster brought to the forefront the barriers to accessing telehealth services for populations affected by SUDs. Service providers realize that there is a need to develop innovative and novel treatment options. The *tele-SUD-care* is here, and we must fully come to grips with our understanding of what teletherapy for individuals experiencing SUDs means. Most importantly, whatever *tele-SUD-care* strategies are deployed, the implementation must be based on an individual's level of techno-literacy, techno-access, clinical, demographic, and socioeconomic factors.

Public health social work professionals who work in the mental health and substance use arena must work to reduce the fragmentation of resources and activities by providing a more seamless disaster response. This should be incorporated across four stages of the disaster continuum:

mitigation, preparedness, response, and recovery (Nojavan, Salehi, & Omidvar, 2018). Hence, we recommend that the SUD profession consider the following activities and resources across the disaster continuum:

Mitigation

- Develop an advisory committee on insurance coverage for mental health and SUD services
- Mandate standards like the National Association of Social Workers, Association of Social Work Boards, Council on Social Work Education, and Clinical Social Work Association Standards for Technology in Social Work Practice (2017) be reviewed and adopted in all agencies (https://www.socialworkers.org/includes/newincludes/homepage/PRA-BRO-33617.TechStandards_FINAL_POSTING.pdf)

Preparedness

- Convene a Task Force that includes individuals impacted by SUD lived experiences to assess our response to the COVID-19 pandemic disaster and address strengths and weaknesses so that we can develop standardized response strategies moving forward
- Implement advocacy campaigns to increase access to technology (e.g., computers, tablets, viable data plans, adequate internet speed and bandwidth, and 24/7 technical support) for individuals experiencing SUDs
- Develop a public health social work disaster management plan that includes ways to address access to SUD treatment services during disasters
- Create a disaster management and technology use and ethics curriculum for the SUD educational 0programs at colleges and universities.

Response

- Train SUD peer support specialists as contact tracers
- Add technostress assessments for SUD clients and providers to SUD treatment regimen as there has been a sudden and often forced move to increased use of technology for treatment services and treatment provision (Ragu-Nathan et al., 2008)
- Partner with the ASAM Caring for Patients During the COVID-19 (CPDC) Task Force to provide public health social work expertise for sustainable treatment for individuals experiencing SUD currently in treatment with public health social workers.

Recovery

- Conduct comprehensive SUD screening and treatment need as part of the COVID-19 pandemic disaster recovery strategy with a focused effort on African Americans impacted by SUD, who are at a greater risk of the adverse outcomes of the COVID-19 pandemic disaster
- Develop trauma-informed SUD assessments in preparation for the imminent negative psychological impact of the COVID-19 pandemic disaster

A more integrated disaster response can help reduce the chance of any adverse reactions to the disaster by individuals impacted by SUD-induced substance use or relapse. When considering such resources and activities, it is important to remember that there are many challenges experienced by individuals impacted by SUD while managing the disaster-exposure. There must be a comprehensive plan to minimize the trauma and stress associated with the short-term response and long-term recovery efforts. The activities and resources recommended above may assist in optimizing the integration of mental health and substance use planning into the overall disaster management planning process. Pre-post-disaster planning must include consultations with mental health and substance use professionals to address the mental health and substance use risks and needs associated with individuals with SUD. Implementation of these activities and resources may also provide opportunities to advance healthier communities post-disasters.

References

Alexander, A. C., & Ward, K. D. (2018). Understanding post-disaster substance use and psychological distress using concepts from the self-medication hypothesis and social cognitive theory. *Journal of Psychoactive Drugs*, *50*(2), 177–186. https://doi.org/10.1080/0279 1072.2017.1397304

Alexander, A. C., Ward, K. D., Forde, D. R., Stockton, M., & Read, M. C. (2019). Do current smokers use more cigarettes and become more dependent on nicotine because of psychological distress after a natural disaster? *Addictive Behaviors*, *93*, 129–134. https://doi.org/10.1016/j.addbeh.2019.01.030

American Psychiatric Association. (2013). *Diagnostic and statistical manual of mental disorders*, 5th ed. Arlington, VA: Author.

American Society of Addiction Medicine. (2020). COVID-19 Resources. Retrieved from https://www.asam.org/Quality-Science/covid-19-coronavirus

Archibald, P., & Thorpe, R. (2021). Chronic medical conditions as predictors of the likelihood of PTSD among Black adults: Preparing for the aftermath of COVID-19. Health & Social work, 46(4), 268–276. https://doi.org/10.1093/hsw/hlab025

Berenz, E. C., Roberson-Nay, R., Latendresse, S. J., Mezuk, B., Gardner, C. O., Amstadter, A. B., & York, T. P. (2017). Post-traumatic stress disorder and alcohol dependence: Epidemiology and order of onset. *Psychological Trauma: Theory, Research, Practice, and Policy, 9*(4), 485–492. https://doi.org/10.1037/tra0000185

Bhutta, N., Chang, A. C., Dettling, L. J., & Hsu, J. W. (2020). *Disparities in wealth by race and ethnicity in the 2019 survey of consumer finances, FEDS notes.* Washington: Board of Governors of the Federal Reserve System, September 28, 2020. https://doi.org/10.17016/2380-7172.2797.

Brooks, S. K., Webster, R. K., Smithy, L. E., Woodland, L., Wessely, S., Greenberg, N., & Rubin, G. J. (2020). The psychological impact of quarantine and how to reduce it: Rapid review of the evidence. *The Lancet (Rapid Review)*, *395*(10227), 912–920. https://doi.org/10.1016/S0140-6736(20)30460-8

Brod, C. (1984). *Technostress: The human cost of the computer revolution*. Addison-Wesley.

Brown, B. L. V., Kopak, A. M., & Marie-Hinkel, H. (2019). A critical review examining substance use during the disaster life cycle. *Disaster Prevention and Management: An International Journal*, *28*(2), 171–182. https://doi.org/10.1108/DPM-07-2018-0206

Capasso, A., Jones, A. M., Ali, S. H., Foreman, J., Tozan, Y., & DiClemente, R. J. (2021). Increased alcohol use during the COVID-19 pandemic: The effect of mental health and age in a cross-sectional sample of social media users in the U.S. *Preventive Medicine*, *145*, 106422. https://doi.org/10.1016/j.ypmed.2021.106422

Capella, M., & Adan, A. (2017). The age of onset of substance use is related to the coping strategies to deal with treatment in men with substance use disorder. *PeerJ*, *5*, e3660. https://doi.org/10.7717/peerj.3660

Cerdá, M., Tracy, M., & Galea, S. (2011). A prospective population-based study of changes in alcohol use and binge drinking after a mass traumatic event. *Drug and Alcohol Dependence*, *115*(1–2), 1–8. https://doi.org/10.1016/j.drugalcdep.2010.09.011

Cerdá, M., Vlahov, D., Tracy, M., & Galea, S. (2008). Alcohol use trajectories among adults in an urban area after a disaster: Evidence from a population-based cohort study. *Addiction)*, *103*(8), 1296–1307. https://doi.org/10.1111/j.1360-0443.2008.02247.x

Daley D. C. (2013). Family and social aspects of substance use disorders and treatment. *Journal of Food and Drug Analysis*, *21*(4), S73–S76. https://doi.org/10.1016/j.jfda.2013.09.038

Flory, K., Hankin, B. L., Kloos, B., Cheely, C., & Turecki, G. (2009). Alcohol and cigarette use and misuse among Hurricane Katrina survivors: Psychosocial risk and protective factors. *Substance Use & Misuse*, *44*(12), 1711–1724. https://doi.org/10.3109/10826080902962128

Gibson, James J. (1977). The theory of affordances. In Shaw, R., & Bransford, J. (eds.), *Perceiving, acting and knowing,* pp. 67–82. Lawrence Erlbaum.

Grant, B. F., Saha, T. D., Ruan, W. J., Goldstein, R. B., Chou, S. P., Jung, J., Zhang, H., Smith, S. M., Pickering, R. P., Huang, B., & Hasin, D. S. (2016). Epidemiology of DSM-5 drug use disorder: Results from the national epidemiologic survey on alcohol and related conditions-III. *JAMA Psychiatry, 73*(1), 39–47. https://doi.org/10.1001/jamapsychiatry.2015.2132

Grossman, E. R., Benjamin-Neelon, S. E., & Sonnenschein, S. (2020). Alcohol consumption during the COVID-19 pandemic: A cross-sectional survey of US adults. *International Journal of Environmental Research and Public Health, 17*(24), 9189. https://doi.org/10.3390/ijerph17249189

Hirst, A., Miller-Archie, S. A., Welch, A. E., Li, J., & Brackbill, R. M. (2018). Post-9/11 drug- and alcohol-related hospitalizations among World Trade Center Health Registry enrollees, 2003–2010. *Drug and Alcohol Dependence, 187,* 55–60. https://doi.org/10.1016/j.drugalcdep.2018.01.028

Jackson, J. S., Knight, K. M., & Rafferty, J. A. (2010). Race and unhealthy behaviors: chronic stress, the HPA axis, and physical and mental health disparities over the life course. *American Journal of Public Health, 100*(5), 933–939. https://doi.org/10.2105/AJPH.2008.143446

Khantzian, E. J. (1997). The Self-Medication hypothesis of substance use disorders: A reconsideration and recent applications. *Harvard Review of Psychiatry, 4*(5), 231–244. https://doi.org/10.3109/10673229709030550

Khantzian, E. J. (2003). Understanding addictive vulnerability: An evolving psychodynamic perspective. *Neuro-Psychoanalysis, 5*(1), 5–21. https://doi.org/10.1080/15294145.2003.10773403

Khantzian, E. J., Mack, J. F., & Schatzberg, A. F. (1974). Heroin use as an attempt to cope: Clinical observations. *American Journal of Psychiatry, 131*(2), 160–164. https://doi.org/10.1176/ajp.131.2.160

Kopak, A. M., & Brown, B. V. (2020). Substance use in the life cycle of a disaster: A research agenda and methodological considerations. *American Behavioral Scientist, 64*(8), 1095–1110. https://doi.org/10.1177/0002764220938109

Lai, J., Ma, S., Wang, Y., Cai, Z., Hu, J., Wei, N., Wu, J., Du, H., Chen, T., Li, R., Tan, H., Kang, L., Yao, L., Huang, M., Wang, H., Wang, G., Liu, Z., & Hu, S. (2020). Factors associated with mental health outcomes among health care workers exposed to coronavirus disease 2019. *J.A.M.A. Network Open, 3*(3), e203976. https://doi.org/10.1001/jamanetworkopen.2020.3976

Lazarus, R. S. (1991). *Emotion and adaptation.* Oxford University Press.

Lazarus, R. S., & Folkman, S. (1984). *Stress, appraisal and coping.* Springer.

Levran, O., Peles, E., Randesi, M., Correa da Rosa, J., Shen, P. H., Rotrosen, J., Adelson, M., & Kreek, M. J. (2018). Genetic variations in genes of the stress response pathway are associated with prolonged abstinence from heroin. *Pharmacogenomics, 19*(4), 333–341. https://doi.org/10.2217/pgs-2017-0179

Makwana N. (2019). Disaster and its impact on mental health: A narrative review. *Journal of Family Medicine and Primary Care, 8*(10), 3090–3095. https://doi.org/10.4103/jfmpc.jfmpc_893_19

McCarthy, B., Carter, A., Jansson, M., Benoit, C., & Finnagan, R. (2018). Poverty, material hardship, and mental health among workers in three front-line service occupations. *Journal of Poverty, 22*(4), 334–354. https://doi.org/10.1080/10875549.2017.1419532

McFarlane, A. C., & Norris, F. H. (2006). Definitions and concepts in disaster research. In Norris, F. H., Galea, S., Friedman, M. J., & Watson, P. J. (eds.), *Methods for disaster mental health research,* pp. 3–19. Guilford Publications.

Mervosh, S., Lu, D., & Swales, V. (2020, April 20). See which states and cities have told residents to stay at home. *The New York Times.* Retrieved from https://www.nytimes.com/interactive/2020/us/coronavirus-stay-at-home-order.html

Mezuk, B., Abdou, C. M., Hudson, D., Kershaw, K. N., Rafferty, J. A., Lee, H., & Jackson, J. S. (2013). "White box" epidemiology and the social neuroscience of health behaviors: The environmental affordances model. *Society and Mental Health, 3*(2). https://doi.org/10.1177/2156869313480892

Moise, I. K., & Ruiz, O. M. (2016). Hospitalizations for substance abuse disorders before and after Hurricane Katrina: Spatial clustering and area-level predictors, New Orleans, 2004 and 2008. *Preventing Chronic Disease, 13*(E145). https://doi.org/10.5888/pcd13.160107

National Association of Social Workers, Association of Social Work Boards, Council on Social Work Education, and Clinical Social Work Association (2017). NASW, A.S.W.B., C.S.W.E. and C.S.W.A. standards for technology in social work practice. Washington, DC: NASW Press. Retrieved from https://www.socialworkers.org/Practice/NASW-Practice-Standards-Guidelines/Standards-for-Technology-in-Social-Work-Practice

Niles, J. K., Gudin, J., Radcliff, J., & Kaufman, H. W. (2021). The opioid epidemic within the COVID-19 pandemic: Drug testing in 2020. *Population Health Management, 24*(S1), S43–S51. https://doi.org/10.1089/pop.2020.0230

Nojavan, M., Salehi, E., & Omidvar, B. (2018). Conceptual change of disaster management models: A thematic analysis. *Jamba, 10*(1), 451. https://doi.org/10.4102/jamba.v10i1.451

Nordløkken, A., Pape, H., Wentzel-Larsen, T., & Heir, T. (2013). Changes in alcohol consumption after a natural disaster: A study of Norwegian survivors after the 2004 Southeast Asia tsunami. *BMC Public Health, 13*(1), 58. https://doi.org/10.1186/1471-2458-13-58

Norris, F., Friedman, M. J., Watson, P. J., Byrne, C., & Kaniasty, K. (2002). 60,000 disaster victims speak: Part I. An empirical review of the empirical literature: 1981–2001. *Psychiatry, 65*, 207–239.

North, C. S., Nixon, S. J., Shariat, S., Mallonee, S., McMillen, J. C., Spitznagel, E. L., & Smith, E. M. (1999). Psychiatric disorders among survivors of the Oklahoma City bombing. *JAMA, 282*(8), 755–762. https://doi.org/10.1001/jama.282.8.755

Overdose Detection Mapping Application Program (ODAP). (2020). The consequences of COVID-19 on the overdose epidemic: Overdoses are increasing. Retrieved from http://www.odmap.org/Content/docs/news/2020/ODMAP-Report-May-2020.pdf

Parslow, R. A., & Jorm, A. F. (2006). Tobacco use after experiencing a major natural disaster: Analysis of a longitudinal study of 2063 young adults. *Addiction, 101*(7), 1044–1050. https://doi.org/10.1111/j.1360-0443.2006.01481.x

Perry, R. W. (2018) Defining disaster: An evolving concept. In Rodríguez, H., Donner, W., & Trainor, J. (eds.), *Handbook of disaster research: Handbooks of sociology and social research*, pp 3–22. Springer. https://doi.org/10.1007/978-3-319-63254-4_1

Polcin, D. L., & Henderson, D. M. (2008). A clean and sober place to live: Philosophy, structure, and purported therapeutic factors in sober living houses. *Journal of Psychoactive Drugs, 40*(2), 153–159.

Pouget, E. R., Sandoval, M., Nikolopoulos, G. K., & Friedman, S. R. (2015). Immediate impact of Hurricane Sandy on people who inject drugs in New York City. *Substance Use & Misuse, 50*(7), 878–884. https://doi.org/10.3109/10826084.2015.978675

Ragu-Nathan, T. S., Tarafdar, M., Ragu-Nathan, B. S., & Tu, Q. (2008). The consequences of technostress for end users in organizations: Conceptual development and empirical validation. *Information System Research, 19*(4), 417–433.

Rogers, J. P., Chesney, E., Oliver, D., Pollak, T. A., McGuire, P., Fusar-Poli, P., Zandi, M. S., Lewis, G., & David, A. S. (2020). Psychiatric and neuropsychiatric presentations associated with severe coronavirus infections: A systematic review and meta-analysis with comparison to the COVID-19 pandemic. *Lancet Psychiatry*, S2215-0366(20)30203-0. Advance online publication. https://doi.org/10.1016/S2215-0366(20)30203-0

Samuels, E. A., Clark, S. A., Wunsch, C., Jordison Keeler, L. A., Reddy, N., Vanjani, R., & Wightman, R. S. (2020). Innovation during COVID-19: Improving addiction treatment access. *Journal of Addiction Medicine, 14*(4), e8–e9. https://doi.org/10.1097/ADM.0000000000000685

Schmidt, R. A., Genois, R., Jin, J., Vigo, D., Rehm, J., & Rush, B. (2021). The early impact of COVID-19 on the incidence, prevalence, and severity of alcohol use and other drugs: A systematic review. *Drug and Alcohol Dependence, 228*, 109065. https://doi.org/10.1016/j.drugalcdep.2021.109065

Substance Abuse and Mental Health Services Administration (SAMHSA). (2019). Key substance use and mental health indicators in the United States: Results from the 2018 National Survey on Drug Use and Health (H.H.S. Publication No. PEP19–5068, N.S.D.U.H. Series H-54). Rockville, MD: Center for Behavioral Health Statistics and Quality, Substance Abuse and Mental Health Services Administration. Retrieved from https://www.samhsa.gov/data/sites/default/files/cbhsqreports/NSDUHNationalFindingsReport2018/NSDUHNationalFindingsReport2018.pdf

Substance Abuse and Mental Health Services Administration. (2020). Opioid Treatment Program (OTP) Guidance. Retrieved from www.samhsa.gov/sites/default/files/otp-guidance-20200316.pdf

The White House. (2020, March 13). Letter from President Donald J. Trump on Emergency Determination Under the Stafford Act [Letter]. Retrieved from https://trumpwhitehouse.archives.gov/wp-content/uploads/2020/03/LetterFromThePresident.pdf

Vlahov, D., Galea, S., Resnick, H., Ahern, J., Boscarino, J. A., Bucuvalas, M., Gold, J., & Kilpatrick, D. (2002). Increased use of cigarettes, alcohol, and marijuana among Manhattan, New York, residents after the September 11th terrorist attacks. *American Journal of Epidemiology, 155*(11), 988–996. https://doi.org/10.1093/aje/155.11.988

Volkow, N. D. (2020). Collision of the COVID-19 and addiction epidemics. *Annals of Internal Medicine*, *173*(1), 61–62. https://doi.org/10.7326/M20-1212

Von Rosenberg, W., Chanwimalueang, T., Adjei, T., Jaffer, U., Goverdovsky, V., & Mandic, D. P. (2017). Resolving ambiguities in the LF/HF Ratio: LF-HF scatter plots for the categorization of mental and physical stress from hRV. *Frontiers in Physiology*, *8*, 360. https://doi.org/10.3389/fphys.2017.00360

Wainwright, J. J., Mikre, M., Whitley, P., Dawson, E., Huskey, A., Lukowiak, A., & Giroir, B. P. (2020). Analysis of drug test results before and after the US declaration of a national emergency concerning the COVID-19 outbreak. *JAMA*, *324*(16), 1674–1677. https://doi.org/10.1001/jama.2020.17694

Wakeman, S. E., Green, T. C., & Rich, J. (2020). An overdose surge will compound the COVID-19 pandemic if urgent action is not taken. *Nature Medicine*, 26, 819–820.

Walker, E. R., & Druss, B. G. (2017). Cumulative burden of comorbid mental disorders, substance use disorders, chronic medical conditions, and poverty on health among adults in the U.S.A. *Psychology, Health & Medicine*, *22*(6), 727–735.

Wang, Q. Q., Kaelber, D. C., Xu, R., & Volkow, N. D. (2021). COVID-19 risk and outcomes in patients with substance use disorders: Analyses from electronic health records in the United States. *Molecular Psychiatry*, *26*(1), 30–39. https://doi.org/10.1038/s41380-020-00880-7

Wisner, B., Blaikie, P., Cannon, T., & Davis, I. (2004). *At risk: Natural hazards, people's vulnerability and disasters*, 2nd ed. Routledge.

Yeeles, A. (2018). Unequal exposure. *Nature Climate Change*, *8*, 359. https://doi.org/10.1038/s41558-018-0166-1

14 How Deliberate Planning and Improvisation Shaped Our Response to COVID-19

Len E. Clark

In light of the ongoing Coronavirus-19 (COVID-19) pandemic, it would be easy to say that the emergency management and public health systems in the United States failed the population. Much like the military, these functions often base their decisions through the lens of the last disaster. When we look at the battles fought, not against a military foe, but against something unseen such as a virus, we look toward the "successes" containing Ebola, Severe Acute Respiratory Syndrome (SARS), and others. So, how did the 2019 Coronavirus Pandemic get such a rapid foothold and spread across the planet with relative ease? In the United States, a combination of factors can be identified. Our Federalist system of government with a shared set of delineated duties among and between the levels of government challenge our ability to coordinate efforts easily. The interrelationship between emergency management and public health, although present and developing, may not have been as fully developed as the nation needed. The keynote is that while this is still evolving, positive work continues to protect the population. The last two areas that were found to be lacking in response to the pandemic were the inclusion of the private sector resources and the, now known, limits of a fragile supply chain and resource management system. Although set against the backdrop of a global pandemic, this essay identifies elements that are applicable to any large-scale emergency that requires the integration of emergency management and the public health systems.

Many of the traditional ideas in emergency management focus on hazards and threats from a variety of sources – natural, manmade accidents, and intentional events – that threaten public safety, health, and welfare. Every emergency management plan contains a section that evaluates the potential hazards that may impact an area. While many of these hazards are bound by the laws of chemistry and physics, each disaster contains an element that is difficult to measure and understand. Certain recent events have caused us to change our understanding. Once we incorporate humans into the disaster, we tend to venture into the unknown. Events from our recent past reveal how much we do not know about human reactions and interactions following a disaster. Fortunately, we continue to witness more pro-social than anti-social behaviors. Our emergency plans are attempts to predict human behaviors and decision-making. To achieve success, emergency managers have to know and understand the composition of the community members and how their conditions tend to shape and define their ability to cope and survive.

Often, we think of emergency response and disaster management as government-focused events. For a large portion of our history, this was true. In 2011, the Federal Emergency Management Agency (FEMA) introduced the Whole Community Approach. This Approach sought to

DOI: 10.4324/9781003140245-14

leverage resources and capabilities from throughout the community with the understanding that the private sector possesses many of the resources needed to counter a disaster. According to FEMA,

> As a concept, Whole Community is a means by which residents, emergency management practitioners, organizational and community leaders and government officials can collectively understand and assess the needs of their respective communities and determine the best ways to organize and strengthen their assets, capabilities and interests
>
> (2011, p. 3)

This concept is intended to outline the methods to incorporate ideas, insights, and expertise from throughout any community. But even with this shift in doctrine, emergency management remains one of the essential government functions.

As part of any government function, the U.S. Constitution and any implementing legislation set the operating parameters. The 14th Amendment of the U.S. Constitution states, "nor shall any state deprive any person of life, liberty, or property, without due process of law; nor deny to any person within its jurisdiction the equal protection of the laws" (U.S. Const., Amend. XIV). The Robert T. Stafford Disaster Relief and Emergency Assistance Act, Public Law 93–288 is the keystone piece of legislation that formed modern U.S. emergency management practice. Within the Stafford Act, the process to declare a disaster ultimately rests with the President of the United States. At the direction of the President, the federal government provides physical, technical, and monetary resources to support local and state response and recovery efforts. These activities are coordinated through the FEMA, but may include resources from throughout the Executive Branch and the American Red Cross. Outside of the Stafford Act, other executive agencies possess the authority to declare disasters within the scope of the respective department or agency such as the Department of Agriculture, Small Business Administration, etc. The Public Health Service Act, P.L. 117–58, provides the authority for the Secretary of Health and Human Services "to declare a public health emergency (PHE) and take such actions as may be appropriate to respond to the PHE consistent with existing authorities; to assist states in meeting health emergencies; to control communicable diseases" (HHS, 2021).

When warranted, both authorities under the Stafford and Public Health Service Acts can be employed to protect the nation. For the COVID-19 pandemic, the President authorized a disaster declaration for all 50 states and U.S. territories under the Stafford Act effective from January 20, 2020 (FEMA, 2021). The Stafford Act requires that the President issue disaster declarations for each respective state and territory, as warranted (P.L. 93–288). This is the first time in U.S. history that all areas under U.S. jurisdiction have been issued a disaster declaration for the same disaster. Following the President's declaration, the Secretary of Health and Human Services issued a disaster declaration under the Public Health Service Act for the COVID-19 pandemic on January 31, 2020 (HHS, 2021).

Other federal laws including the Americans with Disabilities Act, the Rehabilitation Act, the Civil Rights Act and others, provide much of the legal basis for nondiscriminatory practices in the United States. Based upon these laws, one would expect that all members of society are eligible to receive disaster assistance, as demonstrated by need. Although a disaster may dispassionately impact an area, the outcomes experienced by the disaster victims are not spread equally among the population. Although all may experience challenges in the population, certain members of any population may face greater challenges based on their individual circumstances.

Emergency management and public health have been intertwined for many years. According to the FEMA,

> emergency management protects communities by coordinating and integrating all activities necessary to build, sustain, and improve the capability to mitigate against, prepare for, respond to, and recover from threatened or actual natural disasters, acts of terrorism, or other man-made disasters
>
> (FEMA, n.d.)

These disasters include those associated with public health emergencies as we have seen in recent years concerning Ebola, Avian Flu, Sudden Acute Respiratory Syndrome, anthrax releases, and other natural or manmade incidents. The Model State Emergency Health Powers Act identifies PHE as "an occurrence of imminent threat of an illness or health condition" from a variety of natural or manmade sources and "poses a high probability of ...harm..." (AAP, 2001, §104). The recent and continuing pandemic centered around the Coronavirus, SARS-CoV2, has increased the tie between emergency management and public health.

Public health emergencies pose challenges that are unique among the hazard types. Since these are biological threats, the agent causing the harm is microscopic and may manifest itself days or weeks after the initial contact. Similar to many other public health hazards, COVID-19 required an exposure and incubation time and possessed many of the typical cold and flu symptoms. This is not the first time we have witnessed this type of event. The Influenza Outbreak of 1918 (often erroneously referred to as the "Spanish Flu") served as the precursor of COVID-19's spread and its early intervention techniques. Although certain aspects are similar between the two events, there are two major differences. The first is the use of social media as a major tool to share information and allows almost everyone to serve as the "media" or an "information source". The second difference is the development and distribution of viable vaccines. The United States did not possess a viable influenza vaccine until the 1940s, almost twenty years after the 1918 outbreak (CDC, 2019). Contrast this with the COVID-19 pandemic, which had viable vaccines in public distribution within 12 months of the first U.S. case.

In recent years, biological threats have caused alarm across the globe. David McEntire (2015) wrote, "The ease of travel and international economic relations could easily trigger a pandemic in other nations. In other words, disease spreads at the speed and extent of travel and commercial activities" (p. 426). In addition to the presence of disease, a variety of other factors come into play. To understand the spread of any particular disease, one must know the route of transmission and the virulence (Stilp and Bevelaqua, 1997, pp. 378–381). At the onset of CoViD-19, researchers did not understand this factor. The Peoples' Republic of China reported cases of what became known as CoViD-19 on December 31, 2019 and the first U.S. case was reported on January 20, 2020 (Holshue et al., 2020). The National Academy of Science published a report in June 2020 that identified the method of transmission as airborne (Zhang, Zhang, Li, Wang, & Molina, 2020). Virulence is defined as "the amount of a particular microorganism that causes an effect in the host. The smaller the dose needed to infect a patient, the virulent the organism is" (Stilp and Bevelaqua, 1997, p. 379). According to research published by the *Journal of Medical Virology*, although the virus that causes COVID-19 has many similarities to other Coronaviruses, it also possesses characteristics of certain flu strains. This increases the virulence of the Coronavirus (Kumar et al., 2021). Although this is not a chapter on any particular disease, it is important to understand how the recent pandemic will shape emergency management and public health responses in the future.

Perhaps the most chilling idea came from Claire Rubin, a noted expert in the field of emergency management. Ms. Rubin (2007) wrote concerning the previous H5N1 Influenza Outbreak, "The emergency manager must prepare for systemic failure due to widespread illness and deaths from the flu. But until an actual outbreak occurs, the precise nature of the emergency manager's role will remain uncertain" (p. 42). Although the precise pathogen may be incorrect, the prediction is accurate.

Within our communities, many of the public health resources exist outside, but they are an integral part of the response and recovery to disasters. The healthcare infrastructure consists of hospitals, private practice physicians, pharmacies, allied healthcare operations, such as diagnostic centers, visiting nurses, home health care, long-term care facilities, and emergency medical services (EMS). A community's EMS providers may be found in the public sector as an agency combined with another emergency service, typically the fire department, or as standalone agency, or as a private sector service provider in either a for-profit or non-profit structure.

The challenge for managing the healthcare system during a disaster in the United States lies in the ability to coordinate these various service providers into a cohesive organization. Although many of these providers operate under a license granted by the state, usually through its respective Health Department, some providers operate under the license granted by independent boards or departments within the state outside of the Health Department.

For those agencies that operate under the jurisdiction of a State Health Department, the Model State Emergency Health Powers Act contains provisions that the Governor, by edict of declaring a PHE, has the powers to compel private sector healthcare resources under their jurisdiction to provide assistance. Section 502(b) of the Act states,

> To require a health care facility to provide services or the use of its facility if such services or use are reasonable and necessary to respond to the public health emergency as a condition of licensure, authorization or the ability to continue doing business in the state as a health care facility

> (AAP, 2001)

If a community possesses a federal health provider, such as the Veterans' Administration, these facilities may operate under their federal jurisdiction without oversight of a state licensing body.

The decentralized organizational structure of the United States may complicate the nation's efforts to provide a coordinated response to a disaster. According to the U.S. Census (2019), the United States consists of over 90,000 local government units including counties, municipalities, and independent school districts. Each of these have varying levels of involvement and responsibility for disaster management. Sylves and Waugh (1990) identified both vertical fragmentation of actions and responsibilities at the federal level and horizontal fragmentation at the state and local levels of government. Sylves and Waugh wrote, "State and urban areas are by their very nature complexes of jurisdictions with overlapping and conflicting responsibilities, some containing functional areas in which no government has clear responsibility" (1990, p. 233).

Concurrently with the local units of government, the United States possesses almost 6,100 hospitals containing over 55,000 intensive care beds (AHA, 2021). Under normal conditions, each of these organizations operates independently of the other, even if they are in close proximity. The challenge in managing the COVID-19 response and recovery efforts lies in the coordination of these many moving parts under disaster conditions. Erik auf der Heide identified "many organizations continue to act independently in disasters, focusing on their own organizational tasks and sometimes failing to see or find out how their role fits into the overall response effort" (1989, 57).

Massive U.S. disasters since the turn of the 21st century have shifted the attention of public health and organized healthcare toward emergency preparedness. Prior to many of the major events of this century, planning and operational considerations were conducted within specific "silos". This partitioning limits the ability to share information outside of a specific discipline or organization. Auf der Heide identified this as an issue when he wrote, "…the various organizations that have a role in disaster response have carried out their planning individually with little attempt to meld their plans together into a coherent overall strategy" (1989, p. 57). The Center for Medicare and Medicaid Services, the agency that establishes rules and regulations to protect patient safety in a variety of healthcare facilities, stipulates that healthcare facilities must participate in emergency planning activities that involve members of the emergency management community outside of the facility. Facilities must demonstrate that they participate in jurisdictional or regional emergency planning organizations, identify, and share their facility's Hazard Vulnerability Analysis, maintain or have the ability to obtain supplies for a 96-hour period, and train and exercise their emergency plans with the community at-large (42 CFR 482.15). These requirements are further supported by healthcare accrediting bodies, such as The Joint Commission and Det Norsk Veritas, evaluate facilities periodically to ensure compliance with the CMS and other accrediting standards.

Most discussions in emergency management and mass casualty contexts focus on large numbers of trauma-related injuries – blunt force, penetrating, and crush injuries. Often, these are visible and require some type of mechanical intervention, such as surgery and splinting. Alexander (2002) discusses the strain on resources associated with these types of mass care incidents. Disasters are disruptive to the normal resource patterns and may impact availability of pre-hospital and acute care resources. Alexander identifies this shift in resource capability as "Normal procedures… will not work…New protocols and methods are required to allocate resources and services to maximize the number of lives saved, induce the best and most rapid aggregate improvement in patients' prognoses…" (2002, pp. 189–190). What Alexander and others have missed in this discussion is what are the options when all of the healthcare system is overwhelmed at the same time. Some emergency managers have developed plans and resources to address these matters, but the solutions are focused on localized or smaller-scale emergencies. The states and federal government have created deployable medical teams and these have proven invaluable in many instances. Compared with the current pandemic, even something of the scale of hurricane Katrina had the advantage of utilizing resources from outside the immediately impacted area.

Federal policy for emergency management resources can be tracked to Homeland Security Presidential Directive #5, "Management of Domestic Incidents" (dated February 28, 2003) and the incorporation of the National Incident Management System (NIMS). This document required all federal executive agencies and states and localities that received federal preparedness funding to adopt NIMS. Many states mandated their respective state and local emergency management agencies to adopt NIMS as their organizational management baseline tool. Included in NIMS is a section dealing with resource management.

As part of the federal guidance, FEMA issued the 3rd edition of its "National Incident Management System" Manual in October 2017. The guidance identifies the typical methods of acquiring resources – stockpiling, mutual aid agreements, ensuring that vendor duplication does not hinder supplies, and vendor contracts that provide for expedited processing and shipping. The Manual cites the example of "hospitals in the same city relying on one supplier's stock of surge medical supplies that may be adequate for only one hospital" as a potential shortfall in the supply chain (FEMA, 2017, p. 9). All of these points are well-taken, but failed to identify issues associated with an incident spreading beyond the local area.

To remedy these shortfalls required some creative thinking. With the understanding that CoViD-19 may be spread by droplets, public health experts reverted back to the tools used in the 1918 Influenza Outbreak. The use of masks to protect the respiratory system is not a new or novel idea. Many industries and service providers wear some type of respiratory protection. Based on the recent history of various respiratory illnesses, it was not unusual to see members of the general population wearing masks in certain cultures. However, the American experience is different. We witnessed some similarities between the 1908 Influenza Pandemic and current COVID-19 pandemic. Hesitancy to wear a mask in public, maintain social distancing, and closure of schools and public events were concerns in both pandemics. Some organizations mandated the use of masks within their properties or for their staff and visitors. Healthcare organizations required masks in certain situations as a means to limit infections as part of their routine order of business before COVID-19. As part of their response to the virus, most healthcare organizations required everyone entering their facilities to wear a mask. Government organizations, including schools, required similar actions.

This demand for masks created an immense strain on the resource management system. The United Nations International Children's Emergency Fund, UNICEF, estimated that 2.4 billion surgical masks would be required in 2020 (UNICEF, 2021). In response to this demand, manufacturers increased production. According to NonWovens Industry Magazine, Honeywell "delivered more than 225 million facemasks… Medline estimates it will be able produce 36 million face masks per month" (McIntyre, 2021). Private sector production increased to meet demand across the globe.

Although production of personal protective equipment increased to meet the demands, there is a lag between the time the decision is made and the arrival of the product for distribution. Emergency management requires a certain amount of deliberate planning that requires the thoughtful examination of the hazards and application of resources. In some instances, the situation may require innovative and improvised planning to meet the needs. The response to COVID-19 provided many opportunities for improvisation.

To meet this challenge, along with others that appeared as a result of the pandemic, the Food and Drug Administration invoked the Emergency Use Authorization (EUA) provisions of the Federal Food, Drug and Cosmetic Act. This Act operates alongside the Public Health Service Act cited earlier in this essay. The issuance of an EUA may be for medicines, medical devices, and other regulated items, such as personal protective equipment. This is not to be confused with full FDA approvals. The EUA provides for the use of these items after consideration of the risks and benefits when no other alternatives exist (FDA, 2020). To overcome the issues regarding masks, a variety of emergency measures were adopted including the sterilization and re-use of masks, the extension of use time for the masks, and acceptance of alternative standards for the masks. This last measure accepted protection certifications from other countries for certain uses. Some of the more publicly known EUAs cover the medications and vaccines authorized for COVID-19. The current arsenal of vaccines was first made available to adults under an EUA. As research continued, the vaccines were deemed appropriate for teenagers and children. Approvals are only one small part of the chain of events that must occur. The vaccine manufacturers have to be able to produce the vaccine in sufficient quantity. These firms were able to rapidly accommodate the need. The next steps involved transportation, storage, and final dispensing to the public. The ability to dispense the vaccine to the public is a point where emergency management and public health easily intersect. The public health agencies maintained the operational responsibility to administer medications to the public. In the United States, we routinely see this activity associated with the distribution of the annual influenza vaccine. Public health agencies will respond to a variety of emergencies to provide prophylaxis medication. In the recent past, we have witnessed the same mechanisms used for measles, hepatitis A, and other outbreaks. The role of emergency management is to provide support and coordinate efforts. This is the same mission emergency management assumes for other disasters.

A similar activity was tested in 2005 through the Top Officials Exercise Program. The third exercise in the series, TOPOFF 3, simulated an intentional release of a biological agent in New Jersey, along with coordinated simulations in Connecticut, Canada, and the United Kingdom. A variety of after-action reports from the New Jersey portion of this exercise identified concerns with the distribution of medications to counter the simulated biological attack. The Office of the

Inspector General for the Department of Homeland Security (OIG-DHS) identified confusion between federal- and state-level emergency declarations, integration of planning efforts, and coordination among the federal, state, local, and private sector levels (OIG, 2005).

A more pointed review of activities specifically conducted in New Jersey identified planning shortfalls that included the lack of logistics to move large amounts of people through the distribution process, the personnel support needed to maintain operations, and the lack of around-the-clock operations. In any exercise, there are a variety of artificialities. In this exercise, the biological agent was identified at the early onset of the period. The after-action report states, 'The POD [Point Of Distribution] concept also begs the question: "What if the agent was a contagious communicable disease before an individual displayed symptoms"?' (Lioy et al., n.d.). This was the dilemma faced during the distribution of the CoViD vaccines.

By the end of December 2020, the FDA had issued the EUA for Pfizer and Moderna COVID-19 vaccines (FDA, 2020). Governor Philip Murphy (D-NJ) officially toured one of the state's mega-vaccination centers on January 11, 2021 (Alvarez, 2021). Through the combined efforts of the local emergency management and public health departments, many of the concerns expressed in the earlier after-action reports were addressed. Vaccine recipients pre-registered for available timeslots. Recipients were medically screened prior to entering facilities. Organizers had developed queues that provided for safe, but effective access to facilities. Temporary staff members were hired to process recipients and to administer the vaccine. Local law enforcement and National Guard troops were on-site to provide security (Alvarez, 2021). Although TOPOFF3 was conducted 15 years prior, many of the lessons and concerns identified were addressed.

Emergency management officials will state that operations rarely function perfectly. Actions are always nuanced by the conditions of the disaster. Although the plans attempt to take these issues into account, conditions require the plans be amended and adapted. The collective response to CoViD used existing planning, policy, and operational tools. Newly identified issues, such as supply chain concerns, required the creation of new procedures and policies to be created or revisions to existing procedures and policies. Emergency management is an "evergreen" process that is constantly under review and revision as new information is revealed. As we move through this disaster, the community will continue to improve the process of disaster management.

References

Alexander, D. (2002) *Principles of Emergency Planning and Management*. Hertfordshire, UK: Terra.

Alvarez, A. (2021) New Jersey Opens Megasite for COVID-19 Vaccine in Sewell. *Philadelphia Inquirer*. January 11, 2021. Retrieved from https://www.inquirer.com/photo/new-jersey-opens-megasite-covid-19-vaccine-sewell-20210111.html

American Association of Pediatrics (2001) Model State Emergency Health Powers Act. Retrieved from https://www.aapsonline.org/legis/msehpa2.pdf.

American Hospital Association (2021) Fast Facts on U.S. Hospitals 2021. Retrieved from https://www.aha.org/system/files/media/file/2021/01/Fast-Facts-2021-table-FY19-data-14jan21.pdf

Auf der Heide, E. (1989) *Disaster Response: Principles of Preparation and Coordination*. Maryland Heights, MO: Mosby.

Centers for Disease Control (2019) Influenza Historic Timeline. Retrieved from https://www.cdc.gov/flu/pandemic-resources/pandemic-timeline-1930-and-beyond.htm

Conditions of Participation. Code of Federal Regulations – Title 42 (2022). 482.1-482.104. Retrieved from https://www.ecfr.gov/current/title-42/chapter-IV/subchapter-G/part-482/subpart-A#subpart-A

FEMA (n.d.) Emergency Management - Definition, Vision, Mission, Principles. Washington, DC: FEMA. Retrieved from https://training.fema.gov/hiedu/docs/ emprinciples/0907_176%20em%20principles12x18v2f%20johnson%20(w-o%20draft).pdf

FEMA. (2011) A Whole Community Approach to Emergency Management: Principles, Themes, and Pathways for Action. FDOC 104–008-1. Washington, DC: FEMA. Retrieved from https://www.fema.gov/sites/default/files/2020-o7/whole_ community_dec2011__2.pdf

FEMA (2017) National Incident Management System. Washington, DC: FEMA Retrieved from https://www.fema.gov/sites/default/files/2020-07/fema_nims_doctrine-2017.pdf

FEMA (2021) Declared Disasters. Retrieved from https://www.fema.gov/disaster/declarations? field_year_value=2020&field_dv2_state_territory_tribal_value= All&field _dv2_declaration_type_value=All&field_dv2_incident_type_target_id_ selective=All&page=30

Holshue, M., DeBolt, C., Lindquist, S., Lofy, K., Wiesman, J., Bruce, H., Spitters, C., Ericson, K., Wilkerson, S., Tural, A., Diaz, G., Cohn, A. et al. for the Washington State 2019-nCoV Case Investigation Team. (2020). First Case of 2019 Novel Coronavirus in the United States. *New England Journal of Medicine*, 382, 929–936. DOI: 10.1056/NEJMoa200119

Kumar, A., Prasoon, P., Kumari, C., Pareek, Vikas, Faiq, Muneeb A., Narayan, Ravi K., Kulandhasamy, Maheswari, and Kant, Kamla (2021). SARS-CoV-2-specific Virulence Factors in COVID-19. *Journal of Medical Virology*, 93, 1343–1350. DOI: 10.1002/jmv.26615

Lioy, P., Roberts, R., McCluskey, B., Lioy, M. J., Cross, A., Clarke, L., Stenton, L. J., Tepfenhart, W., and Ferrara, E. (n.d.) TOPOFF 3 Comments and Recommendations. Retrieved from http://archive.dimacs.rutgers.edu/People/Staff/roberts/topoffsubmission5–18-06.pdf

McEntire, D. A. (2015) *Disaster Response and Recovery: Strategies and Tactics for Resilience*. Hoboken, NJ: Wiley.

McIntyre, K. (2021) Face Mask Market Report. *Nonwovens Magazine*. Retrieved from https://www.nonwovens-industry.com/issues/2021-02/view_features/face-mask-market-report/

Public Health Service Act, P.L. 117–58 as Amended. Washington, DC: HHS, 2021.

Robert T. Stafford Disaster Relief and Emergency Assistance Act, P.L. 93–288 as Amended. Washington, DC: FEMA, 2021.

Rubin, C. (2007). *Emergency Management: The American Experience 1900–2005*. Fairfax, VA: PERI.

Stilp, R. and Bevelacqua, A. (1997) *Emergency Medical Response to Hazardous Materials Incidents*. Clifton Park, NY: Delmar.

Sylves, R. and Waugh, W. (1990) *Cities and Disaster – North America Studies in Emergency Management*. Springfield, IL: Thomas.

United Nations International Children's Fund [UNICEF] (2021). Medical Masks during the CoViD-19 Pandemic. Retrieved from https://www.unicef.org/supply/stories/ world-mask-week-during-covid-19-pandemic.

U.S. Census (2019) From Municipalities to Special Districts, Official Count of Every Type of Local Government in 2017 Census of Governments. Washington, DC: US Census Bureau. Retrieved from https://www.census.gov/content/dam/ Census/library /visualizations/2019/econ/ from_municipalities_to_special_ districts_ america_counts_october_2019.pdf

U.S. Const. amend. XIV.

U.S. Department of Homeland Security – Office of the Inspector General [DHS-OIG] (2005). A Review of the Top Officials 3 Exercise. OIG-06–07. Retrieved from https://www.oig.dhs.gov/assets/Mgmt/OIG_06-07_Nov05.pdf

U.S. Food and Drug Administration [FDA] (2020) Emergency Use Authorizations for Vaccines Explained. Retrieved from https://www.fda.gov/vaccines-blood-biologics/vaccines/emergency-use-authorization-vaccines-explained

White House (2003) *Homeland Security Presidential Security Directive #5 –Management of Domestic Incidents*. Washington, DC: White House.

Zhang, R., Li, Y., Zhang, A., Wang, Y., and Molina, M. (2020, June) Identifying Airborne Transmission as the Dominant Route for the Spread of COVID-19. *Proceedings of the National Academy of Sciences*, 117(26), 14857–14863. DOI: 10.1073/ pnas.2009637117

15 Lessons Learned and Moving Forward from Hurricane Katrina

Emergency Response Planning to Build an Inclusive Response Framework

Nicola Davis Bivens and DeMond S. Miller

Disasters and critical incidents have impacted society since the flooding of the Nile River in Ancient Egypt (Haddow et al., 2021) and before. According to data from the Emergency Events Database (EM-DAT) at the Centre for Research on the Epidemiology of Disasters, from January 2002 to January 2022, there were 12,817 natural and technical hazards affecting communities throughout the world (EM-DAT, 2022). While hazards occur globally, "each hazard affects countries differently" (The World Bank & The United Nations, 2010, p. 32). "The different economic, cultural, and other characteristics of individuals and groups in society affect the distribution of both exposure and vulnerability to hazards and disaster impacts" (Mileti, 1999, p. 122), with low-income persons and racial and ethnic minorities disproportionately affected by disasters (Kellenberg & Mobarak, 2011). At the macro-level, 11% of the world's population lives in countries with a low Human Development Index yet they account for 53% of natural disaster fatalities (Mochizuki et al., 2014). Even dating back to Ancient Egypt and the flooding of the Nile, there was some indication that social and economic stratification may have influenced which persons were more likely to negatively experience flooding (Park, 1992).

According to Birkland and Warnement (2015), critical incidents, such as disasters, catastrophes, and crises, can impact public policy. Kingdon (as cited in Birkland & Warnement, 2015), coined the term, *focusing event*, to describe events and natural disasters, such as hurricanes, which focus attention on problems and solutions. Hurricane Katrina serves as a focusing event (Birkland, 2006). In the aftermath of the storm, a number of policy problems resulting in new legislation, policy, and practice, make it suitable to examine health disparities in post Katrina New Orleans and the importance of emergency management to plan and mitigate future disasters.

Wisner et al. (2004, p. 11) define vulnerability as "the characteristics of a person or group and their situation that influence their capacity to anticipate, cope with, resist, and recover from the impact of a natural hazard." It results from a number of social, economic, and political factors that influence how some persons experience disasters and may end up displaced (Wisner et al., 2004). Vulnerable populations include the elderly, children, women, those persons with disabilities, low-income persons, as well as racial and ethnic minorities (Kromm & Sturgis, 2008). Perhaps one recent reminder that vulnerable persons, especially low-income persons and minorities, are disproportionately affected by disasters is Hurricane Katrina's impact on the city of New Orleans. Although Hurricane Katrina made landfall along the Mississippi Gulf Coast, causing an estimated US$81.2 billion in damage (Levitt & Walker, 2009), its devastation affected approximately 90,000 square miles throughout the Gulf Coast region (Cutter & Gall, 2006), its impact, coupled with the failed levees, is most attributed to the city of New Orleans. Considered to be a "catastrophe, far greater in scale than almost anything in American history" (Solnit, 2009, p. 235), the images of persons pleading for assistance on roof tops, living in ghastly conditions in the Louisiana Superdome and New Orleans Convention Center, in the days after Hurricane Katrina made landfall,

DOI: 10.4324/9781003140245-15

remain etched in our collective memories. In the month prior to Hurricane Katrina's landfall, the city's population was an estimated 455,188 (City of New Orleans, 2015), with just over 23.2% of the New Orleans population at or below the poverty line, with a median household income of US$39,793 [nearly US$20,000 below the national median household income of US$56,832 that year] (Shaughnessy et al., 2010). In 2005, the city ranked in the 97th percentile according to the Social Vulnerability Index (Cutter & Gall, 2006). Furthermore, following Hurricane Katrina, environmental justice was a major concern in the city of New Orleans (Bullard & Wright, 2009; Bullard, et al., 2009; Lieberman, 2006; McDougall, 2008; Miller, 2008; Miller & Rivera, 2011; Rivera & Miller, 2007; Sharkey, 2007). The impacts following Hurricane Katrina were not equally distributed among the different subpopulations in the city in that the disaster's greater and longer-lasting effects were felt among poor populations of color. In addition, neighborhoods inhabited by vulnerable populations made them more susceptible to harmful environmental exposures with limited health screenings and healthcare access.

According to Bakker (as cited in Passidomo, 2014), the conditions described above are structurally inherent in racism and geography in New Orleans at the time of the storm. Decades-old patterns of segregation regulated that the Black working class be forced to find housing in the least desirable geographic locations of the city, which were most vulnerable to flooding and social isolation. In turn, these communities lacked employment, educational and economic opportunities, social services, as well as access to resources (Passidomo, 2014). In post Katrina New Orleans, "communities of color…suffer disproportionately high rates of institutionalized disinvestment and structural inequality—in majority-minority neighborhoods, schools are poorer, access to health services is dismal, and residents have fewer (if any) options for purchasing affordable nutritious food close" (Passidomo, 2014, p. 385).

Unfortunately, Hurricane Katrina and disasters since the storm have illustrated how planning by local authorities and other decision makers is often not enough. Many of the disaster plans for medically dependent persons are often impractical for vital aspects of the response and temporary sheltering of survivors. This chapter is focused on the role of planning in an intentional comprehensive manner that links local government cooperation, city officials, police officers, and other first responders to the overall goal of increasing survivors' long-term health and non-health related recovery outcomes. Health emergency plans for New Orleans were insufficient and the efforts to coordinate comprehensive healthcare access and services for many medically frail collapsed (such as the drowning deaths of 35 seniors in a nursing home and closure of Charity Hospital [Neighmond, 2015; Robinson, 2013]). While there are numerous social disparities to detail, this chapter concerns health and healthcare access disparities, transportation disparities, and food insecurity. The chapter employs a case study approach to understand the intersection of race, disparity, and disaster-related healthcare access during Hurricane Katrina and how the disaster served as a catalyst for change. Finally, the chapter concludes with recommendations for inclusive, recommendations for emergency preparedness operations in the wake of disasters from an interdisciplinary all-hazards inclusive approach. From an inclusive perspective, a need to address the crises and immediate needs of survivors is pressing. This analysis explores the impact of a healthcare infrastructure of New Orleans once pushed to the brink of collapse and now, nearly two decades after the major storm, the healthcare systems are more, as it is seamlessly integrated into emergency management structures and offers insight for policy makers among citizens and community organizations, government officials, and intergovernmental agencies. We maintain that the chaos of disaster situations can provide opportunities to clarify the roles between individual, community, and structural factors and where action can be taken to promote inclusivity. By seeking to build an inclusive emergency preparedness framework, where healthcare and access to healthcare are priorities, we contend that not only can lives and livelihood security be enhanced, but also advance an inclusive approach to all-hazards emergency planning.

Healthcare Disparities in New Orleans – Pre and Post Katrina

> Hurricane Katrina made it evident that natural disasters occur in the same social, historical, and political environment in which disparities in health already exist. The hurricane was only the disaster agent; what created the magnitude of the disaster was the underlying vulnerability of the affected communities.... These communities experienced social disparities in health before Katrina; their health status was linked to the quagmire of poverty, poor housing, lack of economic opportunities, and discrimination in which they lived....
>
> (American Journal of Public Health as cited in LaVeist, 2020, p. 1445)

Hurricane Katrina reignited debates about racial inequality in many facets of American life. Although Hurricane Katrina exacerbated many health problems, New Orleans had some of the highest rates of infant mortality, AIDS infection, and chronic diseases in the country prior to the disaster. Blacks (roughly two-thirds of the city's population and one-third of that in the state) experienced health disparities in that they experienced heart disease, asthma, and diabetes at higher rates than Whites (Rudowitz et al., 2006). The poverty level in the city, limited access to Medicaid, approximately 20% of adults in Louisiana were without insurance. Only 54% of adults had employer-sponsored coverage, which Rudowitz et al. attribute to the number of jobs in the service and hospitality industry, which at the time, was less likely to offer health coverage benefits. Factor in that 19% of the workforce in the Gulf Coast region (which includes New Orleans and surrounding areas as well as parts of Mississippi), worked in the hospitality industry prior to Katrina (Garber et al., 2006), is further evidence that large segments of the New Orleans population were uninsured. The number of low-income and uninsured population were largely served by Charity Hospital, one of the state-funded hospitals. Charity primarily served low-income, minority populations and offered HIV/AIDS care, outpatient clinics, and psychiatric and substance abuse services, and was one of the busiest emergency room departments in the United States (Rudowitz et al., 2006). In fact,

> [Louisiana] numbered among one of the five worst states for infant mortality, cancer deaths, prevalence of smoking, and premature deaths (defined as years of life lost to deaths before age 75 per 100,000 people). Louisianans also had among the nation's highest rates of cardiovascular deaths, motor vehicle deaths, occupational fatalities, infectious disease, and violent crime
>
> (Zuckerman & Coughlin, 2006, p. 2)

As a result of Katrina, jobs in the hospitality and leisure industries were the hardest hit (Garber et al., 2006), which created a greater gap in the number of persons with access to healthcare insurance and coverage. In fact, the greatest job losses in the region as a result of the storm were in New Orleans and surrounding parishes and communities (Garber et al., 2006). With businesses closed, resulting in unemployment, people were now without healthcare due to a lack of insurance coverage. Access to healthcare was further complicated by the number of hospital closures. During and post Katrina, several other hospitals in the New Orleans region closed (Rudowitz et al., 2006). Charity Hospital closed temporarily and when it reopened, it was in a smaller facility. Low-income residents received care through Charity, Tulane University's hospital, and a network of clinics. Despite these healthcare options, the clinics were seldom visited, resulting in Blacks disproportionately presenting with more advanced head and neck cancer (Friedlander et al., 2013).

Hurricane Katrina had adverse effects on diabetes management. Socioeconomic health disparities were further exacerbated by the storm and the disaster had negative health and economic consequences (Fonseca et al., 2009). Women who are vulnerable to natural disasters were also vulnerable to pregnancy outcomes. Natural disasters, such as Katrina, may also have long-term effects on pregnancy outcomes, including low birth rate and the gestational period resulting in pre-term birth (Harville et al., 2015).

Health, Carlessness, Transportation Disparity in Times of Disaster

LaVeist (2020) posits the intersectionality of the myriad of factors, with transportation as a critical factor, in the ongoing concerns of health disparities in New Orleans before and after the storm. "Many fled for safety as the storm grew and barreled toward the Gulf Coast. Others remained, some unwilling to leave, many more unable to leave because of lack of transportation, health concerns, or lack of financial resources" (LaVeist, 2020, p. 1445) During the evacuation phase in response to the storm, a great deal of effort is placed into reconfiguring the transportation infrastructure for easier flow of traffic in New Orleans away from the city. Long-standing plans remain in place for a contra-flow system allowing anyone with the access to an automobile the ability to evacuate; however, it is difficult to evacuate a city with a largely carless population. In fact, community leaders estimate as much as 80% of New Orleans relied on public transportation when Governor Blanco and Mayor Nagin issued the call to evacuate (United States Congress, 2006). The state of Louisiana evacuated approximately 1.5 million people before Hurricane Katrina made landfall. However, approximately 150,000 to 200,000 individuals (accurate numbers were difficult to attain) remained during the storm (Institute of Medicine, 2007, p. 16). Most of those stranded in New Orleans could have been evacuated had a plan been in place (Renne et al., 2009). However, carless people and their healthcare access and medical needs have often been overlooked during previous disasters. Following Hurricanes Katrina and Rita, a need to recognize the inadequacy of existing evacuation plans for carless populations arose. At the time of Katrina, as much as 27% of all households, affecting as much as 80% of the population, were carless and relying on public transportation (Hess & Gotham, 2007; United States Congress, 2006) Moreover, Hess and Gotham (2007) found that most evacuation plans fail to take into consideration multimodal evacuation planning as well as accommodate that segment of the population that does not drive. Although some plans incorporate public transportation, for even those members of the population who have their own vehicles, most people prefer their own vehicles (Renne et al., 2009). "Those without vehicle access, including the poor, elderly, and tourists, had to rely on family, friends, or other social support systems or else they were stranded" (Renne et al., 2009, p. 36). Litman examined failures in the emergency response to Hurricanes Katrina and Rita. While he posits that Katrina's evacuation plan was somewhat effective for motorists, he contends that the plans failed to serve those persons dependent on public transit (or their friends, family, and other forms of transportation). Equitable and compassionate emergency response requires special efforts to address the needs of vulnerable residents. Improved emergency response planning can result in more efficient use of available resources. Litman (2006) identifies various policy and planning strategies that can help create a more efficient, equitable, and resilient transport system. Additionally, Little dialogue exists regarding the medical needs of the carless society as it pertains to evacuation planning. This area of study deserves considerable attention because a significant portion of carless individuals also have serious medical conditions requiring medication, medical attention, or other special support.

Food Disparities in New Orleans – Pre and Post Katrina

The authors recognize the fact that food access is a complex social, political, geographical, economic, and supply chain logistics phenomenon. This intersection of conditions impacts the degree to which health disparities exist and extend well beyond the initial shock of any disaster and past the recovery phase of the disaster. There is little question that there are racial and economic disparities and access to healthy food throughout the United States, including New Orleans pre and post Katrina (Rose & O'Malley, 2020). Inadequate food access is a social justice issue that serves as a catalyst for unhealthy food choices that can increase the prevalence of various chronic diseases (Rose & O'Malley, 2020). When faced with the basic decision of buying food or seeking healthcare or purchasing medications, low-income persons often defer their healthcare, causing medical conditions to fester, often getting worse before they are able to seek or obtain medical care (Friedlander et al., 2013). Couple that with access to food, and the correlation between healthy diet and certain medical conditions, food disparities have a negative consequence in terms of health and food inequalities. In the United States, geographic food access in urban communities is long documented (Mundorf et al., 2015; Rose et al., 2011). In pre-Katrina New Orleans, racial disparities were significant due to a lack of grocery stores, impacting access to fresh and healthy food in primarily Black neighborhoods (Rose et al., 2011). In Black communities, as designated by Census track data, residents were served more so by small food and convenience stores as opposed to supermarkets. Within those stores, more shelf space is allocated for snack foods vs. fruits and vegetables, which no doubt shaped dietary patterns (Bodor et al., 2010) and subsequently health outcomes.

The racial disparities in food access that existed pre-Katrina were exacerbated as a result of the storm (Mundorf et al., 2015). Post Katrina, residents were faced with challenges in securing nutritious food, which impacted those with medical conditions such as diabetes (Fonseca et al., 2009). In fact, it was not until 2009 that access to nutritious food returned to pre-storm levels of access disparity (Mundorf et al., 2015).

Recommended Policy Considerations

The failed preparedness, response, and recovery to Hurricane Katrina in the city of New Orleans became a focusing event as there was significant legislation enacted in response to some of the failures identified post Katrina as some changes in policies and practice. However, many policies and plans still fall short of taking into consideration the challenges. As a result, the authors make the following recommendations.

Consider Multiple Data Sources When Identifying the Number of Low-Income Persons

There is little question that marginalized communities who experience inequalities experience disasters in greater disparity. In response, emergency managers must factor in vulnerable populations in disaster planning. The Social Vulnerability Index is one such measure that could be applied (Schmidtlein et al., 2008). Public schools are a good source of data when considering the number of schools that receive Title I funding (federal funding to support the number of students who are disadvantaged to ensure they meet academic achievement standards) or the students who receive free or reduced lunch per The National School Lunch Program [children whose households receive benefits through the Supplemental Nutrition Assistance Program, Temporary Assistance for Needy Families, or are 130% below the poverty level] (Durham Public Schools, 2022; Feeding America, 2022). In Orleans Parish, nearly 97% are Title I schools and 85% of its students are deemed economically disadvantaged (Hasselle & Lussier, 2021; Zip Data Maps, 2022). Identifying low-income persons from multiple data sources will allow for emergency planners to have a more accurate indicator of the number of impoverished people in the community and make appropriate plans for the same.

Partner with Colleges and Universities

Colleges and universities have a renewed emphasis in promoting social justice. As a result, faculty and students are willing to partner in initiatives to create research and projects that can assist emergency planners with community-based research to collect data, create databases, and other initiatives to help promote equity in disaster planning (Davis Bivens et al., 2022). In addition, given many of these institutions' long-standing histories of community-based participatory research, service-learning projects (including those in New Orleans post Katrina), they may have a wealth of data and historical knowledge that policy planners may use in writing evacuation plans to make experiencing, responding to, and recovering from disasters more equitable (Davis Bivens et al., 2022; Kadlowec et al., 2006).

Medical schools are also viable partners. Medical students have been part of disaster response, dating back to the 1918 Spanish Influenza, natural disasters, such as flooding and earthquakes, as well as the 9/11 terrorist attacks (Mortelmans et al., 2015). Smith et al. (2014) note that the majority of medical schools offer student-run free medical clinics. Student-run free clinics can assist in addressing healthcare disparities in advance of a disaster or critical event, in an effort to mitigate them. By doing so, the critical event will be less impactful on a number of populations, which are typically negatively impacted by disasters, etc. as noted above. In addition, during the disaster and in the recovery phase, these clinics may also serve as healthcare options when hospitals, doctors' offices, etc. are overburdened. A medical student disaster volunteer corps supervised by emergency physicians can help alleviate overcrowded emergency rooms or work in mobile units as qualified manpower (Pong et al., 2019).

Account for and Plan for Persons Who Cannot Evacuate

Poverty is one of the major reasons why many of the evacuees did not manage to leave before Hurricane Katrina made landfall. They lacked the resources to either travel or support themselves once they relocated. Moreover, the evacuees also tended to share one characteristic closely related to both their racial and economic demographics: 55% had no car or any other way to evacuate (Quigley, 2006).

Of the 270,000 New Orleans Katrina survivors whose eventual evacuation began in shelters, 93% were Black. They were predominately poor and unskilled as 77% had a high school education or less, 68% had neither money in the bank nor a usable credit card (which are necessary for making hotel reservations or securing a rental car in the event of an evacuation), and 57% had total household incomes of less than US$20,000 per year. Recognizing the true needs of low-income persons (i.e. inability to evacuate, or book a hotel room in another city), and the extent of the population in this predicament, will help emergency planners to properly account for the same. In New Orleans, officials were unprepared for the large number of people who either chose or were unable to not evacuate, and the Superdome quickly became inadequate to house the large number of people (United States Congress, 2006).

In addition to low-income persons, disabled persons, the elderly, and other special needs individuals may have challenges to prevent them from evacuating. As a result, evacuation plans must consider the unique needs that each of these populations has and plan for the same. By 2050, 21% of the population will be age 60 and older (United Nations as cited in Lee et al., 2019). Elderly people were among the greatest percentage of deaths in Hurricane Katrina and the 2011 East Japan Great Earthquake (60% and 65% respectively) (Lee et al., 2019). Special needs populations, like the elderly, may have challenges, such as cognitive impairment, physical limitations, and lack of transportation (Rosenkoetter et al., 2007). Planners need to take these challenges into consideration when creating evacuation, mitigation, response, and recovery plans. In addition, they should take their input into consideration as noted below.

Create Inclusive Plans Seeking Input from All

The National Preparedness Goal of the Federal Emergency Management Agency (2015, p. 1) is "a secure and resilient nation with the capabilities required across the *whole community* [emphasis added our own] to prevent, protect against, mitigate, respond to, and recover from the threats and hazards that pose the greatest risk." This resilience begins with the whole community contributing to policy planners' efforts in creating disaster evacuation, response, recovery, and/or mitigation plans. Low-income persons and racial and ethnic minorities are disproportionately affected by disasters (Kellenberg & Mobarak, 2011). By ensuring that they are involved in the planning process can serve two purposes. Not only are they providing input from their experiences and perspectives, but their participation also serves as a means to educate them as to the risks they face. By understanding risk, they can then share with other members of their community, who in turn may share with others.

Diversity must be built into disaster planning (Phillips, 1993). By including racial and ethnic minorities, persons of all income levels (especially low-income households), elderly, and disabled citizens will help officials develop plans inclusive of special needs populations. As a result of doing so, communities can avoid having large segments of the population unable to evacuate and can make an appropriate plan for them in terms of assisting them with evacuation, temporary and long-term shelters, and other areas of response and recovery. Successful relationships can have an "…extraordinary, long- term impact on the community" (Kostro & Riba, 2014, p. 37). Kostro and Riba (2014) posit that given the extent of the use of social media and online activity, disaster planners can better engage and educate the public through their own websites, Twitter, Instagram, and Facebook accounts. Communities can also use social media to warn, direct, and inform the public what do to in advance of, during, and after a critical incident through public announcements. For example, New Orleans residents showed up at the Convention Center, based on rumors that buses would arrive there to take people out of the city. The building was overrun with people seeking to evacuate, in which conditions quickly eroded with people living (and in some instances dying) in the building, non-working toilets (due to the lack of running water), and theft. Had social media been in wide use at the time, residents would have been directed to the Super Dome or other shelters in the city and rumors that buses would arrive could have been quashed.

Conclusion

"Katrina was as much a 'social disaster' as a natural one" (Passidomo, 2014, p. 387). Until disaster planners recognize that inclusive plans can help mitigate the loss of lives [because it is inevitable that there in fact will be loss even with good forecasts all people's lives can't be saved because some people will not or can not evacuate out of harm's way. (Lautenbacher, as cited in Alpert, 2005; Rosenkoetter et al., 2007). Viewing disasters and disaster response from an epidemiological approach is the only way for officials to effectively plan for the same. Although we examined and proposed change using Hurricane Katrina as our focusing event, understand that intentional planning, involving, and including the whole community is the only effective strategy to avoid making the same errors Louisiana officials did in August of 2005. Officials must also make efforts to address inequity and disparity in healthcare, poverty, etc. in advance of a disaster. In addition, disaster planners must factor in these challenges in advance of a critical incident. Embracing current trends, such as the ubiquitous use of social media, disaster planners can utilize the same to educate the public, help manage disasters, and promote appropriate response to minimize the loss of life and property. More recently, On January 20, 2021, President Joseph R. Biden, Jr. released Executive Order 13985 on *Advancing Racial Equity and Support for Underserved Communities Through the Federal Government. This Executive order* requires all federal agencies to assess equity with respect to race, ethnicity, religion, income, geography, gender identity, sexual orientation and disability. To this end, FEMA (see FEMA, 2022) is focused on reducing barriers and increasing opportunities so all people, including those from vulnerable and underserved communities, can get help when they need it.

References

Alpert, B. (2005). Hurricane Season Finally Comes to an End, Times-Picayune (New Orleans), Nov. 30, 2005, at A4.

Birkland, T. A. (2006). *Lessons of disaster: Policy change after catastrophic events.* Georgetown University Press.

Birkland, T. A. & Warnement, M. K. (2015). Focusing events in disasters and development. In N. Kapucu & K. T. Liou (Eds.), *Disaster and development: Examining global issues and cases* (pp. 39–60). Springer International Publishing.

Bodor, J. N., Rice, J. C., Farley, T. A., Swalm, C. M., & Rose, D. (2010). Disparities in food access: Does aggregate availability of key foods from other stores offset the relative lack of supermarkets in African-American neighborhoods? *Preventive Medicine, 51*(1), 63–67. https://doi.org/10.1016/j.ypmed.2010.04.009

Bullard, R. D., & Wright, B. (2009). Introduction. In R. D. Bullard & B. Wright (Eds.), *Race, place and environmental justice after Hurricane Katrina: Struggles to reclaim, rebuild and revitalize New Orleans and the Gulf Coast* (pp. 1–18). Westview.

Bullard, R. D., Johnson, G. S., & Torres, A. O. (2009). Transportation matters: Stranded on the side of the road before and after disasters strike. In R. D. Bullard & B. Wright (Eds.), *Race, place, and environmental justice after Hurricane Katrina: Struggles to reclaim, rebuild and revitalize New Orleans and the Gulf Coast* (pp. 63–86). Westview.

City of New Orleans Office of Homeland Security and Emergency Preparedness (2015). *Hazard mitigation plan city of New Orleans.* City of New Orleans.

Cutter, S. L. & Gall, M. (2006). Hurricane Katrina: A failure of planning or a planned failure? In C. Felgentreff and T. Glade (Eds.), *Naturrisiken und sozialkatastrophen [Natural disasters hazards and social disasters].* (pp. 353–366). Springer Spectrum.

Davis Bivens, N., Quick, D. Miller, D. S., Bledsoe Gardner, A., & Byrd, Y. (2022). Community activism and impacting communities through high impact educational practice. In A. Anisah, A. McLetchie, & J. Wesley (Eds.), *Contributions of historically black colleges and universities in the 21st century* (pp. 92–110). IGI Global.

Durham Public Schools (2022). *Title I.* Durham Public Schools. https://www.dpsnc.net/domain/223

Emergency Events Database (2022, February 13). *EM-DAT database.* Centre for Research on the Epidemiology of Disasters. https://public.emdat.be/

Federal Emergency Management Agency (2015). *National preparedness goal* (2nd ed.). United States Department of Homeland Security.

Feeding America (2022). *The national school lunch program.* Feeding America. https://www.feedingamerica.org/take-action/advocate/federal-hunger-relief-programs/national-school-lunch-program#:~:text=Low-income%20children%20are%20eligible,qualify%20for%20reduced-price%20meals.

FEMA (2022). *Equity.* https://www.fema.gov/emergency-managers/national-preparedness/equity

Fonseca, V. A., Smith, H., Kuhadiya, N., Leger, S. M., Yau, C. L., Reynolds, K., Shi, L., McDuffie, R. H., Thethi, T., & John-Kalarickal, J. (2009). Impact of a natural disaster on diabetes: Exacerbation of disparities and long-term consequences. *Diabetes Care, 32*(9), 1632–1638. https://doi.org/10.2337/dc09-067

Friedlander, P., Balart, L., Shores, N. J., Cannon, R. M., Saggi, B., Jan, T., & Buell, J. F. (2013). Racial disparity in New Orleans: A faith-based approach to an age-old problem. *Surgery, 153*(4), 439–442. https://doi.org/10.1016/j.surg.2012.11.010

Garber, M., Unger, L., White, J., & Wohlford, L. (2006, August). Hurricane Katrina's effects on industry employment and wages. *Monthly Labor Review* / U.S. Department of Labor, Bureau of Labor Statistics *129*(8), 22–39.

Haddow, G. D., Bullock, J. A., & Coppola, D. P. (2021). *Introduction to emergency management* (7th ed.). Elsevier.

Harville, E. W., Giarratano, G., Savage, J., Barcelona de Mendoza, V., & Zotkiewicz, T. (2015). Birth outcomes in a disaster recovery environment: New Orleans women after Katrina. *Maternal and Child Health Journal, 19*(11), 2512–2522. https://doi.org/10.1007/s10995-015-1772-4

Hasselle, D., & Lussier, C. (2021, May 15). *Families of nearly 260K Louisiana students expected to get debit cards for food this summer.* NOLA.com. https://www.nola.com/news/education/article_e2cd-0fde-b4c9-11eb-9d8a-6f2fc955e42d.html#:~:text=Approximately%20699%2C000%20students%20%E2%80%94%20or%2087,the%20Louisiana%20Department%20of%20Education.

Hess, D. B., & Gotham, J. C. (2007). Multi-odal mass evacuation in upstate New York: A review of disaster plans. *Journal of Homeland Security and Emergency Management, 4*(3).

Institute of Medicine (2007). *Environmental public health impacts of disasters: Hurricane Katrina.* The National Academies Press.

Kadlowec, J., Schmalzel, J., Miller, D. S., & Weiss, L. (2006). *Katrina recovery clinic project: An engineering service learning project.* Proceedings of the American Society for Engineering Education/Institute of Electrical and Electronics Engineers 36th Conference, USA.

Kellenberg, D., & Mobarak, A. M. (2011). The economics of natural disasters. *Annual Review of Resource Economics, 3*, 297–312. https://doi.org/10.1146/annurev-resource-073009–104211

Kostro, S. S., & Riba, G. (2014). *Achieving disaster resilience in U.S. communities.* Rowman & Littlefield.

Kromm, C., & Sturgis, S. (2008). *Hurricane Katrina and the guiding principles on internal displacement: A global human rights perspective on a national disaster.* The Institute for Southern Studies.

LaVeist, T. A. (2020). Katrina's lesson: Time to imagine an after COVID-19. *American Journal of Public Health, 110*(10), 1445. https://doi.org/10.2105/AJPH.2020.305883

Lee, H., Hong, W., & Lee, Y. (2019). Experimental study on the influence of water depth on the evacuation speed of elderly people in flood conditions. *International Journal of Disaster Risk Reduction, 39*, 1–13.

Levitt, J. I., Walker, M. C. (2009). Truth crushed to earth will rise again. In: J. I. Levitt, M. C. Walker (Eds.). *Hurricane Katrina: America's unnatural disaster* (pp. 2–21). Oxfordshire: Lincoln, NE: University of Nebraska Press.

Lieberman, R. C. (2006) The storm didn't discriminate: Katrina and the politics of color blindness. *DuBois Review, 3*(1), 7–22.

Litman, T. (2006). Lessons from Katrina and Rita: What major disasters can teach transportation planners. *Journal of Transportation and Engineering, 13*(1). https://doi.org/10.1061/(ASCE)0733–947X(2006)132:1(11)

McDougall, H. A. (2008). Hurricane Katrina: Story of race, poverty, and environmental injustice. *Howard Law Journal, 51(3),* 533–564.

Mileti, D. S. (1999). *Disasters by design: A reassessment of natural disasters in the United States.* John Henry Press.

Miller, D. S. (2008). Disaster tourism and disaster landscape attractions after Hurricane Katrina: An autoethnographic journey. *International Journal of Culture, Tourism and Hospitality Research, 2*(2), 115–131.

Miller, D. S., & Rivera, J. D. (2011). Guiding principles: Rebuilding trust in government and public policy in the aftermath of Hurricane Katrina. *Journal of Critical Incident Analysis, 12*(1), 22–32.

Mochizuki, J., Mechler, R., Hochrainer-Stigler, S., Keating, A., & Willeges, K. (2014). Revisiting the 'disaster and development' debate – Toward a broader understanding of macroeconomic risk and resilience. *Climate Risk Management, 3*, 39–54. https://doi.org/0.1016/j.crm.2014.05.002

Mortelmans, Bouman, S. J. M., Gaakeer, M. I., Dieltiens, G., Anseeuw, K., & Sabbe, M. B. (2015). Dutch senior medical students and disaster medicine: a national survey. *International Journal of Emergency Medicine, 8*(1). https://doi.org/10.1186/s12245-015-0077-0

Mundorf, Willits-Smith, A., & Rose, D. (2015). 10 Years later: Changes in food access disparities in New Orleans since Hurricane Katrina. *Journal of Urban Health, 92*(4), 605–610. https://doi.org/10.1007/s11524-015-9969-9

Neighmond, P. (2015, August 24). *Katrina shut down Charity Hospital but led to more primary care.* National Public Radio. https://www.npr.org/sections/health-shots/2015/08/24/432909068/katrina-shut-down-charity-hospital-but-led-to-more-primary-care?t=1660552612861

Park, T. K. (1992). Early trends toward class stratification: Chaos, common property, and flood recession agriculture. *American Anthropologist, 94*(1), 90. https://doi.org/10.1525/aa.1992.94.1.02a00060

Passidomo, C. (2014). Whose right to (farm) the city? Race and food justice activism in post- Katrina New Orleans. *Agriculture and Human Values, 31*(3), 385–396. https://doi.org/10.1007/s10460-014-9490-x

Phillips, B. D. (1993). Cultural diversity in disasters: Sheltering, housing, and long-term recovery. *International Journal of Mass Emergencies and Disasters, 11*(1), 99–110.

Pong, J., Lim, J., Wu, S., Li, A., Wong, X., Tsang, L., & Ponampalam, R. (2019). Improving emergency department surge capacity in disasters - Conception of a medical student disaster volunteer corps. *Prehospital and Disaster Medicine, 34*(S1), S84-S84. https://doi.org/10.1017/S1049023X19001754

Quigley, B. (2006). *Six months after Katrina: Who was left behind then and now.* The Mardi Gras Index. https://katrinareader.cwsworkshop.org/six-months-after-katrina-who-was-left-behind-then-and-now.html

Renne, J. L., Sanchez, T. W., Jenkins, P., & Peterson, R. (2009). Challenge of evacuating the carless in five major U.S. cities: Identifying the key issues. *Transportation Research Record, 2119*(1), 36–44. https://doi.org/10.3141/2119-05

Rivera, J. D., & Miller, D. S. (2007). Continually neglected: Situating natural disasters in the African American experience. *Journal of Black Studies, 37*(4), 502–522.

Robinson, K. (2013, April 29). *Eight years after Katrina: St. Rita's owners 'still feel the stigma.* ABC News. https://abcnews.go.com/US/years-katrina-st-ritas-owners-feel-stigma/story?id=20110312

Rose, D., & O'Malley, K. (2020). Food access 3.0: Insights from post-Katrina New Orleans on an evolving approach to food inequities. *American Journal of Public Health (1971), 110*(10), 1495–1497. https://doi.org/10.2105/AJPH.2020.305779

Rose, D., Bodor, J. N., Rice, J. C., Swalm, C. M., & Hutchinson, P. L. (2011). The effects of Hurricane Katrina on food access disparities in New Orleans. *American Journal of Public Health, 101*(3), 482–484. https://doi.org/10.2105/AJPH.2010.196659

Rosenkoetter, M. M., Covan, E. K., Cobb, B. K., Bunting, S., & Weinrich, M. (2007). Perceptions of older adults regarding evacuation in the event of a natural disaster. *Public Health Nursing, 24*(2), 160–168. https://doi.org/10.1111/j.1525-1446.2007.00620.x

Rudowitz, R., Rowland, D., & Shartzer, A. (2006). Health care in New Orleans before and after Hurricane Katrina. *Health Affairs, 25*(1), w393–w406.

Schmidtlein, M. C., Deutsch, R. C., & Piegorsch, W. (2008). A sensitivity analysis of the Social Vulnerability Index. *Risk Analysis, 28*(4), 1099–1114. https://doi.org/10.1111/j.1539-6924.2008.01072.x

Sharkey, P. (2007) Survival and death in New Orleans: An empirical look at the human impact of Katrina. *Journal of Black Studies, 37*(4), 482–501.

Shaughnessy, T. M., White, M. L., & Brendler, M. D. (2010). The income distribution effect of natural disasters: An analysis of Hurricane Katrina. *The Journal of Regional Analysis & Policy, 40*(1), 84–95.

Smith, S., Thomas, R., 3rd, Cruz, M., Griggs, R., Moscato, B., & Ferrara, A. (2014). Presence and characteristics of student-run free clinics in medical schools. *Journal of the American Medical Association, 312*(22), 2407–2410. https://doi.org/10.1001/jama.2014.16066

Solnit, R. (2009). *A paradise built in hell: The extraordinary communities that arise in disasters.* New York, NY: Viking.

United States Congress (2006). *A failure of initiative: Final report of the select bipartisan committee to investigate the preparation for and response to Hurricane Katrina.* United States Government Printing Office.

Wisner, B., Blairkie, P., Cannon, T., & Davis, I. (2004). *At risk* (2nd ed.). Routledge.

World Bank & United Nations. (2010). *Natural hazards, unnatural disasters: The economics of effective prevention.* World Bank.

Zip Data Maps (2022). *Title 1 status for public schools in Louisiana counties.* https://www.zipdatamaps.com/counties/state/education/map-of-percentage-of-title-1-status-public-schools-for-counties-in-louisiana

Zuckerman, S., & Coughlin, T. (2006). Initial health policy responses to hurricane Katrina and possible next steps. In M. A. Turner & S. R. Ledlewski (Eds.), *After Katrina: Rebuilding opportunity and equity into New Orleans* (pp. 47–54). The Urban Institute.

16 Health Disparities and Promoting a Culture of Preparedness

Building Resilience and Tangible Trust in an Age of Disasters

DeMond S. Miller and Roland J. Thorpe, Jr.

The exploration of the intersections among disaster risks and health disparities illustrates how social determinants help shape exposure and vulnerability to pandemic disasters and crises among different socioeconomic and racial/ethnic groups, to disproportionately impact medically underserved groups' risk of illness or death. Each chapter, in this edited volume, serves as a reminder by offering key insights into the threats to public health during the response to complex disasters as they address problems within our professional and practical understanding of inclusive emergency preparedness in many cultural contexts. Center stage of planning for disasters during, before, and after the event are the lives affected and the promotion of a long-term resilience culture founded on norms of reciprocity, inclusion, and trust that includes a robust emergency preparedness infrastructure that builds healthy, resilient communities. The complexities of the political, environmental, cultural, economic, and public health contexts make each complex disaster unique (Burkholder and Toole, 1995) and create both immediate and prolonged impacts (UNDRR, 2020). When disaster tends to arise more frequently, as crisis gives way to crises (Miller, 2021), the risks associated with complex disasters exacerbate existing social and racial/ethnic inequities in health, with low-income people and members of racial/ethnic minority groups more likely to live in disaster-prone areas and in lower-quality housing that is less safe when disasters occur (Arcaya et.al., 2020; Raker, 2020, p. 2182). Disproportionate vulnerability to hazards varies within and among populations of children, older adults, low-income communities, public housing residents, and communities within the same geographical area. Hence, the need for a more nuanced understanding of disasters and the intersection of health disparities is needed to reckon and address the underlying root causes of health vulnerabilities that decrease the likelihood of positive health outcomes in the wake of disasters. Tierney (2019) and Raker (2020, p. 2182) maintain that "… few disaster studies are adequately powered to explore outcomes for socially vulnerable groups, even though low-income people and members of racial/ethnic minority groups are most at risk for disaster exposure and have fewer resources to buffer against their effects." In essence, by analyzing key intersectionalities among social groups, the challenges these vulnerable groups face and the root causes of complex public health challenges before disasters and employing that knowledge as part of mitigation "investments;" the intersection of public health and emergency managers to plan community-based mitigation efforts will help reduce health disparities and benefit generations in the wake of disasters yet to come.

Each disaster is instructive—and there are many lessons to be learned, yet, the field of emergency management struggles with applying the "lessons learned" to adequately employ those lessons holistically in such a way that engages practitioners, academics, researchers, policymakers, and grassroots organizations in search of sustainable ways to analyze historical and emerging inequalities that fundamentally stymie recovery. And all too repeatedly, when disaster strikes, the health care system immediately has injuries and acute illness needs during the initial surge,

DOI: 10.4324/9781003140245-16

increasing the demand for emergency medical services and overwhelming the medical community. Chronic conditions among the most vulnerable in the initial surge are often exacerbated, leading to poor health outcomes, worsened disease states, or death during the disaster recovery phase (Mokdad et al., 2005). However, while the exact series of events is unpredictable, social science and medical science have been able to document patterns that unfold during the acute emergency phase; this period of crisis can be shortened by preplanning and timely public health interventions (Burkholder & Toole, 1995). In this conclusion chapter, the discussion expands some of the current paradigms within social science to be more inclusive of public health and different populations to help restore trust in institutions and processes that promote a culture of emergency preparedness.

Advancing Concepts and Incorporating Planning Strategies in Emergency Management

We are living in an age of disasters, social disruptions, risks, and dangers in the global community and those phenomena serve as catalysts for other crises (Chapman et al., 2021; Miller, 2021; Miller & Thorpe, 2022). While concepts including disaster landscape, disaster risk reduction, and mitigation may be the topics of the day, we must strive to work together to be more inclusive in addressing intersectional issues that range from pre/post-disaster health outcomes; social services integration and targeted, long-term services for highly impacted survivors. The nature of disasters and interlocking threats are changing. Social scientists who have expertise in disasters have adopted several conceptual typologies to help explain many aspects of disasters. One such disaster typology, the natural disasters vis-à-vis technological disasters or hybrid disasters (Gill & Ritchie, 2018; Ritchie et al., 2019; Miller, 2006, 2016; Miller & Wesley, 2016) is useful to help us understand the social response to disasters within social structures and processes to examine the utility of new typologies wherein various forms of capitals or community assets have the potential to increase our understanding of the embeddedness of hazards, disasters, and effective responses. For example, Gill and Ritchie (2018) cite how Flora and Flora's Community Capitals Framework (CCF) (Flora & Flora, 1993; Flora et al., 2008; Ritchie & Gill, 2011) has been adopted by the National Institute of Standards and Technology for use in its Community Resilience Planning Guide (NIST, 2014). Based initially on research rooted in the community development tradition, the CCF delineates seven forms of capital: natural, built (infrastructure), financial (economic), human, social, political, and cultural.

Other typologies exist that advance the knowledge and understanding of disaster response and help us understand how to integrate emergency management response to hazards, crises, and disasters. For instance, cascading disasters increase the impact well beyond the original temporal and spatial locations. Pescaroli and Alexander (2016) describe the evolution of the term "cascading disaster" and offer the following integrated definition in their conclusion: Cascading disasters are extreme events in which cascading effects increase in progression over time and generate unexpected secondary events of strong impact. These tend to be at least as serious as the original event and contribute significantly to the overall duration of the disaster's effects. These subsequent and unanticipated crises can be exacerbated by the failure of physical structures, the social functions that depend on them, including critical facilities, or by the inadequacy of disaster mitigation strategies, such as evacuation procedures and land use planning and emergency management strategies. In 2006, Mount Tungurahua erupted in Ecuador, spewing ash that impacted the agricultural livelihoods and health of residents. The community lost its social capital as family and friends moved out of the area, and recovery from the cascading disaster continues today. For cascading disasters, one or more secondary events, such as damage to agricultural livelihoods, can be identified and distinguished from the original source of the disaster (Cutter, 2018; Pescaroli & Alexander, 2015).

Lukasiewicz and O'Donnell (2022, p. 8) "highlight, analyze and discuss three types of complex disasters—compound, cascading, and protracted[…]it can be hard to draw clear distinctions between these types of complex disasters, especially once we start talking about hazards and risk" (see Gissing et al., 2021). They draw attention to the time and spatial elements of complex disasters in a way that overlays hazards and risks to these three disaster typologies. For example, compound disasters are variously described as follows (Gissing et al., 2021; Pescaroli & Alexander, 2018; Ridder et al., 2020; see Lukasiewicz and O'Donnell 2022, p. 9):

- two or more extreme disaster events occurring simultaneously or successively
- combinations of extreme events with underlying conditions that amplify their impact; or
- extreme impacts that result from combinations of "average" events.

Whereas, they further explain that the cascading disaster type usually arises from a triggering instance, which in turn exposes critical infrastructure vulnerabilities as part of interdependent systems, ultimately placing society at risk. The cascading disaster scenario arises because of one's ability to trace a direct "causal chain," where one event triggers subsequent events with their own impacts (Cutter, 2018; Gissing et al., 2021; UNDRR, 2019; see Lukasiewicz and O'Donnell 2022, p. 9). And finally, for Lukasiewicz and O'Donnell (2022), the protracted disaster comprises long-duration parameters of risk and exposure that are in flux rather than constant or linear. Thus, the management of protracted disasters is not straightforward or segmented into clear-cut response and recovery phases, and the time-frame is unknown. For example, the current COVID-19 pandemic serves as a clear example of a modern protracted disaster. For Kruczkiewicz et al. (2021), the pandemic is a "protracted crisis" where waves of infectious outbreaks act as shocks with an ongoing, ever-present response; in essence, emergency management and public health systems are always in a state of "ready to mobilize." Few et al. (2020) contend that COVID-19 is a "long-duration hazard event" where transition out of the crisis will take time and vary across scales. For Miller (2021), the model of crisis begetting crises is yet another way to define a protracted disaster. Additionally, the pattern of the protracted disaster:

> …follows Cutter's (2020) centering of temporal and spatial elements of disasters and the complex risk frame that is climate change, in relation to mental health impacts of disasters (Chen et al., 2020) and rising inequalities due to climate change induced disasters (Cappelli et al., 2021). For Staupe-Delgado (2019), there is a focus on the temporal scale: slow-onset, slowly emerging, slow violence, slow-burning, gradually occurring, gradually manifesting, creeping environmental problems, creeping crises, and disasters.
>
> (see Lukasiewicz & O'Donnell, 2022, p. 12)

Initial triggering events force society to focus attention on both crises that are final and favor a foreseeable end, and disasters that may have unforeseeable projected long-term consequences for survivors (Davis Bivens & Miller, 2022). As such, "social actors are able to effect change and implement policies that impact the outcomes of disasters when the policy institutions are able to align policy formation with societal goals in a meaningful way that secure community buy-in and support" (Davis Bivens & Miller, 2022, p. 14). This can be accomplished through many collaborative avenues that work to improve construction; education; policy changes; economic development and stability; and social development. Collaborations among disaster researchers and practitioners must also involve stakeholders at all levels of government and the community.

By adapting to environmental degradation conditions, resilience to increased extreme events, changing landscapes, and rising seas will have far-reaching socio-political and economic implications for human health. However, the effects of climate change are more likely to influence the health of older adults, who typically have low adaptive capacity, thus making them more vulnerable to climate-related environmental changes. The impact of mega-disasters such as Hurricane Katrina on the well-being of older adults is well documented (Adams, Kaufman, van Hattum & Moody, 2011; Filberto, et al., 2009; Fitzgerald, 2010; Henderson, Roberto, & Kamo, 2010; Malik et al., 2018; Prohaska & Peters, 2019), yet, the development of a comprehensive public policy framework for addressing vulnerabilities to compounded, cascading, or projected disasters is lacking. The preceding chapters have all focused on current disasters with an opportunity to explore ways to build an infrastructure that bridged healthcare and emergency management to address the nine determinants of health that are drivers of health inequities: income and wealth, housing, health systems and services, employment, education, transportation, social environment, public safety, and physical environment (National Academies of Sciences, Engineering, and Medicine, 2017). Exacerbation, during a time of crisis, can severely impact physical, mental, and functional health outcomes.

This chapter poses questions specifically focusing on improving health outcomes by incorporating resilience to the impact of disasters, via specific pre-disaster-planning steps that engage community stakeholders, including often marginalized citizens, as part of the major planning considerations for informed policy. All too often, governments and agencies, and even academic disciplines and professions such as engineering or cybersecurity, regard disasters as if they are "a project" to be managed without full regard for the "the diversity of interactions among sectors and system" (Simpson et al., 2021, p. 489). Few et al. (2020, p. 5) note:

> There is an entrenched tendency amongst governments and aid agencies to regard hazards as singular events with clear start and end dates. This tends to arise from a deeply embedded project mentality that determines fund flows, reporting structures, and ultimately, governance. In the case of disasters however, such mentality translates into a risk reduction strategy that focuses only on the tip of the problem, while disregarding longer-term challenges.

As highlighted by Certified Emergency Manager, Len Clark, (personal communication December 10, 2022):

> As we move from a government-centric approach to recovery, we need to develop, build and sustain networks that consist of all levels of government, the for-profit sector (so as to not compete with commerce), the private, and non-profits (including faith-based, community organizations and grassroots efforts).
>
> From a public administration aspect, one of the major social determinants is the relative wealth and availability of funds to support a response and recovery effort. This is especially difficult for small, low-income, and impoverished communities to be able to support the non-federal cost share match required under the Stafford Act (REF). This then requires the increased attention of elected and appointed officials to use their political capital to secure funding to support such efforts.

Clark further notes:

> [W]hen looking at the traditional social determinants from the public health literature, we can examine the effect of race, poverty, socioeconomic status, etc. on response and recovery. Where we fall short on this in the research is that the academic community has looked at each of these categories as discrete elements, but we have less research on the synergistic effect.

The Role of Trust in an Effective Emergency Response

In light of over a century of institutional mistrust in medical, public health, and first responder institutions, minorities, particularly African Americans, tend to cite the Tuskegee syphilis study as a reason for mistrust because of the deception that leads to deaths. However, the history of medical and research abuse of African Americans goes well beyond Tuskegee. Harriet Washington (2006) eloquently describes the history of medical experimentation and abuse. Her detailed, insightful historical analysis demonstrates that "mistrust of medical research and the health care infrastructure is extensive and persistent among African Americans and illustrating that more than four centuries of a biomedical enterprise designed to exploit African Americans is a principal contributor to current mistrust" (Scharff, 2010, p. 880).

There has been a great deal of social scientific work on the role of social capital in disaster social science literature. Social capital comes in different "flavors" (business, neighborhood, faith-based, government). Individual networks of social capital bridge, link, and have a shared (cohesive) purpose. Building and strengthening these networks should be part of a preparedness program rather than a "fire-drill" during or immediately after an emergency (Carty, personal communication, December 9, 2022). Programs like Community Emergency Response Team educate volunteers about disaster preparedness for the hazards that may occur, and groups like Local Emergency Planning Committees, which consist of individuals from diverse occupations across groups of first responders (Law Enforcement, Fire, Emergency Medical Services) and a wide variety of community partner stakeholders establish relationships among various stakeholders to also educate the public and professional responders on how to react to incidents in an "all hazards" environment. Such groups can be helpful if leveraged properly. They work to build institutional trust among members of the community and among stakeholder organizations. Linking and bridging networks pre-disaster allows for community stakeholders to collectively understand capabilities and gaps within networks (Carty, personal communication, December 9, 2022). Mangeri (personal communication December 10, 2022), a career emergency manager, employs the use of Sir Robert Peel's[1] Peelian Principles and asserts that, "Whether it is community policing or community preparedness, many of Peel's principles are designed to integrate community and government as partners in protecting and responding to threats against the community."

Equally important is the work of social scientists on trust as a vital component of an effective response and recovery (see Aldrich, 2012; Giddens, 1990; Miller, 2016; Miller & Rivera, 2006; Misztal, 1996; Thomas, 1998; see Wray et al., 2006). Trust and social capital, therefore, receive increasing attention in the disaster literature on effective response and recovery operations (Aldrich, 2012).

Additionally, the trust relationship among citizens, social institutions, and non-governmental aid organizations is best described as fiduciary, or a relationship held in trust.

The citizen trusts that the agent will perform in his/her (the citizen's) interest and not his/her (the agent) own interests (Thomas, 1998). Trust also develops through mutual relationships and interpersonal exchanges. Mutual trust is also a component of public trust in government. These relationships and the expectations they prompt are particularly important in determining how the public will respond to government efforts and emergency response (Thomas, 1998; see Wray et al., 2006, p. 48). Government officials and emergency responders who interact with the public and develop mutual trust relationships may be more effective sources for communicating emergency risk information.

(Miller, 2016, p. 413)

When the conditions for institutional trust are not galvanized, institutional distrust, referring to an individual or group's lack of confidence in systems, whether they be medical, public health, and/ or governmental (Best et al., 2021, p. 91; Meyer et al., 2018) can arise and undermine a whole-community approach to addressing immediate public health challenges and the root causes that gave rise to the conditions in the first place. Trustworthiness is a requisite condition to foster trust that is frequently overlooked; distrust is only rational in the absence of trustworthiness (Best et al., 2021, p. 91; Warren et al., 2019). Thus, public health practitioners and institutions have an ethical responsibility to meaningfully engage, educate, and inform diverse communities about health issues, particularly during a public health crisis (APHA, n.d.).

Equally important is the "bounce-back" factor and cooperation in the aftermath of disasters. Local disaster-stricken communities, organizations, and survivors tend to look for bonds that help them cope and adapt. Community stakeholders' cooperation may be best suited to local needs (Aldrich, 2012; Carr, 1932; Comfort & Okada, 2013; Drabek, 1985). The effectiveness of self-organization instructs central authorities to hold back (Boin & Bynander, 2015). Such situations are best served by "enabling leadership" (Nooteboom & Termeer, 2015). This leadership is both before and during a disaster.

Key to understanding a more nuanced view of trust and our ability to tangibilize the intangible aspects of trust in institutions to bring about a more inclusive and effective emergency response. For example, in communities where large disparities exist, the bridged interdisciplinary cooperation of emergency managers and public health officials needs to demonstrate a reified tangible trust against a backdrop of centuries of distrust in social structures. As we plan for future events, an integration of institutional trust, mutual respect, and incorporating the value of local knowledge is critical. A *culture of preparedness* demands that we effectively integrate social concepts' tangible and intangible aspects that ultimately drive an effective disaster emergency response that reduces health disparities using social justice to achieve health equity, now and in the decades to come.

Note

1 Emergency management may benefit from examining the principles for modern policing attributed to Sir Robert Peel (a former British Prime Minister considered to be father of the modern police force). The Peelian Principles, which were originally created to define an ethical police force, are founded on the belief that government must be held accountable. Peel also pointed out that the community as a whole shares the responsibility for vigilance. In other words, there must be a shared responsibility for community sustainability and resilience.

References

Adams, V., Kaufman, S. R., van Hattum, T., & Moody, S. (2011). Aging disaster: Mortality, vulnerability, and long-term recovery among Katrina survivors. *Medical Anthropology, 30*, 247–270. https://doi.org/10.108 0/01459740.2011.560777

Aldrich, D. (2012). *Building resilience: Social capital in post-disaster recovery.* Chicago: University of Chicago Press.

APHA American Public Health Association. (n.d.). Public Health Code of Ethics. https://www.apha.org/-/ media/files/pdf/membergroups/ethics/code_of_ethics.ashx

Arcaya, M. C., Raker, E. J., & Waters, M. C. (2020). The social consequences of disasters: Individual and community change. *Annual Review of Sociology, 46*, 671–91.

Best, A. L., Fletcher, F. E., Kadono, M., & Warren, R. C. (2021). Institutional distrust among African Americans and building trustworthiness in the COVID-19 response: Implications for ethical public health practice. *Journal of Health Care for the Poor and Underserved, 32*(1), 90–98. https://doi.org/10.1353/hpu.2021.0010

Boin, A., & Bynander, F. (2015). Explaining success and failure in crisis coordination. *Geografiska Annaler: Series A, Physical Geography, 97*(1), 123–135.

Burkholder, B. T., and Toole, M. J. (1995). Evolution of complex disasters. *The Lancet, 346*(8981), 1012–1015. https://doi.org/10.1016/S0140-6736(95)91694-6

Cappelli, F., Conigliani, C., Consoli, D., Costantini, V., & Paglialunga, E. (2021). The trap of climate change-induced "natural" disasters and inequality. *Global Environmental Change, 70*, 102329.

Carr, L. (1932). Disaster and the sequence-pattern concept of social change. *American Journal of Sociology, 38*, 207–218.

Carty, K. (2022). Personal communication December 10, 2022.

Chapman, C., Miller, D. S., & Salley, G. (2021). Social disruption of the tourism and hospitality industries: Implications for post-COVID-19 pandemic recovery. *Worldwide Hospitality and Tourism Themes, 13*(3), 312–23. https://doi.org/10.1108/WHATT-02-2021-0038

Chen, S., Bagrodia, R., Pfeffer, C. C., Meli, L., & Bonanno, G. A. (2020). Anxiety and resilience in the face of natural disasters associated with climate change: A review and methodological critique. *Journal of Anxiety Disorders, 76*, 102297. https://doi.org/10.1016/j.janxdis.2020.102297. Epub 2020 Sep 13. PMID: 32957002.

Clark, L. (2022). Personal communication December 11, 2022.

Comfort, L. K., & Okada, A. (2013). Emergent leadership in extreme events: A knowledge commons for sustainable communities. *International Review of Public Administration, 18*(1), 61–77.

Cutter, S. L. (2018). Compound, cascading, or complex disasters: What's in a name? *Environment: Science and Policy for Sustainable Development, 60*(6), 16–25. https://doi.org/10.1080/00139157.2018.1517518

Cutter, S. L. (2020). The changing nature of hazard and disaster risk in the Anthropocene. *Annals of the American Association of Geographers, 111*(3), 819–827.

Davis Bivens, N., & Miller, D. S. (2022). Policy for temporary crisis or sustained structural change in an age of disasters, crises, and pandemics. *Studia z Polityki Publicznej /Public Policy Studies, 9*(3), 9–27.

Drabek, T. E. (1985). Managing the emergency response. *Public Administration Review, 45*, 85–92.

Few, R., Chhotray, V., Tebboth, M., Forster, J., White, C., Armijos, T., & Shelton, C. (2020). *COVID-19 crisis: lessons for recovery: What can we learn from existing research on the long-term aspects of disaster risk and recovery?* London: School of International Development, University of East Anglia, UK, The British Academy.

Filberto, D., Wells, N., Wethington, E., Pillemer, K., & Wysocki, M. (2009). Climate change, vulnerability and health effects: Implications for the older population. *Generations, Journal of the American Society on Aging, 33*, 19–25.

Fitzgerald, K. G. (2010). A timely recovery for literature on disasters and older adults. [Review of the books Geriatric mental health disaster and emergency preparedness, by J. A. Toner, T. M. Mierswa & J. L. Howe and Older people in natural disasters by J. Otani]. *Gerontologist, 51*, 132–137. https://doi.org/10.1093/geront/gng107.

Flora, C. B., & Flora, Jan L. (1993). Entrepreneurial social infrastructure: A necessary ingredient. *Annals of the American Academy of Political and Social Science, 529*, 48–58.

Flora, C. B., Emery, M., Fey, S., and Bregendahl, C. (2008). Community capitals: A tool for evaluating strategic interventions and projects. In G. Goreham (ed.), *Encyclopedia of rural America: The land and people* (pp. 1186–1187). Millerton, NY: Grey House Publishing.

Giddens, A. (1990). *The consequences of modernity*. Oxford: Polity.

Gill, D. A., & Ritchie, L. A. (2018). Contributions of technological and Natech disaster research to the social science disaster paradigm. In H. Rodríguez et al. (eds.), *Handbook of disaster research, handbooks of sociology and social research* (pp. 39–61). Springer International Publishing. https://doi.org/10.1007/978-3-319-63254-4_3

Gissing, A., Timms, M., Browning, S., Coates, L., Crompton, R., & McAneney, J. (2021). Compound natural disasters in Australia: A historical analysis. *Environmental Hazards*. https://doi.org/10.1080/17477891.2021.1932405

Henderson, T., Roberto, K., & Kamo, Y. (2010). Older adults' responses to Hurricane Katrina. *Journal of Applied Gerontology, 29*, 48–69. https://doi.org/10.1177/0733464809334287

Kruczkiewicz, A., Klopp, J., Fisher, J., Mason, S., McClain, S., Sheekh, N. M., Moss, R., Parks, R. M., and Braneon, C. (2021). Opinion: Compound risks and complex emergencies require new approaches to preparedness. *Proceedings of the National Academy of the Sciences, 118*(19), e2106795118. https://doi.org/10.1073/pnas.2106795118

Lukasiewicz, A., & O'Donnell, T. (2022). The evolution of complex disasters. In A. Lukasiewicz and T. O'Donnell (eds.), *Complex disasters, disaster risk, resilience, reconstruction and recovery* (pp. 3–19). https://doi.org/10.1007/978-981-19-2428-6_1

Malik, S., Lee, D., Doran, K., Grudzen, C., Worthing, J., Portelli, I., Goldfrank, L., & Smith, S. (2018). Vulnerability of older adults in disasters: Emergency department utilization by geriatric patients after hurricane sandy. *Disaster Medicine and Public Health Preparedness, 12*, 184–193. https://doi.org/10.1017/dmp.2017.44

Mangeri, A. (2022). Personal communication December 11Wes, 2022.

Miller, D. S. (2006). Visualizing the corrosive community: Looting in the aftermath of hurricane Katrina. *Space and Culture, 9*(1), 71–73. https://doi.org/10.1177/1206331205283762

Miller, D. S. (2016). Public trust in the aftermath of natural and Na-technological disasters: Hurricane Katrina and the Fukushima Daiichi nuclear incident. *International Journal of Sociology and Social Policy, 36*(5/6), 410–431.

Miller, D. S. (2021). Abrupt new realities amid the disaster landscape as one crisis gives way to crises. *Worldwide Hospitality and Tourism Themes, 13*(3), 304–311. https://doi.org/10.1108/WHATT-02-2021-0037.

Miller, D. S., & Rivera, J. D. (2006). Guiding principles: Rebuilding trust in Government and public policy in the aftermath of hurricane Katrina. *Journal of Public Management and Social Policy, 12*(1), 37–47.

Miller, D. S. & Thorpe, R. Jr. (2022). COVID-19 and Health inequalities: Lessons for pandemic disasters yet to come. *Sociological Spectrum. 42*(3), 157–161.

Miller, D. S., & Wesley, N. (2016). Toxic disasters, biopolitics and corrosive communities: Guiding principles in the quest for healing in Flint, Michigan. *Environmental Justice, 9*(3), 69–75.

Misztal, B. (1996). *Trust in modern societies: The search for the bases of social order*. Cambridge: Polity Press.

Mokdad, A. H., Mensah, G. A., Posner, S. F., Reed, E., Simoes, E. J., Engelgau, M. M., & Chronic Diseases and Vulnerable Populations in Natural Disasters Working Group (2005). When chronic conditions become acute: Prevention and control of chronic diseases and adverse health outcomes during natural disasters. *Preventing Chronic Disease, 2*(Spec No), A04.

National Academies of Sciences, Engineering, and Medicine. (2017). *Communities in action: Pathways to health equity*. Washington, DC: The National Academies Press. https://doi.org/10.17226/24624

NIST (National Institute of Standards and Technology).(2014). *Community resilience planning guide*, volume II. Retrieved from https://www.nist.gov/el/resilience/community-resilience-planning-guide.

Nooteboom, S., and Termeer, C. (2015). Strategies of complexity leadership in governance systems. *International Review of Public Administration, 18*(1), 25–40.

Pescaroli, G., & Alexander, D. (2015). A definition of cascading disasters and cascading effects: Going beyond the 'Toppling Dominos' metaphor. *Planet@Risk, 3*(1), 58–67. Retrieved from https://planet-risk.org/index.php/pr/article/view/208/355

Pescaroli, G., & Alexander, D. (2016). Critical infrastructure, panarchies and the vulnerability paths of cascading disasters. *Natural Hazards, 82*. https://doi.org/10.1007/s11069-016-2186-3

Pescaroli, G., & Alexander, D. (2018). Understanding compound, intercon-nected, interacting, and cascading risks: A holistic framework. *Risk Analysis, 38*(11), 2245–2257. https://doi.org/10.1111/risa.13128

Prohaska, T., & Peters, K. (2019). Impact of natural disasters on health outcomes and cancer among older adults. The Gerontologist, *59*(Suppl 1), S50–S56. https://doi.org/10.1093/geront/gnz018

Raker, Ethan J., Arcaya, Mariana C., Lowe, Sarah R., Zacher, Meghan, Rhodes, Jean, & Waters, Mary C. (2020). Mitigating health disparities after natural disasters: Lessons from the risk project. *Health Affairs, 39*(12), 2128–2135.

Ridder, N. N., Pitman, A. J., Westra, S., et al. (2020). Global hotspots for the occurrence of compound events. *Nature Communications*, *11*, 5956. https:// doi.org/10.1038/s41467-020-19639-3.

Ritchie, L.A. & D.A. Gill. 2011. Considering Community Capitals in Disaster Recovery and Resilience. *PERI Scope* (Public Entity Risk Institute) *14*(2). https://www.riskinstitute.org/peri/component/option,com_deep-pockets/task,catContShow/cat,86/id,1 086/Itemid,84/

Ritchie, L. A., Gill, D. A., & Long, M. A. (2019). Factors influencing stress response avoidance behaviors following technological disasters: A case study of the 2008 TVA Coal Ash Spill. *Environmental Hazards*. https://doi.org/10.1080/17477891.2019.1652142.

Scharff, D. P., Mathews, K. J., Jackson, P., Hoffsuemmer, J., Martin, E., & Edwards, D. (2010). More than Tuskegee: Understanding mistrust about research participation. *Journal of Health Care for the Poor and Underserved, 21*(3), 879–897. https://doi.org/10.1353/hpu.0.0323. PMID: 20693733; PMCID: PMC4354806.

Simpson, N. P., Mach, K. J., Constable, A., Hess, J., Hogarth, R., Howden, M., Lawrence, J., Lempert, R. J., Muccione, V., Mackey, B., New, M., O'Neill, B., Otto, F., Pörtner, H., Reisinger, A., Roberts, D., Schmidt, D., Seneviratne, S., Strongin, S. van Aalst, M., Totin, E., & Trisos, C. H. (2021). A framework for complex climate change risk assessment. *One Earth, 4*(4), 489–501. https://doi.org/10.1016/j.oneear. 2021.03.005

Staupe-Delgado, R. (2019). Progress, traditions and future directions in research on disasters involving slow-onset hazards. *Disaster Prevention and Management, 28*(5), 623–635.

Tierney, K. (2019). *Disasters: A sociological approach*. Cambridge, UK: Polity Press.

Thomas, C. (1998). Maintaining and restoring public trust in government agencies and their employees, *Administration and Society, 30*, 166–193.

Warren, R. C., Shedlin, M. G., Alema-Mensah, E., Obasaju, C., & Hodge, D. Augustin. (2019). Clinical trials participation among African Americans and the ethics of trust: Leadership perspectives. *Ethics, Medicine, and Public Health, 10*, 128–138. https://doi.org/10.1016/j.jemep.2019.100405

Washington, H. A., editor. (2006). *Medical apartheid: The dark history of medical experimentation on Black Americans from colonial times to the present.* New York: Random House, Inc.

Wray, R., Rivers, J., Whitworth, A., Jupka, K., & Clements, B. (2006), Public perceptions about trust in emergency risk communication: Qualitative research findings. *International Journal of Mass Emergencies and Disasters*, *24*(1), 45–75.

UNDRR. (2020). *Hazard definition and classification review: Technical report*. Retrieved from https://www.undrr.org/publication/hazard-definition-and-classification-review

Index

Note: **Bold** page numbers refer to tables; *Italic* page numbers refer to figures and page numbers followed by "n" denote endnotes.

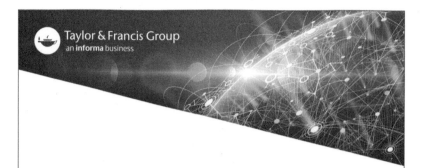